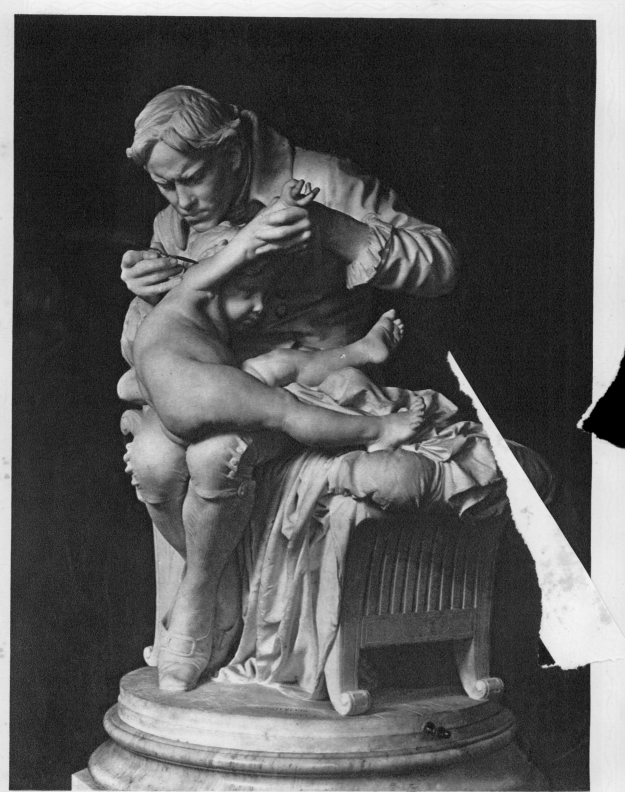

[Group by G. Monteverde.

JENNER INNOCULATING HIS SON.

Fighting disease with its own weapons—a fine group in the Bianco Palace, Genoa, of the pioneer of innoculation at work.

Published under the Auspices of
THE NEW HEALTH SOCIETY

THE
GOLDEN HEALTH
LIBRARY

Edited by
SIR W. ARBUTHNOT LANE

A Complete Guide to Golden Health for Men & Women of all Ages
Written by over **100** of the World's Leading Specialists
with contributions from

The Hon. Sir Arthur STANLEY
Chairman of the British Red Cross Society

SIR THOMAS OLIVER
Professor of Practice of Medicine, Durham

Dr. C.W. SALEEBY
Chairman of the Sunlight League

SIR HARRY BALDWIN
Hon. Dental Surgeon to H.M. the King

SIR RONALD ROSS
Director, Ross Institute for Tropical Diseases

The Viscountess ERLEIGH
The Patron of Baby Welfare

The Rt. Hon. Lord BUCKMASTER
The Eminent K.C. & Ex-Lord Chancellor

Dr. Elizabeth SLOAN CHESSER
Lecturer & Examiner, L.C.C. & British Red Cross Society

SIR BRUCE BRUCE-PORTER
Late Phys. to King Edward VII's Hospital

SIR J. ARTHUR THOMSON
Professor of Natural History, Aberdeen

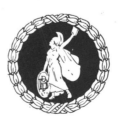

VOLUME   TWO

Published by WILLIAM COLLINS SONS & CO., LTD. for
BRITISH BOOKS LIMITED · LONDON

THE GOLDEN HEALTH LIBRARY

CONTENTS OF VOLUME TWO

VIII. MAN'S PLACE IN NATURE

	PAGE
THE BIOLOGICAL CONTROL OF LIFE	337
by Proefssor J. ARTHUR THOMSON, M.A., LL.D.	
MAN AND HIS ENVIRONMENT	343
by MARY G. ADAMS, M.Sc. (Cantab.).	

	PAGE
THE SPAN OF LIFE	355
by EUGENE LYMAN FISK, M.D.	
THE DEVELOPMENT OF MAN	359
by MARY G. ADAMS, M.Sc. (Cantab.).	
BODY AND MIND	366
by GEORGE SOMERVILLE, M.D., D.P.M.	

IX. HEALTH AND DISEASE

	PAGE
THE MEANING OF ILL-HEALTH	371
by GEORGE SOMERVILLE, M.D., D.P.M.	
PAIN : NATURE'S WARNING	376
by GEORGE SOMERVILLE, M.D., D.P.M.	

	PAGE
THE CAMPAIGN FOR MORE ABUNDANT LIFE	381
by Sir W. ARBUTHNOT LANE, Bart., C.B., M.S., F.R.C.S.	
PERIODICAL MEDICAL EXAMINATION	382
by EUGENE LYMAN FISK, M.D.	

X. THE HUMAN MACHINE

	PAGE
THE HEART AND BLOOD VESSELS	385
by J. H. BARNARD, O.B.E., M.D.	
THE CARE OF THE HEART	398
by G. A. SUTHERLAND, C.B.E., A.M., M.D., F.R.C.P., M.R.C.S.	
THE HEART IN DISEASE	407
by J. H. BARNARD, O.B.E., M.D.	
THE DANGERS OF ACUTE RHEUMATISM	418
by F. JOHN POYNTON, M.D., F.R.C.P.	
DISEASES OF THE ARTERIES	422
by GEORGE SOMERVILLE, M.D., D.P.M.	
HGH BLOOD PRESSURE	430
by G. A. SUTHERLAND, C.B.E., A.M., M.D., F.R.C.P., M.R.C.S.	
THE BLOOD IN HEALTH AND DISEASE	433
by GEORGE SOMERVILLE, M.D., D.P.M.	

	PAGE
BLOODLESSNESS IN GIRLS	439
by C. W. SALEEBY, M.D., Ch.B., F.R.S.E., F.Z.S.	
THE LYMPH VESSELS AND GLANDS	440
by GEORGE SOMERVILLE, M.D., D.P.M.	
THE RESPIRATORY SYSTEM—	
THE PROCESS OF BREATHING	445
by MARY G. ADAMS, M.Sc. (Cantab.).	
THE BREATHING APPARATUS	447
by W. H. HORNIBROOK, F.R.C.S., L.R.C.P., D.P.H. (Irel.).	
DISEASES OF THE RESPIRATORY SYSTEM	451
by J. H. CUTHBERT, M.B., Ch.B., D.P.M.	
THE PREVENTION OF THE COMMON COLD	460
by NATHAN MUTCH, M.A., M.D., F.R.C.P.	

CONTENTS OF VOLUME TWO—*Continued*

PAGE

THE CARE OF THE TONSILS AND ADENOIDS 461
by Sir W. ARBUTHNOT LANE, Bart, C.B., M.S., F.R.C.S.

THE CARE OF THE LUNGS 463
by Sir BRUCE BRUCE PORTER, K.B.E., C.M.G., M.D., M.R.C.S., L.R.C.P.

THE HYGIENE OF THE BREATHING APPARATUS 465
by GEORGES ROSENTHAL, M.D. (Paris), D.Sc.

THE URINARY SYSTEM 472
by GEORGE SOMERVILLE, M.D., D.P.M.

THE DIGESTIVE SYSTEM 481
by GEORGE SOMERVILLE, M.D., D.P.M.

DISEASES OF THE DIGESTIVE SYSTEM 493
by GEORGE SOMERVILLE, M.D., D.P.M.

CANCER OF THE STOMACH 499
by VICTOR PAUCHET, M.D. (Paris).

THE PREVENTION OF CONSTIPATION 507
by ALFRED C. JORDAN, C.B.E., B.A., M.D., B.Ch., D.M.R.E., M.R.C.P.

HUMAN SANITATION 512
by Sir W. ARBUTHNOT LANE, Bart., C.B., M.S., F.R.C.S.

THE PREVENTION OF APPENDICITIS 514
by Sir W. ARBUTHNOT LANE, Bart., C.B., M.S., F.R.C.S.

THE TEETH—
THE STRUCTURE OF THE TEETH 529
by W. H. HORNIBROOK, F.R.C.S., L.R.C.P., D.P.H. (Irel.).

DENTAL DISEASES AND THEIR PREVENTION 530
by C. BOWDLER HENRY, M.R.C.S., L.R.C.P., L.D.S.

DENTAL HYGIENE 538
by Sir HARRY BALDWIN, C.V.O., M.R.C.S., L.D.S.

THE CARE OF ARTIFICIAL TEETH 541
by JOHN CAMPBELL, Ph.D.

TOOTH POWDERS AND PASTES 542
by FRANCIS D. DONOVAN, L.D.S., R.C.S. (Eng.).

DIET AND DENTITION IN THE PUNJAB 545
by Lieut.-Col. H. HALLIDAY, I.M.S., M.B., M.R.C.S. L.R.C.P.

PAGE

THE LOCOMOTORY SYSTEM 546
by GEORGE SOMERVILLE, M.D., D.P.M.

THE FEET 559
by ERIC GORDON FLEMING, D.C. (Universal Chiropract. Coll., U.S.A.), M.C.P.S., M.B.

FOOTWEAR 568
by FREDERICK G. PAGE (Daniel Neal & Sons)

ARTIFICIAL HEELS: THEIR USE AND ABUSE 573
by Sir W. ARBUTHNOT LANE, Bart., C.B., M.S., F.R.C.S.

THE NERVOUS SYSTEM 577
by MACPHERSON LAWRIE, M.A., M.B., B.Ch.

DISEASES OF THE NERVOUS SYSTEM 590
by MACPHERSON LAWRIE, M.A., M.B., B.Ch.

HEADACHES 604
by ROBERT M. MACFARLANE, M.B., Ch.B., D.P.M.

TREATMENT OF ORGANIC NERVOUS DISORDERS 609
by ROBERT M. MACFARLANE, M.B., Ch.B., D.P.M.

THE DUCTLESS GLANDS 615
by GEORGE SOMERVILLE, M.D., D.P.M.

PERSONALITY AND THE DUCTLESS GLANDS 622
by LEONARD WILLIAMS, M.D.

THE SKIN 625
by GEORGE SOMERVILLE, M.D., D.P.M.

COMMON FACIAL DISFIGUREMENTS 634
by W. H. HORNIBROOK, F.R.C.S., L.R.C.P., D.P.H. (Irel.).

THE CARE OF THE NAILS 638
by W. H. HORNIBROOK, F.R.C.S., L.R.C.P., D.P.H. (Irel.).

THE HAIR 639
by W. H. HORNIBROOK, F.R.C.S., L.R.C.P., D.P.H. (Irel.).

THE HYGIENE OF THE BATH 642
by JOHN CAMPBELL, Ph.D.

TOILET SOAPS FOR HEALTH AND BEAUTY 645
by JOHN CAMPBELL, Ph.D.

CONTENTS OF VOLUME TWO—*Continued*

PAGE

ACTINOTHERAPY AND SPECIFIC SKIN DISEASES 648
   by PERCY HALL, M.R.C.S., L.R.C.P.

THE REPRODUCTIVE SYSTEM
THE MEANING OF SEX 652
   by MARY G. ADAMS, M.Sc. (Cantab.).

PAGE

THE REPRODUCTIVE ORGANS 654
   by W. H. HORNIBROOK, F.R.C.S., L.R.C.P.,
   D.P.H. (Irel.).

DISEASES OF THE REPRODUCTIVE SYSTEM 658
   by GEORGE SOMERVILLE, M.D., D.P.M.

THE SOCIAL PROBLEM OF VENEREAL DISEASE 671
   by Mrs. ETTIE A. HORNIBROOK

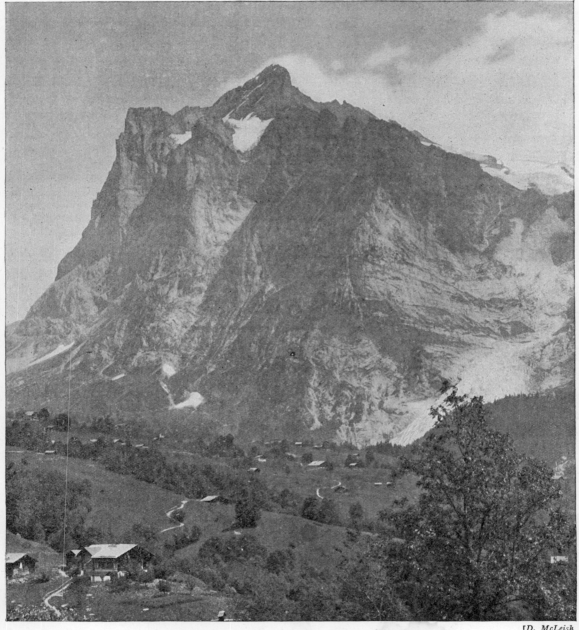

[*D. McLeish*

THE GRINDELWALD VALLEY, SWITZERLAND
A sunny, sheltered, and mist-free resort where sufferers from respiratory diseases benefit from the pure mountain air.

ILLUSTRATIONS
IN VOLUME TWO

The " Golden Health " Chart of Foot Exercises   *facing page* 568
    Daily exercises for maintaining strong and supple feet.

PLATES IN COLOUR

The Human Heart in Section   *facing page* 385

The Digestive System   ,,   481

The Human Skeleton   ,,   529

PLATES IN GRAVURE

Jenner Inoculating his Son   *Frontispiece*

" Convalescent ": H.M. the King Recovering from Serious Lung
    Trouble   *facing page* 433

A Health Resort for Nerve Diseases   ,,   577

The Care of the Skin   ,,   625

Volume Two contains in addition **162** photographs and **142** drawings in black
and white.

Printed in Great Britain at the Press of the Publishers.

VIII
MAN'S PLACE IN NATURE
THE BIOLOGICAL CONTROL OF LIFE

By Professor J. ARTHUR THOMSON, M.A., LL.D., Regius Professor of Natural History at the University of Aberdeen.

IN so far as the art of medicine is based on science—and that takes us back to Hippocrates (born about 470 B.C.)—the biological control of life is theoretically implied in every call on the physician. Yet this is historically too generous, for the art of medicine has not always been scientific ; and the aim of medical treatment has oftener been to effect the cure of a disease than to control the patient's life towards positive health. In his *Instincts of the Herd*, Dr. Trotter defines science as "a body of knowledge derived from experience of its material, and co-ordinated so that it shall be useful in forecasting and, if possible, directing the future behaviour of that material." In a way this links back to Hippocrates : "He will manage the cure best who foresees what is to happen from the present condition of the patient " ; but Hippocrates was a genius, and we

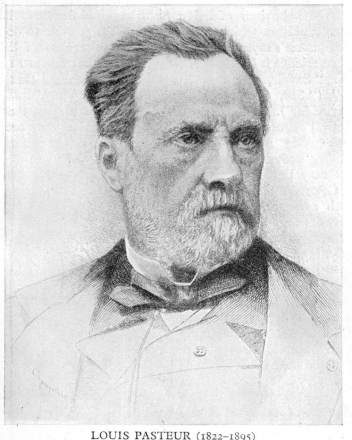

LOUIS PASTEUR (1822–1895)
The French scientist whose discoveries on the action of bacteria marked the beginnings of our biological control of life.

venture to say that the idea of the biological control of life is, apart from pioneer anticipations, a characteristically modern idea, dating from about the time of Pasteur.

The prehistoric domestication of animals and cultivation of plants implied a control of life that has been of fundamental importance, but although we cannot get more than glimpses of what actually happened long ago, there seems little warrant for supposing that the early domestications and cultivations implied a deliberate application of lore, *i.e.* incipient science, to the control of the life of certain useful animals and plants. In any case, it will be granted that the modern scientific breeders, with their Mendelian and other methods, are in a new way focussing scientific principles on practical problems.

And so it has been in modern medicine since Pasteur's day. Biology is being used

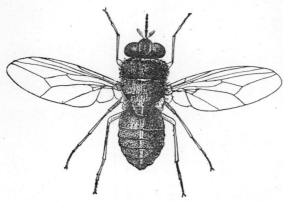

THE DISEASE-CARRYING TSETSE FLY.
The microbe of sleeping sickness is conveyed to humans by the bite of this insect.

for the control of the behaviour of living material—a modern ambition which is expressed in Herbert Spencer's saying : " Life is not for science, but science is for life " ; or in Comte's motto : " Savoir, pour prevoir, afin de pourvoir " (" See, that you may foresee ; and so provide "). Let us try to illustrate the biological control of life.

When disease-producing microbes have got a footing in a living body, such as man's, attempts may be made to baulk them. Counteractives of some sort, such as antitoxins, may be introduced ; antiseptics may be used which directly kill the disease-germs ; the internal defences of the body, such as the phagocytes, may be strengthened ; and, on the principle of setting a thief to catch a thief, a second micro-organism may be introduced that is inimical to the first intruder. The details do not here concern us, for we are simply mapping out the various forms that the biological control of life may take. But the practical outcome is very significant, that in recent years great steps have been taken towards the conquest of many microbic diseases, such as diphtheria, malaria, and syphilis.

Combating Disease.

A battle within the gates is always to be avoided, and for this reason much attention has been given in modern times to various ways of keeping insurgent invaders outside the body. The hookworm is not likely to get into man if he does not walk with bare feet on fouled soil that is densely peopled by the microscopic larvae ; the bilharzia worm is not likely to enter man if he does not wash or wade in water where the microscopic cercariae are swimming about, and does not drink unfiltered water or eat green vegetables that have been " freshened " by careless immersion ; man is not likely to be invaded by guinea-worm, filaria medinensis, perhaps the " fiery serpent " of the Israelites' desert journeys, unless he drinks water containing the water-flea, cyclops, which acts as the first host of this troublesome thread-worm. Similarly, man will not suffer from malaria unless he is bitten by a mosquito which is carrying one of the malaria organisms acquired from a malarial patient. And, again, it is possible to do something at least to lessen the risks of being bitten by the tsetse fly, that serves as the vehicle of the microscopic animal that causes the terrible " Sleeping Sickness." Men are not likely to take bubonic plague, the " black death " of long ago, unless they are bitten by the rat-

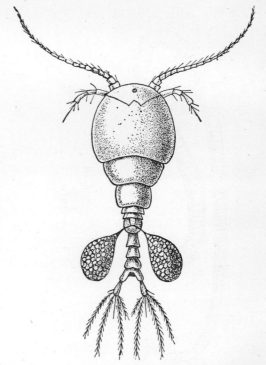

[James's Press Agency

A DANGEROUS WATER-FLEA
Man is not likely to pick up the guinea-worm parasite unless he drinks water containing its first host—the cyclops.

flea which has been feeding on the blood of a rat that is infected with bacillus pestis, the microbe of this terrible scourge. Yellow fever is due to a microbe disseminated by one of the mosquitoes ; and in many places where " Yellow Jack " used to be terribly rife, it is now relatively rare, just because, as in the case of malaria, there has been a vigorous removing or paraffining of the stagnant pools where the larval mosquitoes live. This form of the biological control of life has been rewarded by a great reduction in the number of what may be called gratuitous infections ; and here may be included the familiar methods of securing cleanliness, fresh air, and sunshine, which lessen the risks of repeated infection—formerly so common in households with tuberculous patients.

Students of natural history have been for a long time familiar with the fact that the hedgehog is immune to the venom of the adder. This reptile has no particular grudge against the hedgehog, but it naturally resents being

Increasing Immunity.

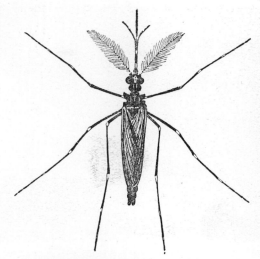

THE YELLOW FEVER MOSQUITO

As in the case of malaria, yellow fever has been brought under control by destroying the microbe-carrying mosquito.

eaten, and retaliates by biting its assailant. But if it succeeds in getting through the hedgehog's guard and plunges its fangs into its enemy's neck, doubtless injecting poison, nothing happens ! We express this fact by saying that the hedgehog is constitutionally immune to the adder's venom. Its blood contains an antitoxin which counteracts the adder's toxin. Similarly, in Egypt and in India, another mammal, the mongoose, immortalised by Kipling, is immune to the bite of the cobra, which is rapidly fatal to a rabbit. But if a fatal dose of cobra poison be mixed with mongoose blood and then injected into a rabbit, nothing happens. The physiological theory of this is extremely difficult, but it is beyond our present purpose, which is merely to illustrate different forms of the biological control of life. By ingenious and meticulously careful methods it is possible to make antitoxin serum preparations which may be used not merely as counteractives against an enemy that has got through the ramparts, but also as an anticipation of the possible consequences of this. A child infected with the diphtheria bacterium may be saved by anti-diphtheritic serum ; but there is more than that, for susceptible children can be forearmed by an anticipatory treatment before there has been any

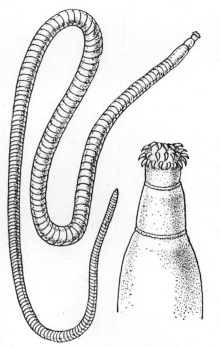

[*James's Press Agency*

A PARASITE OF MAN

The hookworm, a deadly parasite occurring in tropical countries, is picked up by the bare feet of the native.

339

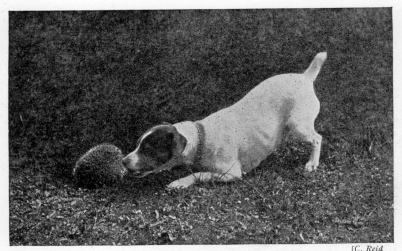

NATURE'S DEFENCE AGAINST ATTACK
[C. Reid

In addition to its prickly armour, the hedgehog is protected by an antitoxin in its blood which renders it immune to the bite of the poisonous adder.

includes the thyroids, the suprarenals, the pituitary body, the islets of Langerhans in the pancreas, and patches of glandular tissue in the ovaries and testes. These are discussed by an expert in a special article; all that is important for our present purpose is the broad fact that a deficiency in the natural production of a hormone, such as the thyroxin of the thyroid gland or the insulin of the pancreas, can be counterbalanced by introducing into the system a supply of the appropriate hormone from elsewhere. This is familiar in connection with cretinism, a pathetic state of arrested development in children, brought about by inadequate activity of the thyroid gland. The child remains infantile, little more than a feeble caricature of humanity, but treatment with the thyroid hormone derived from sheep or calf, or now produced synthetically, may counterbalance the natural deficiency and set development going again. Similarly, in regard to insulin, a hormone probably produced in the islets of Langer-

infection. One of the recent discoveries along this line is the immunising of dogs against distemper, a troublesome and often fatal disease which is due to a filter-passing microbe, invisible under the high-power microscope, and much smaller than ordinary bacteria. We see, then, that strengthening the natural defences of the living body is another form of the biological control of life.

As every one knows, the whole face of physiology has been changed in the present generation by the discovery of

Hormones and Health. hormones or internal secretions of the ductless or endocrinal glands. The hormones pass from their seat of origin into the blood and are distributed throughout the body, regulating and harmonising the functions in a fundamentally important way. Many glands and patches of glandular tissue are concerned in the production of these hormones, which have very intricate uses in integrating, we may perhaps say orchestrating, the activities of the body. The list

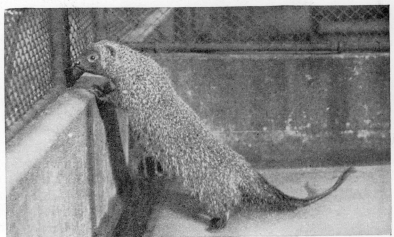

[F. W. Bond, F.Z.S.

THE COBRA'S DEADLY ENEMY
The mongoose of Egypt and India is immune to the bite of the cobra, and is often employed to keep these dangerous reptiles out of the houses.

hans which are included in the pancreas or sweetbread. It has for its rôle the regulation of supply and demand as regards sugar in the body. When the islets of Langerhans are not doing their work properly, the serious disease of diabetes mellitus sets in. But this can be circumvented by the injection of artificially extracted insulin, which compensates for the deficiency.

What brings about the deficiency or the exaggeration of hormone-production is a question still unanswered; perhaps it is simply an instance of the very frequent plus and minus variations in the hereditary equipment of the body. But our present point is that natural deficiency can now be counteracted by artificial control, and every one expects that, as the years pass, the physiologist will give the medical practitioner more and more skill in working these modern miracles. It is important to realise that the hormones, which work like almost magical elixirs, have very specific, and often very subtle, functions. Thus, in the frog, a pituitary hormone has to do with everyday colour-change; in man, a hormone of similar origin has to do with the regulation of growth, one kind of disturbance resulting in an unhealthy giant and another resulting in an unhealthy dwarf.

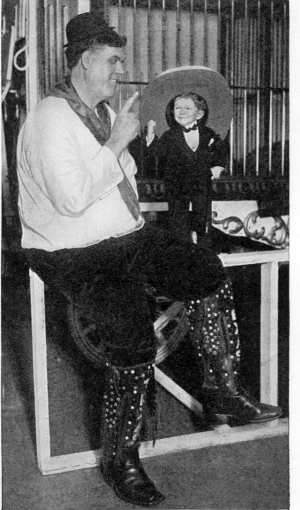

[*Topical*

TWO OF NATURE'S FREAKS

The biologist now knows that the giant and the dwarf are due to disturbances in the glands which produce hormones.

Also of profound importance is the way in which the hormones influence the mental as well as the bodily aspect of life, now exciting and again depressing. On the other hand, it seems that emotions may influence hormone-production, as in the case of anger and the secretion of adrenalin by the suprarenal bodies. We know how the cat's anger starts a concatenation that makes its hair stand on end; and we know how righteous wrath in man starts a concatenation that prepares his body for a fight. We know the physiological aspect of the old observation that the oil of joy makes the face to shine.

The whole trend of the modern study of heredity is towards the conclusion that new hereditary characters cannot be developed after the individual life has begun, that is to say, after the egg-cell has been fertilised by the sperm-cell. Each organism gets its "hand" of hereditary cards, which it can play for better or for worse, but it cannot add to the number. If, to use the language of the immortal parable, there are some men with five different talents and other men with ten different talents, they may duplicate or triplicate each of their several talents, but they cannot introduce a new one. And if

Influence of Nurture.

one of the various talents is a false coin, so to speak—we mean a disease taint, for instance—the organism may find it very difficult to get rid of it. Night-blindness has persisted in the Nougaret lineage since the time when Charles I. was king in England ; and haemophilia or "bleeding" in another lineage for a still longer time.

But while a man with no sense of pitch or tone need not expect to develop a musical talent, a great deal can be done to encourage the expression of any desirable quality that is represented in the inheritance, and contrariwise to inhibit the expression of any deleterious one that is lurking in latency. If we compare hereditary characters to buds, the number of these cannot be increased, but the degree to which they find expression is determined by the sunshine and the soil, the wind and the rain. These influences which determine the development, that is the expression of the inheritance, are summed up in the word "nurture," which Sir Francis Galton made a technical term. In this usage he followed Shakespeare, who made Prospero say of Caliban : "A devil, a born devil, on whose nature nurture will never stick."

It is at present impossible to estimate how far beneficial nurture may go in raising the standard of health ; and this is particularly true in regard to such organisms as mammals and flowering plants where the developing embryo remains for a long time in close physiological partnership with the mother or the parent. We know that ameliorative nurture must always be to the good ; it may greatly increase general vigour ; it may evoke unusual fineness of development in some of the hereditary characters ; and it may also inhibit the development of deteriorative or disintegrative characters, which become like "sleeping buds." Yet there are two limitations to be recognised—(a) that good nurture cannot evoke a new character which is not represented in the hereditary equipment ; and (b) that there is little evidence in support of the view that modifications directly due to peculiarities of nurture can be transmitted even in a representative degree to the offspring.

Under the term "nurture" should be included three sets of factors—environmental, nutritional, and habitudinal. In other words, the degree of development is influenced by surroundings, by food, and by activities or occupations, all of which have a minus as well as a plus sign. The blind newt called Proteus, that lives in the subterranean streams of Carinthia, has no pigment in its wan skin, and its eyes remain small, arrested on their way outwards from the brain. It might be said to have lost the hereditary factors for pigmentation and for vision. But this is far from being the case. If the Proteus is kept for a week or so in a well-lighted laboratory, it becomes spotty, and in a short time it becomes dark like an ordinary newt. The nurtural influence of illumination activates the dormant capacity for producing the pigment called melanin. Moreover, if some Proteus larvae are brought from the caves into a laboratory and reared under red light, the eye recommences its development, it increases in size, it grows to meet the skin, and it becomes so well formed that the animal is said to be able to see. This case shows how careful we should be in saying that this or that factor has entirely disappeared in an individual or a stock, for it may be that what is lacking is merely the appropriate liberating stimulus. We cannot linger to illustrate the form of nurture that is concerned with dieting, but it may be enough to refer to what is said elsewhere in regard to vitamins. Similarly, in regard to habitudinal nurture, we may refer to the articles on exercise.

We have used our available space to map out the main forms of the biological control of life—(1) combating microbic disease ; (2) lessening risks of infection ; (3) increasing immunity ; (4) artificial hormonising ; and (5) encouraging ameliorative and discouraging deteriorative nurture. This remains a very partial survey, yet we cannot do more than try to reduce "the fallacy of omission" by laying emphasis on three points. (a) Conquering disease, and this type of advance is on the whole to the good, but the progress of man-

Selective Breeding.

kind cannot continue unless processes of sifting or selection are also at work. Unless there is breeding from the best, the end will be the prolific worst, even allowing for their high mortality, which the heroic hygienists and physicians continually strive to reduce. It is not easy to make positive eugenic proposals; but every one is agreed that the spoiling of good stock by bad should be severely discouraged. (*b*) The applications of biology are doing wonders in baulking preventable diseases, in effecting cures, in veneering the human body with preventives and counteractives; and we have reason to congratulate ourselves as well as the experts on these achievements. Yet it cannot be denied that modern man has too often fallen far below a reasonable standard of positive health. (*c*) Finally, while unswerving in our loyalty to biology, we must emphasise the imperativeness of keeping always before us—what Hippocrates and Galen saw so clearly—the Unity of the Organism, the thrilling of body to mind, the thirling of the psyche to protoplasm. The ideal must remain, " *Mens sana in corpore sano.*"

MAN AND HIS ENVIRONMENT

By MARY G. ADAMS, M.Sc. (Cantab.), *Tutor in Biology to the Cambridge University Board of Extra-Mural Studies.*

WHEN we think of any living thing, seed or egg or adult organism, we cannot dissociate it from its environment. The manifestation of life is dependent upon the presence of certain external conditions. To see a seed long dormant begin to germinate after the simple device of soaking it in water, or spring vegetation deferred until the appropriate stimulus of warmth and sun, never fails to impress upon one's mind the important part which environmental factors play in developing the latent possibilities of the organism. Many life processes are strictly conditioned by the environment, for instance, human thought is only possible within a narrow range of blood heat, a range not greater than four or five degrees centigrade. It has long been known that most external conditions can be grouped within a limiting range, a range which may be small or great according to the adaptability of the organism. There is nearly always a minimum below which, and a maximum above which, life is not possible. Some internal parasites, for example, have a comparatively small range of temperature and pressure within which their growth is possible, and they will quickly die if exposed to the air.

Many organisms can reproduce only in the presence of certain associated conditions of temperature, moisture, oxygen, etc.

Within the limiting range there is, however, an *optimum* set of conditions which are most favourable to healthy development. Needless to say, few organisms actually live under the optima for all factors in their environment.

The most successful creatures are those which are sufficiently plastic to adapt themselves to constant deviations from their optimum conditions. Free-living organisms have the advantage of being able to roam in search of their particular optima, whereas sessile plants and rooted animals, like anemone or hydra, must make the best of the environment in which they find themselves. This often implies a great plasticity and adaptability in fixed species. Survival for those species with a narrow range of suitable conditions is only possible if they are prepared to wander in search of these conditions. At the same time it is clear that free-living organisms are far less modified by environmental influences than fixed species. A hawthorn tree must bend and grow to suit prevailing winds. But a bird can fly over hundreds of miles seeking good nesting conditions or adequate food. One would also expect greater uniformity in size and vigour among the members of a free-living species; a survey of a few examples from wild life—sparrows, rabbits, butterflies—will convince one of the truth of this statement.

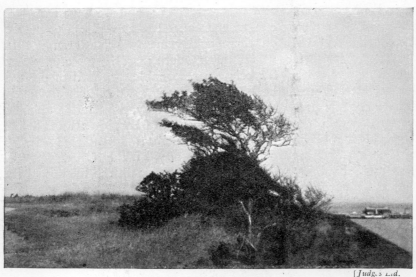

BENT BY THE WINDS

[Judg.s L.d.

Plants and trees must adapt themselves to prevailing conditions. Man and the animals can wander in search of better environment.

negligible in producing individual modifications. We know, for example, that the sun's rays cause pigmentation in the skin, but, at the same time, we know that genetic constitution determines the amount and extent of that pigmentation. Blondes are more susceptible than brunettes.

Man's position, however, is peculiar in one important respect. For the most part, he has stopped wandering in search of good conditions, and has begun to alter existing conditions to suit his needs. This partial control that he has acquired over natural forces has not been entirely satisfactory to himself; it has provoked many unthought-of reactions on the part of other organisms. Man steps in and breaks one link in a chain of associated organisms which has been forged by age-long processes of evolution, and his blundering evokes a menace to himself

Man shares with other free-living creatures this power of resisting the influence of the environment. It follows, therefore, that many of the differences we see between members of the same race are likely to be due to variations in heredity rather than to differences in environment. On the whole, men are tall or short, because they inherited those characteristics, not because food, climate, or occupation hindered growth in one case and promoted it in another. Workers in the Galton Eugenics Laboratory have concluded that " it is five to ten times as profitable for a child to be born of parents of sound physique and of brisk orderly mentality as for a child to be born and nurtured in a good physical environment." This line of argument, although it emphasises the power of heredity, does not mean that surroundings — food, occupation, training — are

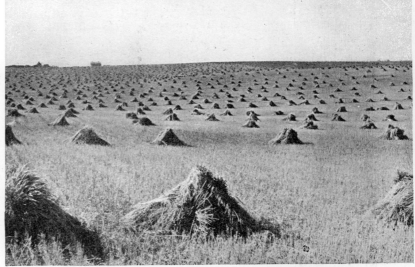

THE WHEAT FIELDS OF CANADA

Although wheat originally came from Mesopotamia, by a long process of selection breeds have been produced which flourish in the colder climate of Northern Canada.

as well as to other animals. By favouring one species he encourages the growth of the undesirable parasites they harbour. Thanks to the peculiar demands of civilisation, he immures himself within a stuffy home; he hoards his food and refines it with cooking and condiments; he piles clothes on his back, domesticates other animals for amusement and profit, and then protests against the emergence of bed-lice, house-flies, clothes-moths, and liver-flukes. To keep himself healthy he has to expend infinite time and labour in defending himself from the consequences of his own interference with Nature's laws and from the blind reaction of Nature's more natural creatures.

"The biological control of life"

Control of Life. is a new phrase—but some understanding of its meaning is essential if healthy living is to be promoted and maintained. It implies a rigging of the market in which natural competition is going on, so that bidders useful to man may be successful. Take an example—ladybirds eat greenfly: greenfly eat useful crops. The biological method of saving a crop in danger from greenfly is to encourage ladybirds to eat the greenfly. When the ladybirds have finished all the greenfly they die, so it is well to keep a spare set of ladybirds for emergencies. The idea underlying this plan is fundamentally different from the idea underlying the plan of walking around with a squirt of soap and water. It is the biological idea. Consider another example: the biological control of disease.

Malaria is caused by a protozoon called plasmodium vivax, which spends some of its life inside a mosquito. The

Bacterial Disease. disease-producing activities of P. vivax can be circumvented by arranging that the right kind of mosquito shall not have any suitable place for breeding. Mosquitoes lay their eggs in water, and the eggs will not hatch properly unless the water is aerated. Therefore, if a little oil is poured on to all the water in which a mosquito can lay eggs, malaria will be reduced to vanishing-point. Where this can be done, it works perfectly. Of course, great care has to be taken to avoid breaking a chain of associations which may at some point be useful to man. A lot has to be known about the relationships of an animal before it is very wise to encourage it or kill it, on a large scale: witness the story of the rabbits in Australia.

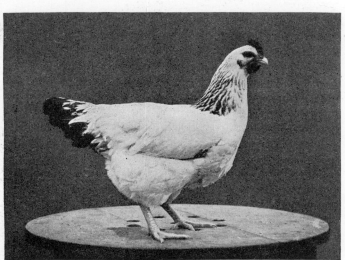

[Newman, Berkhamsted

A RESULT OF CAREFUL BREEDING

The Light Sussex is one of the famous laying strains produced by breeding from the best layers for many generations.

The effective control of many bacterial diseases has been attained by understanding the life-history of the parasites and seeking biological remedies. When harmful bacteria invade man, his blood begins to manufacture chemical substances, called antibodies, which have the effect of counteracting the ill effects of the poisons the bacteria produce, or sometimes of assisting in their destruction by the body. If it is possible to cause the blood to start producing this antibody before the invasion begins, it is evident that the body will have a much better chance of withstanding the attack, since it will be forearmed. This is the biological method underlying vaccination, in which proceeding

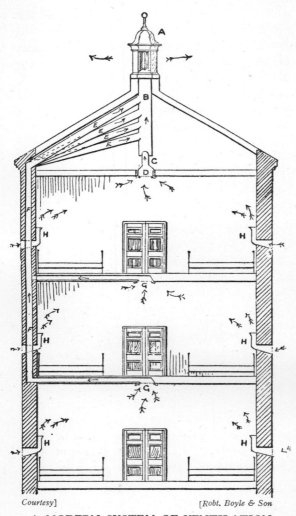

Courtesy]   [Robt. Boyle & Son

A MODERN SYSTEM OF VENTILATION

A building with many air inlets fitted with valves for controlling the air supply. The arrows show the direction of air movement.

plants. Many modern varieties are the result of scientific breeding and careful selection. A hen naturally lays a few dozen eggs a year at most. Simply by selecting the best layers and acting in accordance with the laws of heredity, people have produced hens which lay nearly two hundred eggs a year regularly, and exceptional birds which have produced over three hundred. In the same way, breeds of wheat are now to be had which will yield a good crop in the north of Canada, whereas the original wheat came from the Mesopotamian district.

Health is the normal condition of the human body. By seeking to understand the working of the normal body in appropriate surroundings we are familiarising ourselves with the postulates of health. Let us briefly inquire what are the basic requirements of a healthy body. They are—(1) nutrition; (2) air and sunlight; (3) warmth; (4) exercise and rest. Many of these requirements are inadequately met, some are supplied in excess and few human beings are living under the optima for all four conditions. Nor must it be forgotten that there are psychical demands which must also be satisfied, else the body will not thrive in spite of food and clothes and rest. Food is wasted if eaten in an atmosphere of gloom; rest is impossible in dirt and ugliness; work may become dangerous if poverty whips the brain. Our present purpose, however, is to describe the relationship of the animal body to its environment from two points of view: (1) The demands made by the body for supplies of food, air, sun, and exercise; (2) the responses of the body to such supplies.

Analysis of Environment.

The uses of food are many. Food is needed—(1) for growth; (2) to make good waste and general wear and tear of tissues; (3) to be expended on work as fuel; (4) to maintain a constant temperature in the body; and (5) for storage purposes. It will be clear from this that the diet requirements of a nursing mother and a young child and a

Nutrition.

a mild form of the disease is brought about artificially, and although the patient recovers quickly the antibody produced persists, so that should the man be attacked by smallpox afterwards he has a reserve of protection which may enable him to overcome the disease. In some diseases it is possible to introduce the antibody ready-made into the blood of the infected animal or man. This again adds to the defence against the disease.

Another way in which the biological method can be used to control life is seen in the breeding of animals and

retired elderly man are very different ; they require food for different purposes, and their menus should be varied accordingly. It is customary to measure the energy value of foods in terms of " calories " (a heat measure : 1 calorie = amount of heat required to raise the temperature of a litre of water through 1° C.). The following table shows the energy requirements (in large calories) per day of different workers, each weighing about 10 stone :—

Profession.*	Energy needed in Food.
Clerk	2,410
Tailor	2,510
Cobbler	2,940
Metal Worker	3,290
House Painter	3,500
Carpenter	3,550
Stonemason	4,660
Woodcutter	5,400
Cyclist (racing for 16 hours)	10,240

Foods include :—(1) *proteins*, contained in foods like cheese, eggs, meat, fish, pulses, etc. ; (2) *carbohydrates*, as in sugars, and starchy foods—bread, potatoes, cereals, etc. ; (3) *fats*, as in cream, butter, suet, lard, vegetable fats, etc. ; (4) *salts*, especially sodium chloride, as in most foods, particularly milk, vegetables, and fruit ; (5) *water*, which is a variable constituent of all foods ; (6) *vitamins*, the accessory food factors present in many fresh foods and in some cooked foods.

A suitable diet must contain representa-

* From Haldane and Huxley : *Animal Biology.*

tives of each of the above groups, but as the energy values of the various classes are different, the daily diet should be arranged so that it contains contributions appropriate to the energy requirements of the individual. Energy can be obtained from the oxidation of either proteins, carbohydrates, or fats, in the following proportions :—

1 gram protein	= 4.1 large calories.
1 ,, carbohydrate	= 4.1 ,, ,,
1 ,, fat	= 9.3 ,, ,,

Most of the energy we need comes from fats and carbohydrates ; proteins are mainly required for growth and repair. Within limits, one food can replace another if it yields the same amount of energy. For instance, 100 grams of protein can replace 100 grams of carbohydrate or 50 grams of fat. It should be remembered, however, that the body is constantly in need of repair, so that some protein is always required ; the amount naturally is large in persons engaged in growing, infants, pregnant and nursing women, and athletes in training. Moreover, there are different kinds of proteins of varying body-building value ; vegetable proteins are on the whole less valuable than animal proteins. The other classes of food substances have various uses, *e.g.* calcium is used in bone-making, iron for the red pigment of the blood, common salt for sweat, iodine for thyroxin manufacture. The vita-

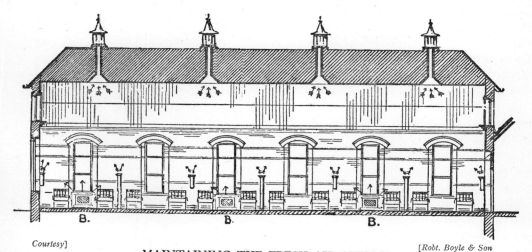

Courtesy] [*Robt. Boyle & Son*

MAINTAINING THE FRESH AIR SUPPLY
Another example of a natural system of ventilation, applied to a hospital for infectious diseases.

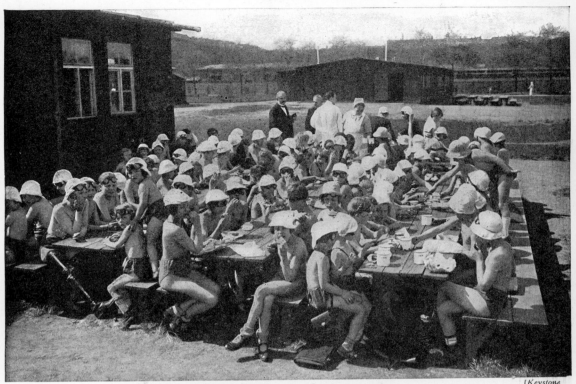

[*Keystone*

A MOVE TOWARDS GOOD HEALTH

School children who are taught that cheerful companionship and fresh air are great stimulants to digestion.

mins are organic substances. Vitamin A is fat-soluble and promotes growth : in fact, it is essential to proper growth ; B is water-soluble, its absence causes nervous troubles ; C is water-soluble and prevents scurvy ; D is allied with A, its absence leads to rickets and unhealthy teeth ; E is oil-soluble, and its absence brings about a condition of sterility. Probably there are other vitamins still undiscovered.

Nutrition is not only a matter of food ; it involves digestion and assimilation ; these in their turn depend on other factors of the environment, on fresh air, rest, and proper elimination of waste products. Man has become accustomed to cooked food, eaten at certain more or less regular short intervals, under social conditions : there is no doubt that such tradition could be greatly modified without much harm.

The tradition of corporate meals is valuable from its social aspect, interesting conversation, and companionship, aiding the digestion in much the same way as palatable flavours and appetising smells.

Fresh Air. The fostering of appetite is part of the science of feeding, for " appetite is juice," and unless adequate supplies of saliva and gastric juices are forthcoming, good food will be ill-used. Unfortunately, however, tradition and climate decree that meals shall be eaten indoors. This is a pity, for a great stimulus to digestion is thereby lost. Fresh, moving air is essential for the proper functioning of the blood, which during digestion has an extra burden of work thrown upon it. Moreover, breathing is affected by the processes of digestion. Soon after the beginning of a meal the breathing is slowed down slightly. Some of the carbonic acid normally breathed out is retained to counteract the alkalinity of the blood which has been caused by the flow of hydrochloric acid into the stomach. Later there is a speeding-up of breathing, for when pancreas and intestine come into action the blood would become too acid unless arrangements were made to restore the balance.

Fresh, moving air is not only highly desirable for good lung breathing, it is also necessary for adequate skin breathing. The skin of civilised man is shamefully treated; the wearing of clothes causes it to be surrounded by a moist, overheated, stagnant atmosphere, saturated by gaseous and watery waste products. There is little chance for its proper functioning. Clothes should be loose in fit and texture and light in weight and colour. Pure lightweight wool next the skin in winter and artificial silk in summer are good materials for permitting the right kind of temperature and air exchanges. Free evaporation from the skin should be encouraged; moist air stops evaporation and the body temperature becomes uncomfortably hot. The oppression felt in a stuffy, poorly ventilated room has apparently little to do with the amount of carbon-dioxide present, and with lack of oxygen. It is due rather to the difficulty of evaporation in a moist, hot atmosphere.

The biology of ventilation is founded Ventilation.on these facts. The air must be kept *moving*. Fresh, moving air (1) regulates the humidity and temperature in the air, promoting evaporation from the skin and keeping the body temperature from stagnating; (2) it prevents the accumulation of dust particles, microbes, or poisonous gases, and removes evil odours; (3) it increases, in some obscure way, the " breathability " of the air. Even poor air can be breathed with less discomfort if it is kept moving. The victims of the Black Hole of Calcutta died, not from lack of oxygen or an accumulation of poisonous carbon-dioxide, but probably from " heat-stroke," caused by a high temperature and excessive humidity. Modern laws regulating the humidity of the air in factories and condemning the practice of artificially increasing the humidity of workshop air for trade purposes, embody a recognition of this fact. On the other hand, there is often a danger of having the air too dry in artificially

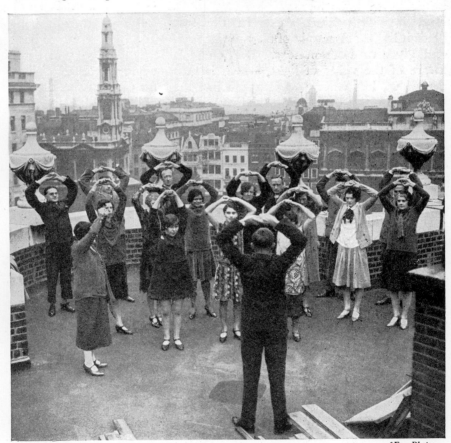

[*Fox Photos*

CLEAN LUNGS FOR WORKERS
Madame Novello Davies, the well-known singer, gives breathing exercises on a roof in Aldwych, London.

heated houses, and evaporation from a free water surface ought to be provided. Ventilation of workrooms and houses, however, must not be allowed to take the place of lung-ventilation. Most people rarely use their lungs to full capacity, and sedentary workers hardly take a really deep breath from one week-end to the next. There should be a regular practice of deep nose-breathing in the open air. There would be fewer drowsy clerical workers if such a practice accompanied the afternoon cup of tea.

Dust is a very important factor in the economy of nature. Its effects are ill-appreciated, yet minute dust particles in the upper air make the sky appear blue, and the sunrise and sunset multi-hued ; make rainbow and fog, and protect us from the intolerable brilliance of the sun. Yet, here, we needs must inveigh against dust. In the first place it limits our supply of ultra-violet rays, and gives us London fogs. Every one is aware of the value of light, which is thus denied us, but fewer people appreciate the disastrous effect of fog upon vitality. During a very foggy fortnight in London some years ago the death-rate is said to have risen from 27 to 48. Occupational mortality figures show that the dangerous trades are the dusty trades. Dust in the form of

Dust.

sharp, hard particles, such as arises in quarrying, in brass-founding, in glass or cement working, scratches the delicate cell membranes lining the air sacs of the lungs, setting up inflammation and allowing access to disease germs. Dust may be due to organic particles, as in printing, grain-handling, jute working, wool and linen spinning ; here it chokes up some of the air passages and reduces the actual breathing surface.* Modern factories supply masks for filtering the air. There are finer particles still which may bring harm, namely, bacteria, pollen, and fungus spores. But the danger from disease microbes floating in air is magnified. Most germs of this nature soon die if exposed to sun and moving air.

The good effects of sunlight in relation to health have only comparatively recently been scientifically explained, although heliotherapy in medical practice has been known from the very earliest times. The biologist never forgets that all food is stored sunlight, for without sun the green plant, mainspring of life on this planet, cannot synthesise carbohydrates from elemental substances in air and soil-water. Nor does man forget that coal and oil, without which modern civilisation would cease to exist, likewise owe their existence to the energy of the sun shining millions of years ago. He has made little attempt, however, until quite recently, to harness the sun for his own particular uses. In fact, the dangers of faded carpets and sunstroke were sufficient excuse to pull down blinds and sit in the shade. All this is changing. We welcome sunlight in home and school and bath. But it is alarming to learn that, in one fair month of June, 54 tons of dirt were deposited from the air in an area of

Sunlight and Warmth.

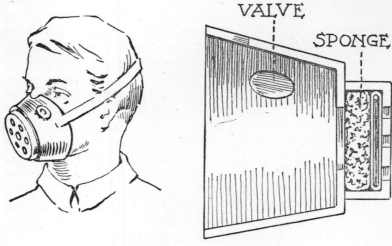

VALVE

SPONGE

A PROTECTION AGAINST DUST

Excess of dust chokes up the air passages and scratches the delicate lung membranes. To prevent this happening in dusty trades, some factories supply the workers with special masks.

* See section on " Industrial Diseases."

one square mile in the City of London. Of these 54 tons, 18 tons were soluble sulphates, chlorates, and ammonia, and 36 tons were insoluble grits, soots, and tars.

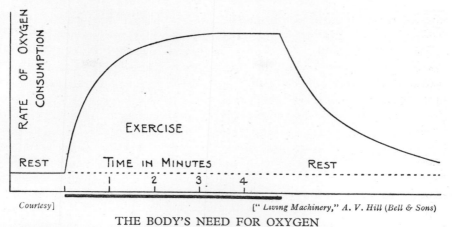

THE BODY'S NEED FOR OXYGEN

The graph shows how much greater is our oxygen consumption during exercise than during rest. The underlined portion represents the time spent in exercise.

Many devices are appearing for capturing sunlight. Special glass lets through the valuable ultra-violet rays which ordinary glass arrests; clothing of artificial silk has the same property; food suitably exposed to sunlight benefits the consumer; fruit allowed to ripen or dry in the sun has a more valuable vitamin content than fruit grown in relatively sunless climates or allowed to ripen in the hold of a ship. Sunlight in moderation encourages metabolism, growth, and development, and acts as a psychological stimulus whose value no one can deny. Disease microbes dislike sun,—sunlit air is as effective as a good disinfectant.

Sunlight and warmth, although often associated in the popular mind, have quite distinct effects. Warm-blooded **Body Heat.** animals have to maintain a constant body temperature and possess elaborate heat-regulating mechanisms for this purpose. If we become cold, orders are sent to the muscles to produce more heat and to the blood-vessels in the skin to contract; if we become too hot we sweat, or pant, or lie down, all of which have the effect of bringing down our temperature. Of course, one puts on clothing, or takes it off, to aid these automatic adjustments, but putting on thick clothing to keep the cold out really means " putting it on to keep the heat in." In spite of great fluctuations in outside temperature, body heat remains remarkably constant except when we are ill. It is interesting that this same thing happens even in cold-blooded creatures; if you take the temperature of a sick banana or invalid orange you will observe a rise so long as it is still alive. Dead fruits are not affected in this way. Most people are in danger from overheating rather than from overcooling. Personal habits make the skin oversensitive to cold; hot rooms and thick clothing put the sweat glands out of normal action with the result that the heart has to do the work they should perform. This is tiring, and it is small wonder that boredom, sleepiness, listlessness, headaches, and irritation result from working in an overheated room. The necessity for ventilation is again apparent. Good healthy sweating, which does not necessarily mean obvious perspiration, makes for a clear brain, responsive muscles, and sound digestion; but when blood has to pulsate through the skin there is not so much of it left for brain, stomach, or muscles. Health cannot be maintained unless the organs of the body are given scope to carry out their *appropriate* function.

Muscular exercise in promoting sweating, as well as deep and frequent breathing, is an important means of regulating **Exercise.** body temperature and of eliminating waste products more quickly through skin and kidneys. Moreover, the co-ordination required between muscles and nerves strengthens the brain, informs the judgment, and maintains equilibrium. " By dint of hammering one becomes a smith." Exercise is essential for the proper functioning of digestive, respiratory, and excre-

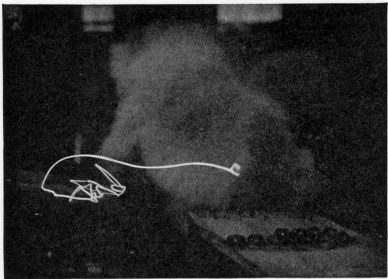

ECONOMY OF MOVEMENT

An ergograph reading showing the movements of the best worker in a chocolate-covering department.

popular opposition of " brain or brawn." The desire for such muscular strength is on the wane, however, and most of us engage in feats of mental or physical endurance against our will. Modern life is full of " tired " folk, victims of overwork in one direction or another. What is the biological meaning of this tiredness, this fatigue? Take a single case in which fatigue is due to excessive muscular effort. When the muscles are tired a chemical substance, lactic acid, accumulates in the muscle fibres and begins overflowing into the blood ;

tory systems as well as for the balanced healthy development of the body from birth to maturity. Muscular exercise seems to *liberate* mental energy in a curious way. The brain-worker will often employ his leisure in some different form of " labour " —golf, perhaps, or gardening ; he returns to his desk or school not merely rested, but stimulated and encouraged. Taken in moderation, muscular exercise is not only an excellent lubricant for the machinery of the body, but it adds to the general store of energy, and increases the total work output.

Great development of muscle, so often regarded as a visible prize by the athlete, is no great advantage in itself. Big muscles have to be fed, and additional work is therefore thrown on the digestive system and on the heart. Energy goes to the muscles which should go to the brain. There is something to be learned from the

when its concentration in the blood has reached a certain value, the individual is forced to stop expending energy. This limiting value depends on the health, training, and physical development of the individual, but it is also conditioned by his resolution and fortitude. This is more obvious when the work is prolonged than

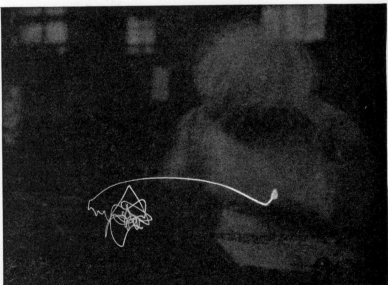

UNNECESSARY LABOUR

A worker of long experience making many unnecessary movements.

when it is short and intense. In order to remove the lactic acid which through the blood affects the nervous system and other organs of the body, oxygen has to be used up. Oxygen can be obtained in two ways, either by increasing the intake, through the lungs, by breathing quickly and deeply, or by running into debt and using up existing oxygen supplies. Fatigue, therefore, means lactic acid poisoning and "oxygen debt." The relation of these two factors to skill and efficiency in muscular effort is discussed by Prof. A. V. Hill in his fascinating little book, *Living Machinery*. With it should be read Prof. T. H. Pears' *Skill in Work and Play*.

Work and Fatigue.

The actual presence of these fatigue poisons can be demonstrated by ingenious laboratory methods. If a muscle taken from the leg of a frog is made to do work (through stimulation by an electric current) until it is too tired to do any more, it may be restored to working power by being washed in salt water. If this same salt water is then injected into a fresh

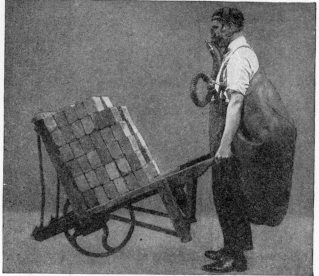

Courtesy] [" *Living Machinery," A. V. Hill (Bell & Sons)*

TESTING FOR MAXIMUM EFFICIENCY

An oxygen consumption experiment to find the best speed and load for a man wheeling bricks.

muscle, working at full speed, the muscle immediately becomes too tired to work.

Conversely, severe mental work tires the whole body. Ergograph tests were made on students before and after an examination, and it was shown that there was an appreciable decline in purely muscular strength at the end of the period.

Fatigue signs do not inevitably appear after physical or mental work—it is the *pace* that kills. Work under pressure, or in unhealthy, cheerless surroundings will leave signs of fatigue and depression when the same amount of work under good conditions will produce no such symptoms. There is a maximum efficiency for the performance of work, clearly related to the conditions of the environment. Much research has been devoted in recent years to this problem of "maxi-

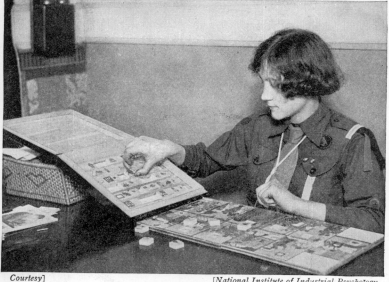

Courtesy] [*National Institute of Industrial Psychology*

A TEST OF INTELLIGENCE

One of a series of intelligence tests devised for helping young people in the choice of a vocation. Small blocks have to be selected in a given time to fill in the cut-outs in the pictures.

THE GOLDEN HEALTH LIBRARY

mum efficiency" which has everyday application in factory and home, in school and on the playing-field. The modern study of industrial fatigue is an investigation, both physiological and psychological, into conditions of work : attention is given to speed and rest pauses in relation to output, to repetition and rhythm, to arrangement of material and handling of tools, and to hours of labour. Already many reforms have been projected if not adopted.

The aim of such alterations in procedure is to establish a pace which will unite the maximum of output with the minimum of fatigue. Anything that will economise effort and lighten monotonous labour—whether it be typing to gramophone music or coal-heaving to the sound of a metronome—is considered worth a trial. Naturally, attention must be paid at the same time to physical conditions of the environment—temperature, humidity, sunlight, proper food, and suitable clothing ; all these are *basic* for happy, efficient work. One of the most important preconditions of good work is adequate leisure and means for the enjoyment of the leisure. A demand for adjustments in hours of work has been one of the most insistent, and one of the wisest of Trade Union demands. The insidious effect of long working days upon the individual and upon society is at last being recognised, and in the overstaffed trades " economic necessity " is no longer called in to bear witness that the industry cannot support a shorter working day. What is true for the factory is true also for the school—many school children suffer from chronic fatigue. Homework should never be allowed to take up the leisure needed for health-giving exercise and sleep. The overworked child displays dangerous signs, restlessness, and irritability, lack of concentration and disturbed sleep, fastidious appetite and " drawn " expression, extreme liability to colds and other infectious diseases, and so on. Unfortunately, man has grown out of or discarded one of his most valuable animal instincts—the ability to recognise the danger signals of fatigue. He has lost, in the market-place of evolution, his instinct for rest.

Chronic tiredness more often arises from distaste for one's job than from any other single cause. There are so many square pegs in round holes in our modern world, so many misfits in society, and so much squandering of human energy. Most people enter on their life's work from economic necessity, parental pressure or advice, or the chance opportunities of time and place. Few are free to choose their work. Consequently many people look upon leisure merely as an escape from unattractive work. Boredom and irritation soon spell fatigue, and fatigue as we know has a physical basis—poisonous waste products. Consequently the worker is in a perpetual state of reduced efficiency and subnormal health. Darwin once said that for him being lazy was working at something he liked.

Contented workers mean healthy workers ; to be contented one must be working at something one likes, and to like one's work is, generally speaking, to be fitted for it. Herein lies the crux of the matter—native ability must be recognised and encouraged. Square holes must be found for square pegs. The possibilities in round pegs must be explored. Psychologists are lending their aid to this task—a task *primarily* psychobiological, but hedged about with economic difficulties of our own making. Methods are being devised whereby children can be guided to their appropriate job by " vocational testing," so that natural skill or ability can find a suitable medium in which to express itself. This is research pregnant with possibilities for personal health and happiness as well as industrial efficiency and peace.

BOOKS OF REFERENCE

Food and Health. A. B. CALLOW.
Organism and Environment, as illustrated by the Physiology of Breathing. J. S. HALDANE.
Sunshine and Open Air. L. HILL.
Health and Environment. L. HILL and A. CAMPBELL.
The Air We Breathe. KERR JAMES.
Industrial Fatigue, with a Section on Vocational Guidance. C. S. MYRES.
Vitamins and the Choice of Food. V. G. PLIMMER and R. H. H. PLIMMER.
Principles of Human Physiology. E. H. STARLING.

THE SPAN OF LIFE

By EUGENE LYMAN FISK, M.D., Medical Director, Life Extension Institute, New York.

INASMUCH as the body is not an inanimate machine but a physiological mechanism—covering waste, maintenance, and repair—the fixation of a limit to its existence by other than natural causes, more or less under scientific control, implies supernatural agencies acting in an arbitrary way. Has it been decreed somewhere, somehow, by somebody, that the tissues of the human body, or of any other living organism, shall become lifeless within a certain length of time?

At once we see the implied and essential fundamentalism of such a view which actually is quite as crude in its aspect as the belief that all existing organisms are descended from those that came out of the Ark. Whether we use the term " nature " or " creator," there is involved in such a belief the inevitable thesis that life cycles of living organisms have been fixed by edict and not through evolution or reaction to conditions in the universe.

Evolution or Edict.

Time and again I have been told by physicians that, whereas some slight extension of human life may be possible through improved hygiene and better scientific control, there is a natural limit to human life which cannot be exceeded. Yet, at a recent meeting of the British Association for the Advancement of Science, it was agreed by the foremost students of these problems that we are ignorant of the real nature of life and its origin. The notion that life arrived on this planet from some other planet simply pushes the problem back but does not solve it, because we must then ask, How did life arise on that particular planet? The trend of present thought seems to be in the direction of spontaneous generation, long discarded as an immediate solution of the origin of existing forms of life, but obviously a necessary explanation of the origin of life in remote geological ages. By spontaneous generation I mean, of course, the interaction of natural forces resulting in life.

With the problem of life and its origin unsolved, we may well be daunted by the problem of death. Sir Arthur Keith sees life as a manifestation of automatism in the universe, and he discusses, as many others have done, the theory of practical immortality through continuity of the germ plasm. We may freely admit this and yet believe in a prolongation of the existence of those discontinuous outcroppings of the germ plasm which we call individuals.

Heretofore, this matter has been left entirely to evolutionary influences. The weight of opinion in the biological field seems to be that there is no natural tendency toward the formation of a superman of higher quality or greater longevity. We must assume, of course, that there was a period during the earth's existence when life of only the lower forms existed ; hence there is precedent in a way for the evolution of higher and higher forms of organisms. This might warrant some hope for the future that if man is left alone subject to evolutionary influence, without conscious control of his development or physical condition, in the natural course of events something in the nature of a superman will be developed.

This, however, is a logical sword that cuts both ways. Highly developed species of organisms have perished from the earth, and while we have abundant testimony to the effect that many causes of human death and illness have been wiped out, there is no evidence available in man's historical period to support the belief that man has shown any marked improvement in the quality of his structure or mental endowment. On the other hand, there is considerable evidence that certain structures have shown a tendency to waste, and lose their function.

Keith speaks of " life as a web on the loom of time," and asks, " Who, then, is in charge of the loom?" It is no answer for the biologists to say that the loom works automatically and that the threads spin them-

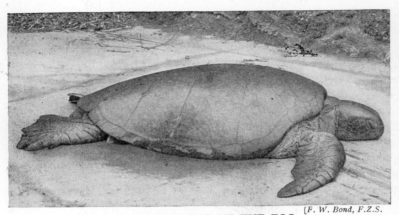

[F. W. Bond, F.Z.S.

A CENTENARIAN AT THE ZOO

The turtle is an example of a highly specialised organism with an extremely long life.

Certainly heredity determines whether an individual shall be a dog, a horse, or a man—and to that extent heredity determines his life cycle. But it is no satisfactory explanation to say that, having the inheritance of a dog, or of a man, or of a horse, this fact alone explains the duration of the life of such an organism. People often speak of heredity as an original and final cause of things, forgetting that whatever constituents there may be in the germ plasm which determine characteristics of any kind, whether of race, structure, personality, or longevity, there must be behind such constituents some

selves. This is a sufficient answer so far as describing the observed mechanism, but it does not define final causes, because such definition is beyond the power of human intelligence. Yet there is merit in ascertaining and outlining the mechanism of life, especially if it leads us to a better understanding of the ways and means of improving life. Keith nevertheless utters the pregnant truth : " The human threads in that web differ from all the other strands within it in one important respect : man alone can alter the spinning and the pattern."

Everything that science knows about the workings of the universe upholds the belief that behind all observed phenomena we must predicate some natural cause. If a turtle lives one hundred and fifty years, a horse thirty-seven years, and a human being rarely a hundred years, it is no final answer to say that these varied life cycles are fixed by nature. That is a wholly unjustifiable personification of nature. In saying it, we are wholly unscientific unless we mean that behind these life cycles there are numerous natural causes, conceivably subject in some degree to human control, that determine them. Weissman perhaps approached the truth, so far as existing forms are concerned, when postulating that each organism shows a life cycle that represents its most favourable adjustment for survival.

Survival Value.

The first cause is unquestionably heredity.

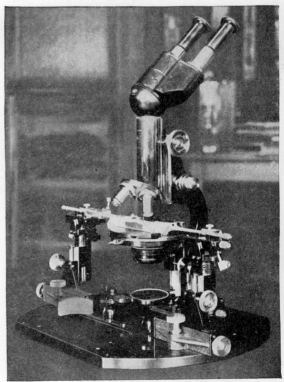

[Keystone

A KEY TO BIOLOGICAL KNOWLEDGE

A micro-manipulator, by means of which operations and dissections can be performed upon the simplest living organisms.

original physical factor. If we hold to any other view, we draw in the supernatural as an explanation of natural phenomena.

Carrel has shown that a living organism —of simple structure, it is true—has been endowed, through scientific control, with practical immortality; that is, as long as science does control the condition of the connective tissue cells which he secured under aseptic precautions from the heart of a chicken embryo, they will keep on living and multiplying.

Tissue Culture.

The natural answer of the laboratory biologist to such a statement is that this is a very simple and undifferentiated organism, and it proves nothing with regard to so complex an organism as the human body. It has been claimed that a shortened existence is the price that man pays for his highly differentiated organism; yet other highly differentiated organisms have had much longer life cycles—witness the turtle, the elephant, and the dinosaur.

If this principle of the non-fixity of the life cycle of even a simple organism has been once demonstrated, we may assume that it is a possibility in a highly differentiated and complex organism, granted only an adequate amount of knowledge and competent technique.

The experiments with the fruit-fly, whereby a mere change in temperature has brought about a prolongation of the normal life cycle of that organism to nine hundred times the normal, is another case in point, dealing with a more or less complex organism.

Inasmuch as nothing is really fixed in nature, even the movements of the heavenly bodies, and there is constant flux and change, I contend that it is wholly contrary to the law of probabilities that the life cycle of any organism should be so fixed that no outside influence could possibly change it. No one questions the possibility of shortening the life cycle of an organism. Why, then, should the opposite concept of lengthening it be considered illogical or fantastic? The truth is that the thesis of a changeless limit to the life cycle of any type of organism is a fantastic conception, dogmatic in the extreme, without justification in scientific principle, and implying absolute omniscience on the part of the person postulating it; while the negation of the fixity of the life cycle is a far more modest claim, confessing to limitation of scientific knowledge and also its possible expansion.

If we have successfully cleared the way to this point of view, I feel that we have relieved certain inhibitions which tend to limit the activity of scientific men and of those interested in preventive medicine. I am able to say, from a fairly broad experience in this field, that one of the greatest obstacles to prolonging human life lies in the acceptance, at least tacitly and subconsciously, of the thesis that such effort is more or less futile, that the years of man are threescore and ten, and that it is more important for him to study ways and means of having a good time during that period than in attempting the impossible in endeavouring to work against nature— whatever that may mean—in attempting any emphatic prolongation of the human life cycle.

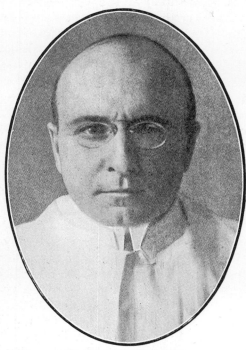

DR. ALEXIS CARREL

The French surgeon who, in 1912, was awarded the Nobel prize for his wonderful work in growing living tissues on microscope slides.

In going over the literature on this subject, and in discussing it with various men of science, I have been impressed by the fact that there is usually some one-track road to relief suggested or some one-track explanation offered of the cause of the breaking down of the human organism either through disease, old age, or death. It would seem to me desirable to present a statement of the possible causes of human breakdown so that we may avoid falling into error or dogma in regard to any particular cause, but rather through research and experimentation ultimately fairly evaluate the various factors that must of necessity have something to do with the disintegration and death of the organism. Loeb has suggested that natural death of the organism may be due to the accumulation of poisons within it or to the loss of some hormone essential to the maintenance of health.

Causes of Death.

I have grouped these factors of causation as follows, making no claim, of course, for finality as to existing knowledge under each category, but rather emphasising the enormous gap yet to be covered :

Heredity.
Infection.
Poisons.
Food deficiency or excess.
Air deficiencies or defects.
Hormone deficiency or excess.
Physical trauma (or strain).
Physical apathy (or disuse).
Psychic trauma (or strain).
Psychic apathy (or disuse).

Dr. Charles H. Mayo has stated that, in his experience, 85 per cent. of deaths are due to some form of infection. He has also stated that there are probably more forms of organisms menacing to the human race yet to be discovered than there are now known to exist.

If we consider Carrel's experiment with the connective tissue cells of the chicken embryo and attempt to present the reasons why these cells have continued to exist, I think the phenomenon may well be brought under complete explanation through the categories I present. These cells were endowed with structure of a certain form through heredity. They were protected from poison, from infection, from food inadequacy, from food excess ; they were protected from injury. The only gap in this symposium is the question of hormone deficiency or excess. In so simple an organism, the organs do not exist for the formation of hormones, so far as we know. Yet there may possibly have been in this simple mechanism—even in the nucleus of the cells—some provision for a hormone that would stabilise the organism in a state of health, provided the other factors I have mentioned were fully excluded as unfavourably influencing the individual.

Carrel himself has said that these organisms were apparently relieved of any influence of time. This, of course, is a mere figure of speech. Time never had anything to do with influencing these or any other organisms, because time is a mathematical abstraction and not a physical entity, as philosophers long before Einstein have pointed out.

The idea of time having an influence over ageing and decay exerts an enormous influence and may be found in practically every text-book of medicine, but it is as baseless as the jargon of a voodoo savage. Old age is a disease. Death is always due to morbid changes in the body. The things that happen in the course of time are the influential factors. Given sufficient knowledge and power, these things can be brought in some degree under human control, as Sir Arthur Keith has stated.

I am willing to admit that only a comparatively limited extension of human life, say ten or fifteen years, can be attained by simple adjustment of personal hygiene and the correction of physical defects found on periodic health examinations. It may well be that any great extension of human life, say beyond a hundred years, must be attained by some specific means, especially by control of the endocrine glands. Nothing can hold back human effort in that direction.

Extension of Life.

The endocrine cycles of childhood and

growth, puberty, maturity, and the climacteric have been advanced as proof of the fore-ordained fixity of the life cycle itself, but these subsidiary cycles are subject to the influence of external factors and are determined by them, and, so far as we know, by nothing not conceivably subject to some modification or control by scientific means.

When I am asked, therefore, as to the probable duration of human life in the remote future, I am compelled to answer that science has no present data upon which to determine this, but that the prolongation of human life, far beyond the present most favourable life cycle, lies within the legitimate bounds of scientific effort.

Of course, actually, life cycles have been prolonged, and even the human life cycle, within the last hundred years, has been extended about thirty-seven years—if we deal only with the average lifetime. It is quite true that this extension has been due largely to the saving of young lives, and that the ultimate span of human life has not been greatly extended. Yet, in certain populations, there has been a material reduction in the death-rate in the older age periods, and, in the experience of the Life Extension Institute, direct scientific control over individuals of middle age taking periodic health examinations has resulted in a reduction in the death-rate among them of more than 50 per cent.

When results of this kind, even in small degree, are scientifically demonstrable, results in much larger degree may be justifiably predicted—limited, as I have implied, only by the boundaries of human science and the degree of human interest in seeking such objectives.

THE DEVELOPMENT OF MAN

By MARY G. ADAMS, M.Sc., Tutor in Biology to the Cambridge University Board of Extra-Mural Studies.

WERE Shakespeare to rewrite his estimate of man's life, he would perhaps add to the famous seven ages an eighth of equal if not of greater importance than the rest. Instead of regarding man's birth as his beginning, he would know that it is but the second stage. The life of the individual begins with the fertilisation of the egg-cell in the body of the mother by the sperm-cell of the father. The result of this union is that the embryo develops in the body of the mother until the new individual is ready for an independent existence.

This first period is for nine months in man ; in other animals gestation varies, roughly, with their size. During the whole of this time there is an intimate partnership between mother and unborn child, which is effected by means of the placenta. The embryo derives fluid food, oxygen, and stimulating hormones (secretions from ductless or endocrine glands) from the blood-vessels of the mother, and carbon-dioxide, waste products, and hormones pass back to her. After birth, follow infancy, childhood, and adolescence, during which

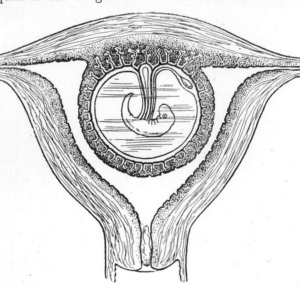

The Human Embryo.

THE HUMAN EMBRYO
A stage in the development of the child reminiscent of our evolutionary history—the foetus with a tail and gill-slits in the neck.

periods the individual gains in size, strength, and experience ; the building-up forces are stronger than those of decay. Manhood sees the gradual equalisation of these two forces, and finally the oncoming of old age witnesses the ascendancy of the latter.

Table of Gestation Periods in some Common Domestic Animals (compared with Man—270 days.)

Mare	. .	11 months.
Cow	. .	9 months.
Ewe	. .	about 5 months.
Sow	. .	112–116 days (about 4 months).
Bitch	. .	60–63 days.
Cat	. .	56–63 days.
Rabbit	. .	30 days.
Guinea-pig	.	62 days.
Tame rat	.	21 days.

In view of the tremendous influence of the first stage upon the subsequent life of the individual, and the light which it throws on man's animal ancestry, it is worth while examining it in a little more detail. The fertilised egg-cell, about $\frac{1}{125}$ inch across, divides until a cluster of cells is formed—the embryo. This surrounds itself by two membranes—the amnion and the chorion. The inner one, the amnion, is filled with a clear liquid, in which the embryo is suspended, thus receiving an equal pressure on all sides. The outer one, the chorion, gives rise to the placenta, which is attached to the womb of the mother, and which conveys both food and oxygen to the embryo, now called the foetus. Two cavities are then formed, containing the lungs, heart, and viscera. The foetus has a blood circulation of its own, supplied with oxygen from the placenta, but forced round by its own heart, a simpler structure than when it is mature. The organs which will have to deal with digestion—the stomach, kidneys, intestines, etc.—are more rudimentary, since their work, as well as that of the lungs, does not begin until birth.

A curious reminiscence of our evolutionary history is seen in the tail, a structure which generally disappears before birth, and in the four grooves which appear in the neck during the third week. These gill-slits, so called because they occur in the same position as the gills of a fish, give rise to the ear, the lower jaw, and part of the throat. Occasionally, however, the slits may not be completely obliterated, and one or more of them may occasion, in adult life, a discharging fistula in the neck. The limbs become evident last of all. The main feature of this stage is that, within the first few weeks after conception, the foetus is formed with rudiments of every organ, suspended in a clear fluid, and obtaining its food and oxygen from the mother's blood through the placenta. By the end of the third month development proper is over. The remaining time till birth is spent in developing those parts already present.

Although we may regard birth as a second stage in the life cycle, the

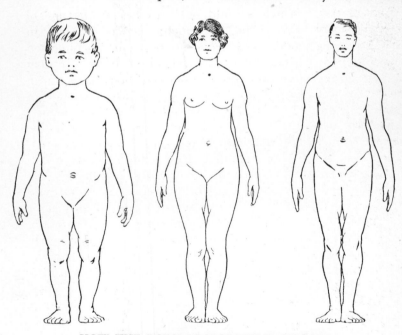

HOW THE BODY PROPORTIONS CHANGE
The three figures are drawn the same size for the sake of comparison. Notice the large head and short limbs of the child.

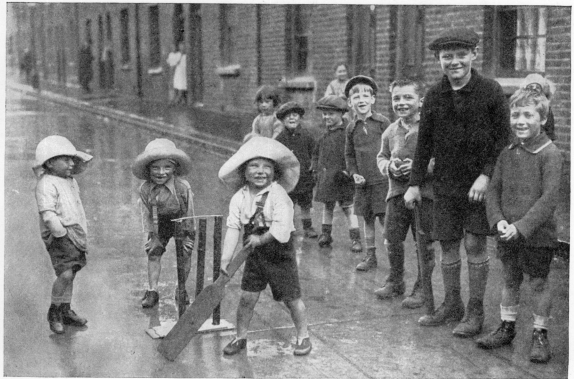

[*Photopress*

DEVELOPING STRAIGHT LIMBS AND QUICK WITS

The natural instinct of play is an important factor in the development of Man's most recently acquired possessions
—brain power and erect gait.

change in the environment is so marked —from a liquid to the air—that important changes occur, especially in the breathing apparatus. The lungs are now to be used : the blood must pass into them once during every complete circulation so that the oxygen may be taken up, and some carbon-dioxide got rid of. To arrange for this fresh circuit the heart has to change from a two-chambered to a four-chambered organ. Occasionally this change is not completed, and a malformed heart is the result.

Other malformations due to imperfect development in the foetus are " hare-lip " —the three segments of the upper lip not fusing together ; extra toes or fingers, due to an extra division of the cells forming the foot or hand ; cleft palate, and cloacal opening. It is noticeable that though so much development occurs before birth in man, yet lower animals are generally much more advanced. The brain of a gorilla at birth is already developed to the point

which a child only reaches at the age of five : the subsequent increase in size in both cases seems to be quite unconnected with any increased mental activity. In man his most recently acquired possessions, brain power and erect gait, are perfected late in his development—after, and not before, birth, and in bringing this about the native instinct of play must not be underestimated.

During infancy and childhood there is a rapid growth of the limbs and body ; the first set of twenty teeth is erupted Infancy and and discarded, and twenty-eight Childhood. of the permanent teeth usually appear at about the age of 12. In the early years the head grows rather faster than the rest of the body. Although the sex of a child is determined before birth, yet it is not before puberty—between 11 and 15—that specially marked sexual growth takes place. Then the sex organs become active ; the male produces sperms and the female ripe egg-cells. This stage represents the beginning of a fresh cycle for the race—since fertilisation and conception could now occur, and the whole process begin again. In the individual it merely marks a further stage, made more noticeable by such characteristics as the distribution of hair, change of voice, and development of the mammary glands. The body

Maturity. fills out as manhood is reached.

Until maximum physical activity is attained the individual is termed adolescent. During this time the jaws grow larger and bolder in outline, and this is necessarily accompanied by further growth of the facial muscles. The round-faced child becomes the strong-featured man or the piquant-featured woman. The neck muscles grow considerably in size, not so much to carry a heavier head as to steady it during the much more powerful movements of the jaw.

The body is at its best at about the age of 25 for men—a little earlier for women ; the skin is still elastic, and the arteries are capable of their most violent fluctuations ; the athlete can perform his greatest feats of speed and sheer physical prowess at this age. The co-ordination of brain and muscle, however, is most perfect at about 35, so that this is the age of maximum efficiency. After 25, there is a slight decrease in the elasticity of the skin and arteries. Movements are slower, and middle-age begins to show itself in the less clearly cut features, wrinkles in the skin round the eyes and temples ; the lines of the mouth are less firm. Some of the natural fat is absorbed, to be replaced sometimes by an unequal and ungraceful deposition of it elsewhere. In women there is a decline of sexual activity, sometimes accompanied by a tendency to a more masculine type. Middle-age merges imperceptibly *via* the elderly age into old age, when

Old Age. the joints become stiff, the backbone bent, the muscles shrunken, and veins and ligaments are no longer buried in the flesh, but stand in ridges beneath the skin. Naturally, the phases of this life-curve are variable, and we are just beginning to know something of the conditions which " time " the phases. Different kinds of hormones probably act as " accelerators " or as " brakes " to developmental activity, and it seems possible that more knowledge of the activities of the endocrine glands will suggest methods of controlling the growth phases of mammals.

AVERAGE HEIGHTS AND WEIGHTS
(For men of thirty, with clothing.)

Height. ft. in.	Weight. st. lb.	Circumference of Chest, in inches.
5 0	8 0	33½
5 1	8 4	34
5 2	9 0	35
5 3	9 7	35½
5 4	9 13	36
5 5	10 2	37
5 6	10 5	37½
5 7	10 8	38
5 8	11 1	38½
5 9	11 8	39
5 10	12 1	39½
5 11	12 6	40
6 0	12 10	40½
6 1	13 0	41

Add 3 lbs. for every four years over 30.

THE BODY'S RELICS OF ITS ANCESTRY

Besides the malformations brought about by some failure or arrest in embryonic developments to which reference has been made, man normally carries about with him curious, apparently functionless, structures— glands, muscles, membranes—which throw light on his evolutionary history. The appendix is one of the best known of these " vestigial " structures, but from the crown of his head to the soles of his feet man is a museum of similar anachronisms. The reader will think of many parallels in his social life, evidences of ancient history in his clothes, his language, his customs.

The distinguishing characters of mammals are hair and milk. One of these, at any rate, man has begun to discard—the hair on his body is scant, unprotective, and dirt-harbouring. The hairy man has, on the whole, been the unsuccessful suitor in mate selection. Woman, the more conservative partner, still possesses a body covering of fine embryonic lanugo. There are not wanting champions of the theory, also, that man's mammalian milk-secreting habit may be lost in the course of time. Modern civilisation makes it an inconvenient habit, it is true, but inconveniences are acquired characteristics, and as such are probably not inherited.

In the inner corner of the human eye is a little pulpy mass which in birds is a well-developed third eyelid. We have other methods of keeping the eye free from dust. Some reptiles of the remote past possessed a third eye in the top of the head. Comparative anatomy shows that the pineal gland in man has some connection with this third eye. The great philosopher Descartes thought that it was the seat of the soul; nowadays it is difficult to assign any such definite function to the pineal gland. The ability to twitch ears and scalp is the possession of a select few—but it is a primitive characteristic, and adults lose their admiration for it. Most of us put forth a hand to flick off a fly—we cannot use for that purpose the surface muscles which served many of our lesser mammalian ancestors. One quarter of our muscles are in our face and neck, and by means of them we express emotion—of a kind denied to ape or dog. There are many functionless muscles in trunk, head, and limbs which have a history full of effort.

The "vermiform appendix" is a narrow tube, 3 or 4 inches long, which forms a blind alley at the junction of the small and large intestine. It undergoes muscular contraction, but seems to play no valuable part in digestion, although food may enter its cavity. Some progressive individuals have only a rudimentary appendix; in others it is large, as in the gorilla, and although apes are not known to suffer from appendicitis when living in a state of nature, man appears to have become increasingly liable to it when living in a state of civilisation. Appendicitis may be a kind of revolt against the modern menu.

There are other vestigial structures—structures best termed rudimentary, like the mammae of males, which are the expression of a different type of inheritance, and can be thought of as due to the activity of a set of hormone "inhibitors." And, again, there are the numerous vestigial structures connected with the adoption of an erect posture.

MAN'S BONY SKELETON AND ERECT POSTURE

Most animals walk on all fours; man stands and walks erect: yet, when we compare the bony framework of a man with, say, that of a horse, we find that they correspond almost bone for bone. Has the

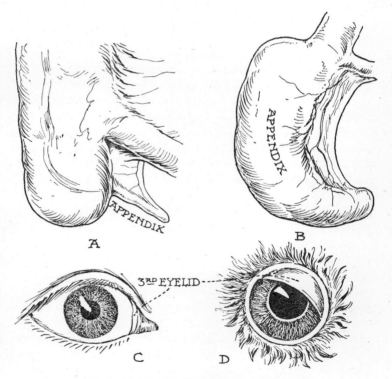

THE BODY'S LINKS WITH THE PAST

Man's appendix (A) is a now useless relic of an earlier structure (B), while the third eyelid (now reduced to a rudimentary form (C)) is well developed in birds (D).

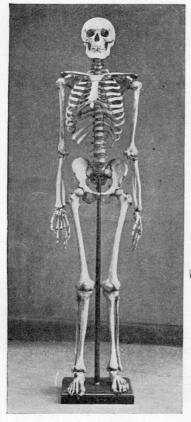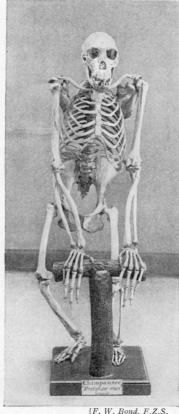

[*F. W. Bond, F.Z.S.*]

MAN'S UPRIGHT POSTURE

Skeleton of a human being and of a chimpanzee (reduced to the same size for comparison), showing the changes produced in Man's skeleton by upright posture.

legs. The limbs are really a series of different types of levers, with joints. Joints may be either of the ball-and-socket type, as in the shoulder and the hip, or the kind of joint we have at the wrist consisting of a number of small bones, capable of movement in any direction. Through the length of the backbone runs the *spinal cord*, which enlarges in the skull, forming the brain. Although the other bones of the skeleton do not contain this nervous tissue, yet we should realise that they are living ; they supply an essential part of the blood, the red corpuscles, which are formed in the marrow of the bone, and under certain conditions can form new bone material. Normally the bones do not increase in size after maturity.

Attached to all the limbs are muscles, and it is the contraction and relaxation of these which move the levers—or bones. These muscles are composed of bundles of fibres, generally surrounded by a thin membrane, and ending in an inelastic tendon. The muscles of the hand, for instance, are in the forearm, and only the tendons are in the hand itself, thus avoiding a very clumsy and bulky limb. This type of muscle is known as striped muscle, and is voluntary, *i.e.* it only acts under a direct impulse through the nerve from the brain. The muscles of the intestines (smooth muscle) are not under a direct control, but contract and relax almost automatically under stimuli from various digestive juices.* The movements of the heart muscle are practically automatic and unceasing during life.

* See " Digestive and Nervous Systems."

change of posture been a gain or loss : and what are the gains or losses ?

The bones of the skeleton fall naturally into two groups—those of the trunk and those of the limbs. Of the first group the backbone is the most important : this is made up of 33–35 segments, or vertebrae, connected by an elastic ligament, and with a cushion of cartilage between each pair of vertebrae. The whole is thus quite firm, and can yet give in any direction. The skull is set on the top, the ribs are fastened to some of the upper vertebrae, and to the breastbone in front, forming a protected cavity for the thorax. Above the ribs is a girdle of bones, the collar and shoulder bones, to which the arms are attached. Towards the lower end of the backbone is the pelvic girdle, supporting the lower organs, and also serving as a pivot for the

MAN'S PLACE IN NATURE

Man's habit of standing and walking in an erect position has caused many changes,

Changes due to Posture. not only in bone and muscle, but in lungs, circulation, and abdominal organs. The thighs and trunk now form one column instead of being roughly at right angles to each other : the contents of the trunk can no longer be supported by flat muscles on the surface : the viscera tend to sink towards the pelvis. Even the expansion of the chest, in breathing, has now to be between back and front, instead of from side to side. The backbone has a sigmoid curve, instead of being arched from end to end ; and the skull, instead of continuing the line of the backbone, is set at an angle to it. The muscles of the neck, trunk, leg, and foot all have to be adapted to this new position. The lungs are now partly supported by the diaphragm, stretched across the body beneath them. An extra part, the azygos lobe, seen in apes, which normally lies at the end of the lung, has disappeared entirely in most men ; a rudimentary lobe may occasionally persist. The muscles which move the tail in animals are spread out across the pelvis to support the viscera. Muscles have developed to set the shoulders square ; the one in the upper part of the arm, used by monkeys in climbing, has generally disappeared.

But the most important weakening effect occurs in the pelvic region where the organs are partially crushed together already. The lengthening of the thigh stretches the abdominal wall : there is no other animal so susceptible as Man to the rupture of this wall either before or after birth. The hernia which cripples the strength of so many men is then part of the price to be paid for an upright posture.* The existence of prolapse of the uterus and certain childbirth difficulties is another such sign that the body is as yet imperfectly adapted to its position.† The joints in the foot have been stiffened since it now has to bear the whole weight of the body, and an arch is formed. It is common knowledge that

* See section on " Diseases of the Digestive System."
† See section on " Woman and Her Health— Gynaecology."

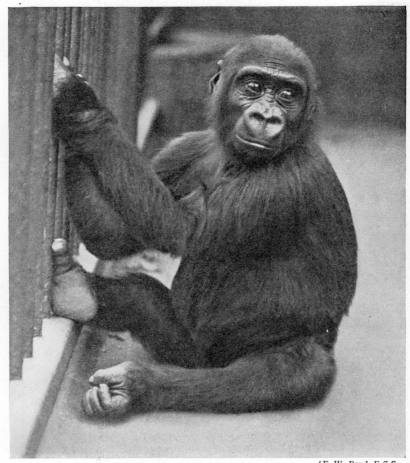

[F. W. Bond, F.Z.S.

A YOUNG GORILLA

Showing the prehensile foot which was a useful possession of Man's ancestors.

occupations involving much standing cause " flat-foot "—the arch is not strong enough for its new task, and breaks down at the mid-tarsal joint, which was flexible in the four-footed monkeys. A high instep arch, such as is found in Europeans, necessitates powerful calf muscles to make up for the smaller, less efficient heel, so that a well-

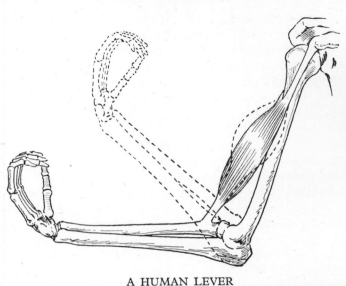

A HUMAN LEVER

The contraction and relaxation of the voluntary muscles move the levers or bones with the joints as fulcrum.

developed calf is another progressively human characteristic. We see, therefore, that this great advance in evolutionary progress was brought about without the appearance of any really new structure — instead, there was wholesale adaptation and conversion of pre-existing structures and the consequent retainment of many elements no longer useful.

BOOKS OF REFERENCE

Man and Woman. HAVELOCK ELLIS.
Sex. P. GEDDES and J. A. THOMSON.
Nerves. FRAZER HARRIS.
Glands in Health and Disease. B. HARROW.
The Human Body. Sir ARTHUR KEITH.
The Engines of the Human Body. Sir ARTHUR KEITH.
Romance of the Human Body. R. C. MACFIE.

Body and Mind. W. MACDOUGALL.
An Introduction to Sexual Physiology. F. H. A. MARSHALL.
The Integrative Action of the Nervous System. C. S. SHERRINGTON.
Internal Secretion and the Ductless Glands. SWALE VINCENT.
The Structure of Man. R. WIEDERSHEIM.

BODY AND MIND

By GEORGE SOMERVILLE, M.D., D.P.M., Deputy Medical Superintendent, West Ham Mental Hospital.

IF we accept that the highest object of medical science and the best means to complete and happy living lie in the attainment and preservation of a *sound mind* in a *sound body*, it is a necessary corollary that we should possess a clear understanding of the nature and relationship of body and mind.

There has lingered long a tendency to view the mind as a mystic entity or as an intangible essence, independent and aloof from the body it inhabits. Now this belief is an unfortunate legacy of theological speculations concerning the soul. Even in the centuries of scientific enlightenment it hindered rational investigation of the phenomena of mind—a happening which was reflected in the barbarous cruelties inflicted on the insane.

For the body was looked down upon with contempt as vile and unclean, to be despised and castigated : it was the sordid earthly prison from whose bourne the pure and ethereal mind desired to escape. In harmony with this doctrine of mind and body, insanity was not ascribed to disease but to enslavement by a supernatural agency of diabolical nature, and the treatment to be adopted was that which was appropriate for the devil, namely, chains and scourges.

Happily, with the advances in knowledge of the physiology of the animal body in the nineteenth century, it became clear that the manifestations of the mind take place through the medium of the nervous system and that its derangements are a result of nervous disease, able to be investigated and treated as other disease. The mind was liberated from the bondage of false theology and the science of psychology was born. Thus only in the last century was regained the standpoint concerning the relation of mind to body which was in vogue among the Ancient Greeks four hundred years before the birth of Christ.

The human brain is the apex of the evolutional process. Its development, in unbroken chain, can be traced from **The Mind Machinery.** the earthworm up through the lower to the higher animals till it reaches its highest exhibition in man. The brain is the essential organ of the body, for the sake of which all others exist. It consists of a mass of special cells arranged in groups which link up, co-ordinate, and control all organic activities. Situated on the surface or cortex of the brain is the " grey matter," a layer of delicate nerve cells arranged in a most complicated fashion, and this portion is devoted to the all-important function of the mind.

The working of a nerve cell may be compared to a minute electric battery. The cell, through its vital activity, evolves nerve force and sends it out by way of its attached fibres in the same way as the battery, by chemical activity, evolves electricity and sends it out. " Mind may be regarded as the highest form of nerve force. It is not ' created ' in the brain, but it is

absolutely conditioned by that organ " (T. S. Clouston).

The physiological foundation of mind lies in the reactions of the individual to his surroundings and to stimuli arising from within his body. Stimulation of a sense organ, such as the eye by a bright light, causes an impulse to travel to the brain *via* a *sensory* nerve fibre—where, by means of an association fibre, a new impulse is generated, and this passes *via* a *motor* nerve fibre to certain muscles—in the example given, to the eye muscles, causing blinking and constriction of the pupil. This event—the motor response to sensory stimulation—is known as a " simple reflex," and it is a protective mechanism very necessary for the survival of the individual.

The brain is essentially a system of connections between the in-going sensory fibres and out-going motor nerve fibres, and these connections are correlated and co-ordinated in a tremendously complicated manner. But the working of the entire nervous system, including the brain, is organised on the basis of the reflex, and a great deal of mental activity, revealed by conduct, is occasioned by a *chain* of reflexes *conditioned* by associated experiences.

The brain cells of the newly born child, the vehicle of mind, possess infinite potentialities. It is chiefly in childhood that development of those cells takes place, as a result of impressions or stimuli which are constantly received from the various sense organs — eyes, ears, nose, etc.— and, in addition, from the working of the internal organs—heart, lungs, intestines, etc. Sense im-

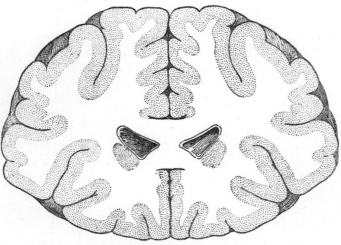

THE THINKING MACHINE

The function of the mind is performed by the " grey matter " of the brain—a layer of delicate nerve cells arranged around the outer surface.

pressions are recorded in the nerve cells as sound waves are recorded in the gramophone record, and, given certain conditions, are capable of reproduction.

The reception within the brain cells of stimuli from the self and the surroundings produces what is called " sensation," and *consciousness* is simply awareness of such stimuli. Thus all mental functioning is founded primarily on sensation, and consciousness is best regarded as the most highly developed stage of the irritability, or power to respond to stimuli, which characterises the protoplasm of all animal cells. Upon the healthy functioning of the highly developed cells of the brain cortex (grey matter), therefore, consciousness depends, and should these cells be injured, as by a blow on the head, or poisoned as by alcohol or disease toxins, then consciousness may be limited or actually suspended.

In order to have healthy and vigorous brain cells and consequently a vigorous mind, it is necessary that these **Mental Activity.** cells should be plentifully supplied with nourishment. Thinking or feeling uses up brain energy, and the body meets this demand by increasing the blood supply to the brain. Hence arises the necessity for pure and abundant blood and a strong heart—with elastic vessels to circulate it to the brain. Many disorders of the mind result entirely from poisons floating in the blood stream.

Another important factor essential to the continued development and attainment of vital brain cells is a steady and varied stimulation obtained from the sense organs. Absence of such stimulation, such as may result from defect of the sensory apparatus, may be productive of mental impairment ranging from slight deficiency to actual idiocy. The cases of Laura Bridgman and Helen Keller are instructive examples of how mental development may be reached through sensory stimulation.

" Both girls lost their sense of hearing and sight and the faculty of speech in early life. They both from this cause remained for years in a condition of virtual idiocy through brain arrestment. The only sense available for their development was that of touch. By a marvellous process of teaching, touch was made to take the place of the other lost senses, and they both became intelligent members of society. They were restored to the enjoyment of intellect, emotion, imagination, inhibition, morals, and the social contact of their fellows." *

It is thus clear that the attainment of a keen, intellectual, emotional, and happy life, in other words, mental health, is fundamentally dependent upon healthy nutrition of the brain cells and upon a sufficiency and variety of impressions derived from stimulation of the senses.

Although the brain is pre-eminently the mind centre, it is nevertheless impossible to **Brain, Mind and Body.** limit the study of mental activity to the solitary study of that organ, for it receives impressions *via* the nerves from every part of the body and, at the same time, exerts an influence, beneficial or harmful, on every element of it. All parts of the body, from the most simple to the most complex, are linked in a sympathetic contact of which mind, through the brain, is the crown and consummation. Brain function is indissolubly bound up with bodily function, and mind comprehends the whole of bodily life.

Subtle but continuous influences act on the brain and mind from the healthy or unhealthy working of the lungs, heart, digestive organs, skin, and ductless glands. The background of mental feeling is plainly determined by the state of the internal organs, and in this respect we need only consider how our moods depend upon hunger, repletion, the state of the bowels, fatigue and rest, cold and warmth, pure and impure air, stimulants and drugs.

In our daily life our bodily routine is the counterpart of our mental routine. In health we rise vigorous and energetic : our breakfast reinforces this state, and our mental powers approach their maximum as the day advances. With the using up of energy they gradually fade, but are renewed by

* *The Hygiene of Mind :* T. S. Clouston.

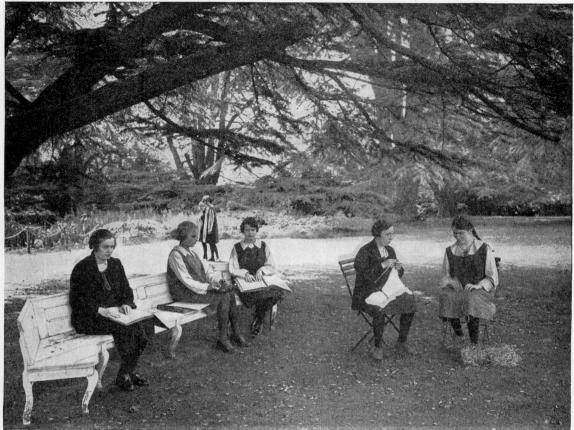

Courtesy] [National Institute for the Blind

TEACHING THE HANDS TO SEE

Blind girls learning to replace their sight by the sense of touch. A defective sense organ impairs the development of the brain unless another can be made to take on its duties.

fresh nourishment and remission of work. Towards the end of the day, fatigue sets in and fades into the oblivion of sleep.

The Viennese psychologist, Adler, attributes an extreme significance to the occurrence of physical (organic) inferiorities. He believes that the development of the child's personality is influenced to a very large extent by the unconscious desire to compensate for the sense of inferiority aroused by contact with the world, and that the childish attitude to life persists into maturity affecting all the thoughts, feelings, desires, and actions.

The influence of bodily afflictions or diseases upon the mind furnishes evidence of the intimate connection between **Bodily Afflictions.** mind and body. The consumptive patient is well known for his sanguine optimism : affections of the heart are often accompanied by anxious dread and apprehension : liver troubles engender a gloomy, spiteful mood, and dyspepsia leads to irritability and querulity. A diminished blood supply to the brain from thickened arteries may produce premature senility, and the poisons from a fever, circulating in the blood stream, may cause delirium. Physicians realise only too well how every bodily ailment has its mental counterpart.

The effects of the endocrine or internal secretory organs—the "glands of personality"—upon mental activity are very remarkable. Should the thyroid gland become feeble in function or fail altogether, consciousness is blunted, power of concentration is diminished, and initiative almost disappears. (Physical changes of a degenerative type accompany the mental deterioration : myxoedema.) Removal or disease of the sexual glands similarly leads to profound mental changes : the eunuch is morally and intellectually debased as well as physically emasculated.

Thus, there can be no doubt that any variation in the body will produce a variation in the mind, and on every side there are facts revealing to us at every moment of our existence "how at the mercy of material happenings our spirit is."

All health is ultimately mental health, for the mind is the supreme function of the **Mental Health.** body. A sound mind and a sound body are mutually dependent : the one cannot exist without the other. Already it has been demonstrated how a sick organ affects the mind, and it

teaching people the laws of correct functioning of mind and body, and rational hygiene must rest solely on a sound physiological conception of the true relation of the brain and mind to each other and to the rest of the human organism.

All scientific evidence points to the futility of studying mind apart from body. **Essential Unity.** Although we cannot at present form any conception of the way in which mind processes originate from the chemical and physical changes in the molecules of the protoplasm of the nerve cells, with the advancement of our knowledge, the interrelation between mental and bodily processes becomes more clearly understood, and we realise their inseparable nature

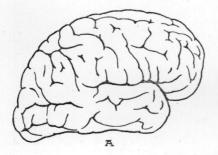 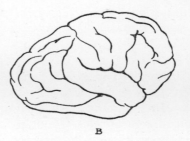 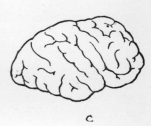

A   B   C

A COMPARISON OF BRAIN POWER

A is the brain of a normal adult ; B shows the smaller and less complex structure of an adult idiot's brain ; C is the brain of a new-born child.

can likewise be shown how a sick mind affects the body. Severe and protracted mental depression enfeebles the vitality of all the organs, disturbs the balance of the endocrine glands, and increases the susceptibility to germ infection. Anxiety and fear cause an inhibition of the digestive function with all its attendant evils. Hysteria may lead to various muscular paralyses or to the development of insensitive patches on the skin (anaesthesia). All mental diseases have their physical accompaniments — some obvious, some hidden.

To enjoy health is the right of every man, and for a happy, efficient, and full life, a healthy mind is the prime necessity. It is the purpose of mental hygiene to prevent disease, and to reveal the way to health by

—a very practical issue, for it is the basis of the science of mental hygiene. "The metaphysician may, for the purposes of speculation, separate mind from body, and evoke the laws of its operation out of the depths of self-consciousness ; but the physician who has to deal practically with the thoughts, feelings, and conduct of men ; who has to do with the mind, not as an abstract entity concerning which he may be content to speculate, but as a force in nature, the operations of which he must patiently observe and anxiously labour to influence—must recognise how entirely the integrity of the mental functions depends on the integrity of the bodily organisation— must acknowledge the essential unity of body and mind." *

* *Body and Mind :* H. Maudsley.

IX

HEALTH AND DISEASE

THE MEANING OF ILL HEALTH

*By GEORGE SOMERVILLE, M.D., D.P.M., Deputy Medical Superintendent,
West Ham Mental Hospital.*

THOUGH all of us know what we have in mind when we speak of health and disease, so long as human knowledge is incomplete, all efforts to define these terms in full must be in vain. We may regard health as the perfect balance of the changing equilibrium in the life of an organism : disease signifies something less than this perfect balance. Health is not a quiescent state : it indicates a continual and successful striving to adjust and maintain the organism in its ever-varying environment. Disease implies a failure in this relationship : it must not be looked upon as an entity apart—as something imported and subsequently possessed by the body, which can be expelled by drug or knife ; it is a disturbance which contains no elements essentially different from those of health.

Health and disease are best regarded as relative *conceptions* in harmony with contemporary knowledge, necessary and useful —as convenient as the ether of the physicist or the atom of the chemist.

"The healthy know not of their health but only the sick." Disease in human beings, sooner or later, reveals

Symptoms and Signs. itself in a consciousness of something wrong. The body is empowered to respond to disease : we "complain" ; in other words, we describe our "symptoms"—the subjective evidence of disease. If we are observant or visit a physician, certain "signs" are detected— the objective evidence of disease. For example, if we have heart disease we may complain of shortness of breath and pain : these symptoms direct the physician to examine our heart, and he may detect certain signs—murmurs or enlargement.

Symptoms and signs do not present themselves in a disorderly array, but tend to arrange themselves in groups with a certain degree of constancy ; they form "syndromes" which *pari passu* with the advances of medical science, have become correlated with certain morbid bodily processes, and have given rise to a classification of disease. From a study of symptoms and signs it thus becomes possible to "diagnose" a disease entity. Classification is a measure of our knowledge of the pathology of all organisms : diagnosis is the recognition of a disease already classified, and the reference of it to its place.

It is necessary to emphasise that symptoms and signs do not constitute the disease. Though occasioned by the presence of disease, they are merely the altered reactions of the organs and tissues to the various stimuli of life, both from within and without. An example will make this clear : if a lobe of the lung is put out of action by pneumonia, the symptom of breathlessness will arise ; but increased respiration is necessary to maintain a sufficient oxygen supply in the circulating blood—hence the symptom is the normal or correct reaction to the demands of life occasioned by the abnormal stimuli from the diseased lung.

This distinction is of more than theoretic interest : it leads to an important principle in the science of therapeutics or the treatment of disease. Although symptoms and signs are the outward and indirect flourishes of disease, the primary aim of therapeutics is to eradicate the causal factors of disease and to place the organism in the best possible circumstances which will allow the natural recuperative powers of the body to assert themselves. It is incidental that the symptoms and signs disappear : to remove symptoms and signs *per se* is not the object of therapeutics ; in fact, to do so may react adversely on the diseased person. For example, to diminish the breathlessness of lung disease by a drug would lead to deficient aeration of the blood with its evil consequences ; to check the nose bleeding, which acts as a safety-valve when the blood-pressure is high and the arteries hardened, is to run the risk of inducing a cerebral haemorrhage.

The symptom of pain deserves special comment. The object of pain is to draw attention to the existence of something wrong. Without pain many deep-seated diseases would go unnoticed, and herein lies one aspect of the tragedy of cancer, for, in its early and possibly recoverable stages, it is painless, and consequently either ignored or unperceived. Yet the symptom of pain may overstay its useful purpose, and then it becomes necessary to adopt methods to relieve it—though this is in no sense an attempt to treat the underlying disease, and has in it an element of danger. For should pain be the only or predominant symptom, the diseased person is apt to imagine that he has recovered from his disease, whereas only its outward manifestation has been removed.

Concerning the causation or " etiology " of disease, as a rule, many factors are in operation. Aristotle said that " Men are called healthy in virtue of the inborn capacity of easy resistance to those unhealthy influences which may ordinarily arise ; unhealthy in virtue of a lack of that capacity." It is well known that members of certain families and races are peculiarly liable to suffer from certain diseases. To this inborn proclivity is applied the term " diathesis." Gout is a striking example of a diathetic disease. Members of gouty families are prone to suffer attacks on the slightest provocation, whereas a combination of all the known exciting influences is powerless to affect a member of an immune family. Haemophilia, or the tendency to bleed on

Causation of Disease.

slight cause, affords another good example of a diathetic disease. Similarly with tuberculosis : although the presence of the tubercle bacillus is essential, the tissues of certain individuals appear predisposed to invasion, and the occurrence of disease. Certain persons are predisposed to attacks of skin disease, notably psoriasis, and the rheumatic diathesis is well defined. In the realm of the mind, diathesis has its counterpart in the pre-psychotic personality.*

The ultimate nature of diathesis is a scientific problem yet unsolved : in a general way it may be presumed to imply the inheritance of various physico-chemical modifications of the complex molecules of the body cells. It is believed to be transmitted according to the Mendelian Law— sometimes as a dominant and sometimes as a regressive tendency. It is interesting to note that the study of diathesis is one of the most ancient and, at the same time, has been one of the most sustained in medical history. Although the revelations of bacteriology in the last century eclipsed the factor of diathesis, to-day the subject is being scientifically investigated on all sides—statistically, anthropologically, and bio-chemically—with promising results.

Closely related to diathesis is " idiosyncrasy "—a hypersensitiveness to certain proteins, which occurs in related individuals in different generations. In this condition the ingestion of the albumen of milk or eggs, or the flesh of shell-fish, is followed by gastro-intestinal disorder (vomiting : diarrhœa) and nettle-rashes. No doubt idiosyncrasy is also dependent upon aberrations in cellular structure.

Diathesis represents the " soil." To understand the soil is to be in a position to remedy its deficiencies or guard against its contamination. Herein lies an important and far-reaching aspect of diathesis, for when scientific knowledge is such that it is possible to diagnose diathesis with certainty, to know its dangers, and to prevent its diseases, the applications of preventive medicine will be greatly extended. Already

* See section on " Mind in Health and Disease."

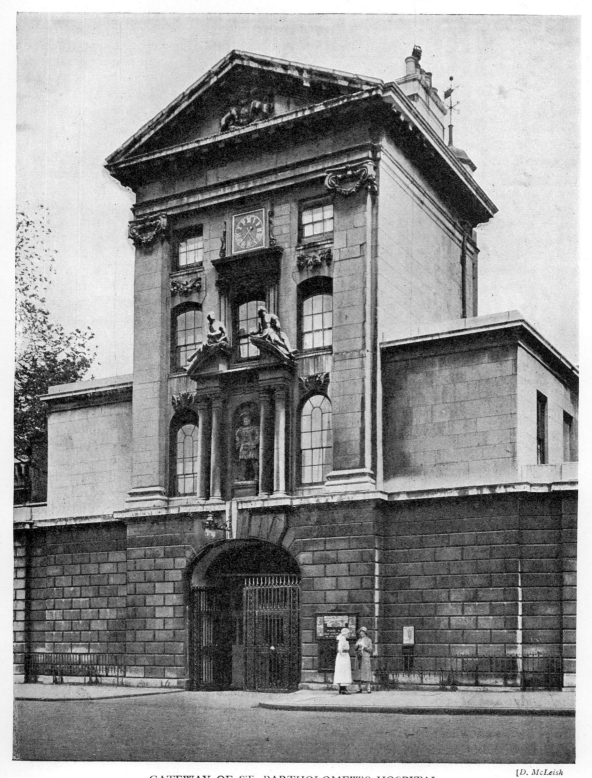

[D. McLeish

GATEWAY OF ST. BARTHOLOMEW'S HOSPITAL

London's oldest hospital was originally founded in 1123 by Rahere, a canon of St. Paul's. The fine gateway dates
from 1702.

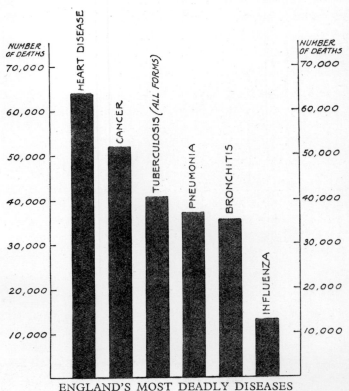

NUMBER OF DEATHS
70,000
60,000
50,000
40,000
30,000
20,000
10,000

HEART DISEASE
CANCER
TUBERCULOSIS (ALL FORMS)
PNEUMONIA
BRONCHITIS
INFLUENZA

NUMBER OF DEATHS
70,000
60,000
50,000
40,000
30,000
20,000
10,000

ENGLAND'S MOST DEADLY DISEASES
Showing the proportion of deaths due to the chief fatal diseases in England and Wales in one year.

similarly with the bacilli of influenza and pneumonia. In contrast, however, it seems certain that infection with organisms of anthrax or syphilis will in all cases result in disease. Thus bacteria vary in their potentialities as disease-producers : the presence of some is inevitably followed by disease : with others, disease may or may not follow. In the case of the latter, one or other or both of two factors may be at work : either the organisms have a wide range of virulence or there is bodily resistance or susceptibility to the infection. High virulence of the bacteria and low resistance of the body make disease certain : low virulence of the organisms and high resistance of the body make health certain.

Resistance and susceptibility to bacterial disease is an anthropological problem of considerable magnitude which is yet far from solution.‡ Susceptibility may be inborn (constituting diathesis), or it may be acquired by allowing the body vitality to become lowered by neglect of the laws of hygiene. Injuries, deficiency of sunlight and fresh air, insufficient exercise, diet which is unsuitable in quality and quantity, self-poisoning from constipation—all contribute to diminish the body resistance to bacterial disease.

headway has been made in this direction. The rheumatic diathesis has been the subject of much research : knowledge is now available by which it is possible to detect the pre-rheumatic child and, by the application of suitable measures, to prevent the manifestations of this disease.*

If diathesis is described as representing the " soil," then bacteria may be regarded as representing the " seed." The Bacteria.† presence within the human body of certain bacteria is related to the occurrence of certain diseases, but although the occurrence of such disease necessitates the presence of the specific bacteria— certain of these bacteria *may* be present in the body *without* producing the disease. Thus, in diphtheria, the diphtheritic bacilli are present somewhere in the body (usually in the throat), but some persons may harbour the bacilli without evidence of the disease :

It is necessary to emphasise that a proper perspective should be maintained regarding the relationship of bacteria to disease. The advances of bacteriology during the latter half of the last century focussed scientific attention on bacteria as the preponderating factor in disease. More and more it is being realised that although in certain bacterial diseases the specific bacteria are the sole factors in their causation, in many others (it may be most) the factor of bacterial infection must be viewed in conjunction with other factors of relatively greater significance.

* See section on " Rheumatism."
† See section on " Bacteriology."

‡ See " Protective Powers of Blood."

The factors of diet and self-poisoning in the production of disease are of far-reaching importance and are considered in detail in the sections on " Diet and Nutrition," " Human Sanitation," " Skeletal Changes and Pathological Principles," " The Teeth in Health and Disease," and " Chronic Rheumatism."

The influence of disease may interfere with any of the three types of cellular activity—namely, nutrition, reproduction, and special function. Injurious agents may attack the cells by various channels : they may act *directly* as on a free body surface, or they may be transmitted *via* the blood or lymphatic circulations : they may act *indirectly* through the mechanism of the nervous system, or by undermining the activity of an organ, such as the thyroid, which is vital to the health of other cells.

Disease Processes.

The harmful influence may produce retrogressive changes such as *degeneration*, which is characterised by the transformation of the cell protoplasm into inert material ; or *infiltration* where inert material, which may arise elsewhere, is accumulated in excessive amounts in the cells. Actual death of cells may result—to which the term "necrosis" is applied, and should this condition be complicated by putrefaction from subsequent bacterial infection, it is defined as " gangrene."

When there is a diminution of the number of active specialised cells of an organ or tissue with their replacement by a lower tissue of a fibrous nature, this retrogressive process is described as " atrophy." In old age, where the reparative capacity of the tissues to make good the waste due to metabolism is lost, general atrophy or wasting supervenes. Similarly, in starvation due to deprivation of food or some of

its essential elements, in absence of nerve control or the internal secretions, in the presence of specific bacterial poisons or the absorption of noxious substances generated in the alimentary canal—general atrophy of tissue and organ cells ensues. In some instances the atrophy may be local : it affects individual organs or a group of allied tissues. Such an atrophy may occur as a physiological process, as in the involution of the thymus gland in childhood, and in the female reproductive organs at the climacteric. It may result from defective nutriment, as when an artery is narrowed by disease, from diminished functioning or

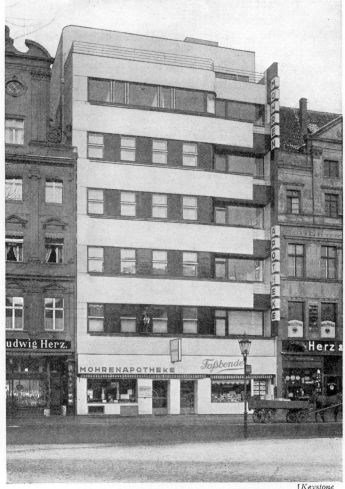

[Keystone

EUROPE'S ONLY " MEDICAL HOUSE "

Built to the latest designs, this house in Breslau contains the consulting rooms of nine physicians, with a chemist's shop on the ground floor.

disuse, from prolonged excessive use, from continuous pressure, and from a local failure of nerve control.

A group of body cells may proliferate in an unlimited manner, independent of the needs of the body, and uncontrolled by the factors which govern normal growth. This aberrant activity results in the formation of a " tumour " or " neoplasm," and disease is occasioned by its pressure on or infiltration of bodily organs and tissues, thus impeding their function or causing destruction of their component cells.

Anything which causes damage or irritation to the tissues—bacteria and their toxins, mechanical, chemical, and thermal irritants—excites body reactions for the prevention and repair of that damage. These reactions are classed under the term " inflammation." The phenomena of inflammation are a series of events occasioned by the *health* resources of the body in response both to the irritant factor and the damaged cells. By means of inflammation the irritant is got rid of and the damage repaired. Fever is a common accompaniment of inflammation—almost constantly present in severe inflammation of bacterial origin—and is a normal protective reaction on the part of the body, for high temperature is inimicable to the activities of disease-producing organisms. Closely allied to inflammation, in fact, forming an aspect of this process, are the protective powers of the blood. These are health responses to the process of disease. On the same principle, in order to meet a demand for an increased functional activity, an

Health Processes.

organ may increase its essential component elements : it is then said to " hypertrophy." A common example of this process may be seen in the greatly increased size of the muscle of the left ventricle of the heart in cases where there is increased resistance to the blood circulation such as results in arterio-sclerosis. Hypertrophy is an attempt on the part of the body to compensate for or neutralise the effects of disease.

From these observations it is evident that the state of health is a peculiarly active process. Not only does it signify an equilibrated functioning on the part of every organ or collection of cells in the body to maintain a maximum of organ efficiency, it also implies potential resources for the combating of disease and for the reparation of the results of disease. And to *maintain* health is similarly an active process. Health is a state of being which is largely within the control of individual persons, and is a state to be attained only by the continued striving towards the ideal implied by a " health conscience " founded on scientific knowledge. Man has created a civilisation through the activities of his mind which has placed his body at many disadvantages. On the survival of the body depends man's future : therefore he must create a way to health. Education is a preparation for complete living—and complete living signifies health. Instruction in the form and functioning of the human body in relation to its environment, the effects of disease and its prevention—guides to the golden road to health—is the educational right of every man.

PAIN: NATURE'S WARNING

By GEORGE SOMERVILLE, M.D., D.P.M., Deputy Medical Superintendent at the West Ham Mental Hospital.

AS human beings, with minds conscious of our bodies and of the outside world, we are all sensitive to pain ; indeed, pain may be regarded as a condition of life, necessary and ultimately beneficent, for pain is Nature's indication that all is not well with the human machine. Pain is the

body's message to the mind, calling attention to defect or injury ; it is the signal of distress demanding an immediate response in the interests of bodily safety and health.

Fundamentally, our mental consciousness is dependent upon the reception within our brains of sensations derived from stimulation of our sense organs, and all our sensations are accompanied more or less by a feeling of pain or of pleasure. Painful sensations arise from harmful stimuli, and cause us to avoid them. Hence it is clear, from the biological point of view, that our ability to perceive pain is a special sense which our bodies have evolved in order that they may protect themselves by avoiding injurious conditions.

Pain is a mental phenomenon; in other words, it only exists in our minds.

Pain and the Mind. If our conscious minds are obliterated by means of chloroform inhalation, a state of unconsciousness ensues which is characterised by *anaesthesia*, a condition of inability to perceive all sensations—painful or otherwise. To say that we feel pain in a certain area of our body is strictly speaking inaccurate; we *feel* the pain in our mind but *localise* it in the special area of our body. This is easily demonstrated: the intense pain of facial neuralgia can be eliminated by severing or blocking (by means of injected drugs) the nerve conveying the impulses which are to be interpreted in the mind as painful sensations, but which in consequence never reach the mind, and so cannot arouse pain; similarly, a person whose leg has just been amputated may complain that he "feels" a pain in his toe.

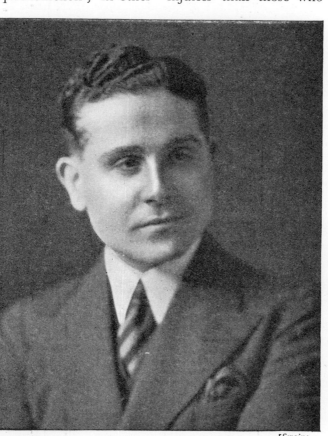

DR. GEORGE SOMERVILLE　　*[Swaine*

Pain, therefore, is a mental state dependent upon the condition of the nervous system, varying in accordance with the power of the nerves to conduct, the brain to receive, and the mind to interpret a certain kind of impression. That all pain is really mental pain is in harmony with common experience. It is well known that some individuals can bear pain much better than others, and that the healthy are less affected by painful injuries than those who suffer chronic ill health, and whose nervous systems are in a state of irritability. By mental effort, persons with a determined will can bear pain well and, in varying degree, may even inhibit the painful impressions so that they feel less pain or actually no pain at all. In the same way, if the mind is dominated by a powerful emotion, painful impressions will be inhibited for a time. This is illustrated in the case of soldiers wounded in the heat of battle, the injured player in the exciting rugby match, and, in bygone days, the martyr at the stake.

Conversely, persons with disordered minds, hysterics, may suffer pain in a localised portion of the body which is perfectly healthy. The body pain is an outward expression of an inward mental conflict. A soldier, facing the awful experiences of the battlefield, develops intense headaches which incapacitate him from active service. Within his mind wages the conflict between the stern call of duty and the natural instinct of self-preservation. He does not, in cowardly fashion, turn tail ; his mind compromises and gains its end by the unconscious subterfuge of the incapacitating headache, in this way maintaining his feeling of self-respect. Such hysterical pains are curable by means of mental exploration or, in less scientific manner (and well known to " faith-healers "), by suggestion and persuasion.

Sufficient has been written to demonstrate the importance of relating pain to the functioning of the mind. Let us now investigate the sense of pain and its association with injury and disease.

The sense of pain is specific in character, being due to stimulation of certain anatomically distinct sensory nerve-endings. "Pain Spots." These special endings or " pain spots " are not distributed evenly throughout the skin, but are more thickly collected in certain areas. It is a common experience that skin sensitiveness to pain varies in different parts of the body. Special nerve-fibres exist for the conduction of painful impressions up the spinal cord, and eventually they reach a special reception centre in the brain. In the spinal cord the pain-fibres run separately from those of touch, and this is clearly revealed in the disease, " syringomyelia " (affecting the central portion of the spinal cord), where there is destruction of the sense of pain without impairment of the sense of touch. This condition of loss of power to feel pain while the power to feel touch remains is termed " analgesia." In " anaesthesia," which may result from disease or injury to the brain, spinal cord, or special nerves, *all* sensations, including pain, are absent.

Although pain is the most widely distributed sense in the body, it is not accurately localised in the internal organs. The brain, bowel, muscles, and bones are comparatively insensitive, and may be cut or burned in a conscious person without pain being experienced. This is quite natural when we consider that pain has evolved as a protection from injury and, in contrast with the skin, the internal organs are relatively immune to damage by external objects. Nevertheless, disorders of our organs are associated with pains in some distant area of the skin, and these so-called " referred " pains play an important part in ascertaining the position of internal maladies.

Referred pain may be felt on the skin surface overlying the diseased organ, as is often the case with the heart, stomach, liver, and bowel, or it may be referred to a distant point. In certain heart disorders (*e.g.* angina pectoris) severe pain is often experienced running down the inner side of the left arm to beyond the elbow ; in dyspepsia and stomach irritation, pain may be experienced in the pit of the stomach or in the middle of the back ; in liver affections, pain is often experienced in the region of the right shoulder ; in conditions affecting the lower end of the bowel, pain is commonly experienced in the back of the thighs, especially the left thigh ; in disorders of the uterus (womb), pain is seldom felt internally, but is usually experienced in the lowest part of the back and thighs and, when the ovaries and Fallopian tubes are affected, the pain has often a very wide distribution, including the small of the back, groins, fronts of thighs, and occasionally the hip or knee joint and the heel ; in peritonitis the pain and tenderness often extend not only all over the abdomen, but also into the chest and thighs ; in ordinary intestinal colic the pain depends on the part of the bowel affected by spasm ; in gallstone colic, very acute pain is felt above the navel to the right, and often to the left side also ; in renal colic, severe pain commences in the small of the back, and radiates to the lower part of the front of the abdomen, and in both these last cases the pain is often agonising, and may be succeeded by such extreme tenderness that the sufferer can scarcely bear to allow his clothes to touch his body.

The explanation of referred pain lies in the fact that the sympathetic nerve-fibres, which are distributed to the internal organs, are connected with the sensory fibres of the same segment of the spinal cord and the passage of excessive nerve impulses (from organic disorder) up the sympathetic nerve-fibres leads to stimulation of the sensory nerves, which results in pain and tenderness in the skin, supplied by these latter nerves. Each organ appears to be associated with a definite patch or band of skin, and these areas have been mapped out as already indicated,* and prove of great advantage to the physician in the diagnosis of internal maladies.

Inflammation occurring in deeply seated structures, especially when the tissues involved are dense, is capable of producing severe pain owing to the congested blood-vessels pressing upon the nerves. In bone inflammation the pain may be of a "boring" character, and is accompanied by a throbbing sensation. Tumours infiltrating surrounding tissues tend similarly to produce a "gnawing" pain. Excessive muscular activity from irritation, as in the spasm of colic in the bowels, bile-ducts, or ureters, results in intense "griping" pain.

Kinds of Pain.

* See Diagnosis Chart.

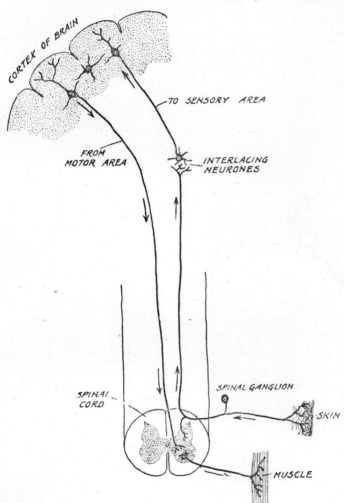

THE HUMAN TELEGRAPH SYSTEM

When trouble attacks the body machine at any point, a warning message is flashed to the brain by the nervous system, pain is "felt," and the brain sends immediate orders for defence.

Prolonged overaction of weak muscles, probably from the accumulation of the chemical waste products of fatigue, leads to continuous "aching" pain. Any source of irritation in the course of a nerve is liable to produce the severe pain known as "neuralgia." "Shooting" or "darting" pains are experienced in neuritis or nerve inflammation, and also very characteristically in loco-motor ataxia, where they are described as "lightning" pains. In certain forms of dyspepsia, owing to the excessive secretion of acid in the gastric juice, a "burning" pain may arise, and this is due, as in skin burns, to the irritation of the sensitive nerve endings exposed through the erosion of the mucous membrane.

It is necessary to refer to what is termed "mental" pain. Already it has been indicated that *all* pain is really mental pain, but by common usage the expression "mental pain" has been specially reserved for the anguish of purely mental suffering. Such pain is probably the most severe of all pains, and it characterises the mental disease known as "melancholia." In this condition

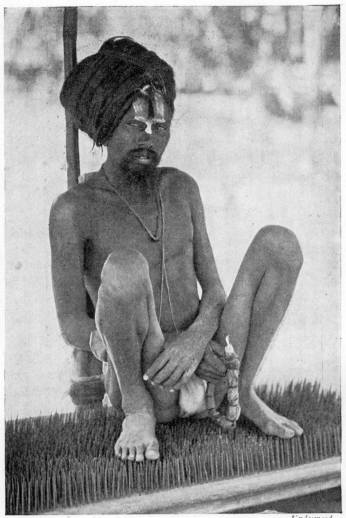

OBLIVIOUS TO PAIN

Underwood

The Hindu fakir has so learnt to control the sensation of pain that he can endure long periods of physical torment.

produce cessation of movement or the state of *rest*, which is the fundamental object aimed at by the physician in the treatment of all disease.

Pain is obviously of great importance as a guide to the physician in the detection and diagnosis of disease. It is also a guide to the individual in the preservation of health. When pain occurs, its seat, character, duration, tendency to recur, and its relationship to any other symptom or event should be accurately noted. Also attention should be directed to any happening which appears to cause, excite, or aggravate its occurrence. For example, burning pain in the stomach occurring almost immediately after taking food, sometimes accompanied by a feeling of sickness and relieved by vomiting, would be strongly suggestive of the presence of a gastric ulcer.

In discussing pain as a diagnostic agent of great value, it is necessary to mention that hysterical and hypochondriacal persons are liable to experience pains which originate from mental conflict, and which do not have any organic cause.

Finally, it must again be insisted on that as soon as a pain is experienced its origin should be sought : to remove the pain by drug or other means should be a secondary consideration, for pain is Nature's warning, and to remove the warning without knowing the cause is to court disaster. Herein lies a danger of "faith-healing," Couéi m, and hypnotism. By such methods it is possible to eradicate pain, but this only creates an unjustified and dangerous feeling of security, for the causal disease remains operative. We may cheat our minds, but we may not cheat our bodies with impunity.

the depression or mental pain is so intolerable that the sufferer tends to find in suicide the only method of escape.

It has been already emphasised that in a general way pain is a warning symptom of injury or disease ; pain is also a stimulus to muscular contraction or rigidity, the object of which is to retain the damaged or affected tissues at *rest*—a condition essential to promoting healing. Thus, in pleurisy, the pain checks the respiratory movements and so tends to limit the spread of the inflammation. Pain, therefore, through the medium of the muscles, tends to

THE CAMPAIGN FOR MORE ABUNDANT LIFE

By Sir W. ARBUTHNOT LANE, Bart., C.B., M.S., F.R.C.S.

THE outstanding success of the modern practice of medicine is in the direction of preventive measures based on a wider knowledge of the natural history of disease. This is far more evident in the case of the Public Health Services than in the everyday relation between the individual citizen and the practising physician, even though in the former case the new knowledge is being but imperfectly utilised.

The public continue to regard the doctor as one who heals rather than one who teaches, and to seek his aid only in times of trouble.

The American nation, always practical, has in the past few years realised the fact that as one approaches the age of middle life there are many diseases, slow, insidious, and often painless, which exact a heavy toll, but which may be greatly mitigated, if not altogether prevented, by a thorough, regular, and systematic "overhaul" by an able and experienced physician.

Diet, muscular exercise, occupation, intellectual and social habits, etc., peculiar to this age, are also taken stock of as part of such examination.

The American insurance companies have already realised the advisability of having their clients medically "overhauled" from time to time.

"The advantages," says Sir William Milligan, M.D., " of such a system applied to such persons past middle age have been proved (where it has been tried already) to be so great that it is conceiv-

able that some such system may one day be insisted upon by legislative enactment." Many other eminent medical men in this country have expressed their appreciation of the value of this regular overhaul for the clients of American insurance companies, and their regret that English life assurance companies, with two partial exceptions, have not so far seen their way to follow the good lead of America.

It is almost too much to expect that any great number of our English people of, or over, middle age will consult a medical man about their health if the latter happens to be more or less satisfactory to themselves. They only want the doctor when it is not. So the great hope for this medical " overhaul " must lie with our big life assurance companies.

After six years' experience, during which

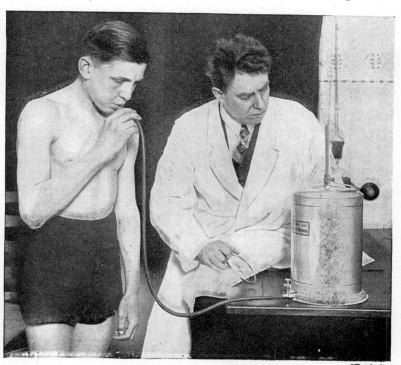

[Topical]

A PRECAUTIONARY MEASURE

A lung test during periodic medical examination—a branch of preventive medicine which is growing rapidly in importance.

the Metropolitan Life Insurance Company of America used the service, its statistical department, under Mr. Dublin, cast up accounts. The results were so astonishing that the actuarial department and the medical department refused to believe them, until forced to do so by going over the records for themselves. The three departments then united in a report showing that as a consequence of expending $60,000 on medically examining 6000 people within six years, the Metropolitan had gained through premiums of people whose lives were extended, $120,000.

In other words, the life insurance company had made 100 per cent. on its investment. . . . After this record, 44 other life insurance companies joined the service.

Physicians are trained to treat the sick. They must also learn how to treat the well.

Defects in habits of living were found in 99 per cent. of those examined.

" The favourable results of the Metropolitan Life statistics confirm, and are confirmed by the similar statistics of the Guardian Life and the Postal Life. The Guardian Life finds an average reduction of 23 per cent. in the death-rate of policy-holders affected."

In the highly complicated and differentiated structure of the human machine there are many parts to get out of order. Merely to examine a man with regard to his physical condition is not enough. It also implies, or should imply, the heightening of all the powers of the personality. The chief trouble with regard to health is that it is human nature not to seek advice until you feel ill. If that is carried to its logical conclusion one would not consult the dentist until the tooth had already decayed.

Such a policy as we have described might also cover, above an agreed figure, special medical and surgical expenses incurred by the family. There is a very large family class to whom the expense of expert medical services is very crippling and often prohibitive. Such investigation, advice, and treatment would thus be secured in the early stages of trouble. The usual course adopted is to seek such aid as a last resort—generally too late to be of any use. It would serve also to encourage timely visits to the family practitioner.

The insurance companies could do much in this way to promote a better understanding on the part of the public as regards the value of preventive treatment and advice.

PERIODIC MEDICAL EXAMINATION

By EUGENE LYMAN FISK, M.D., Medical Director, Life Extension Institute, New York.

" THAT they may have life and have it more abundantly."

Though the term " life extension " is a necessary one from the standpoint of convenience and public appeal, the real objective is not merely the addition of a few years to the average lifetime, but rather an increase in the capacity to live and to enjoy life to the full. In attaining this objective, the extension of the span of human life is a necessary by-product. This may, to some, seem like stating the obvious, but, as a matter of fact, some eminent physicians and scientific men have criticised the life extension movement because of a lack of understanding of its true objectives. It has been questioned as to whether there is any great advantage in adding a few years to a life that is perhaps none too happy or comfortable. This is a crude and superficial and, of course, a mistaken view both of the aims of life extension and of its actual workings.

At a recent public health meeting, Dr. Louis I. Harris, Health Commissioner of New York City, stated that we have passed through the age of sanitation, through the age of personal hygiene, and we have now reached the age of periodic health examinations. Such a statement by a physician charged with the heaviest responsibility for community health is significant of the change in sentiment that has taken place within the past ten or fifteen years.

HEALTH AND DISEASE

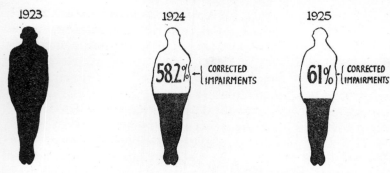

INCREASE OF HEALTH IN INDUSTRIAL WORKERS

The figures show the reduction produced in the initial number of 594 impairments in health by the system of periodic medical examination in a group of 596 industrial workers (expressed here as a single figure).

The first public health activities were concerned with community abuses and deficiencies. About fifty years ago the Health Department of New York City was a subordinate branch of the Street Cleaning Department and it was occupied with little else than the abatement of nuisances and the removal of garbage. Health inspectors were often recruited from the ranks of saloon keepers.

Community Health Measures.

The tremendous impetus given to sanitary science by the discoveries of Pasteur led us, as Dr. Harris stated, to the age of sanitation, where communicable disease was brought under control and food and water supplies were safeguarded. The opinion has been expressed by one eminent authority that only 20 per cent. of what can be accomplished in the improvement of public health can be attained through sanitation and community health measures. The balance must be accomplished through personal hygiene and the ways of living of the citizen himself.

The appeal for a programme of healthful living as adapted to individual needs was largely an after-development of the work carried on by President Roosevelt's Conservation Commission and the Committee of One Hundred,

of which Prof. Irving Fisher, of Yale University, was Chairman. This Committee issued its Report on National Vitality in 1909. There was assembled in this report existing information as to the prevalence of disease and physical disability and the consensus of scientific judgment as to what could be accomplished by reasonable application of scientific knowledge in the improvement of public health and the prolongation of human life. Predictions were made as to the probable reduction in the mortality rate from various diseases, and it was stated that at least fifteen years could be added to the average lifetime. It was concluded that 40 per cent. of American mortality was preventable or postponable, and that there were constantly three million people ill in the country, some 50 per cent. of this illness probably being preventable.

Since this Report on National Vitality was issued, in 1909, nearly fifteen years actually have been added to the expectation of human life as then shown from the death-rates in Massachusetts for 1893 to 1897. The expectation of life at that time was 45 years; it is now 58 years.

Extension of Human Life.

At the time it was issued this Report was looked upon by many conservative scientific

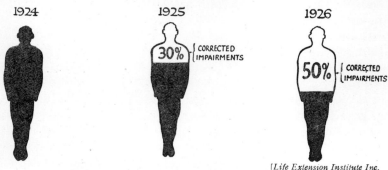

[*Life Extension Institute Inc.*]

INCREASE OF HEALTH IN POLICYHOLDERS

Showing the reduction produced in 1189 instances of impairments in health by the system of periodic medical examination in a group of 1000 policyholders (expressed here as a single figure).

men as radical, imaginative, and unsound ; yet its conclusions have been justified in a remarkable degree. The possible influence of periodic health examination was not considered in that Report, and there was then lacking the wealth of information that has since come to hand with regard to the influences of chronic infections, of diet deficiencies, and of other faults in personal hygiene. An additional possible ten years' extension of human life has been predicted by Dr. Louis I. Dublin on the basis of the experience in existing groups in the population. The leaders in public health are now predicting a twenty years' extension as the probable outcome of progress in health education.

The Report on National Vitality prepared the way for the campaign for periodic health examinations, although this was not a part of its programme. Periodic health examinations were made possible in a widespread way through the business interests of life insurance companies in this matter.

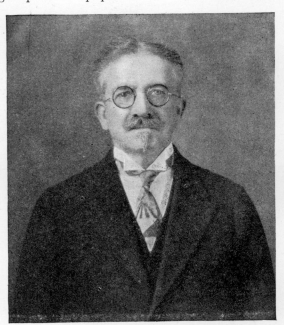

DR. EUGENE L. FISK

In 1913, the Life Extension Institute was organised on a semi-philanthropic but self-supporting basis. At the present time this Institute is serving forty-five American life insurance companies and is examining about twenty thousand people annually. The Institute also offers its service to the public at a moderate cost and has gradually developed various types of intensive and comprehensive examinations that include elaborate laboratory and X-ray research.

It should be thoroughly understood that the Institute offers nothing in substitution for ordinary clinical supervision and clinical contact. The work is wholly in the pre-clinical field, where the individual can secure an impartial, critical examination, made from no standpoint other than a desire to protect his future. With the report assembling the data contributed by such a study, the individual seeks his own physician or surgeon for treatment and correction of disabilities.

As this work has gone forward, certain basic principles have been revealed. Old age, disease, and death are shown to be due to definite causes such as heredity, infection, poisons, food or hormone deficiency or excess, air deficiencies or defects, and physical or psychic strain or disuse.

A considerable amount of work has been done among industrial employees, where the problem of fatigue is an ever-present one. Most studies of fatigue have been approached from the wrong angle—that of assuming that no other causative factor can be responsible for fatigue except work. We raise the question in our contact with industrial workers as to whether the man is tired because he is ill or ill because he is tired ; and in the majority of instances we find that he has disabilities or infections or disturbed functions of the body that are not in any way related to his work.

Periodic medical examination is well worth while as a measure to be recommended to the individual, to employers for their employees, or to insurance companies for their policyholders. If an insurance company can make two dollars profit on every dollar expended, it is a measure that is more than self-supporting. It costs the policy-holder nothing, it costs the company nothing, and the net result is that the people have life and have it more abundantly.

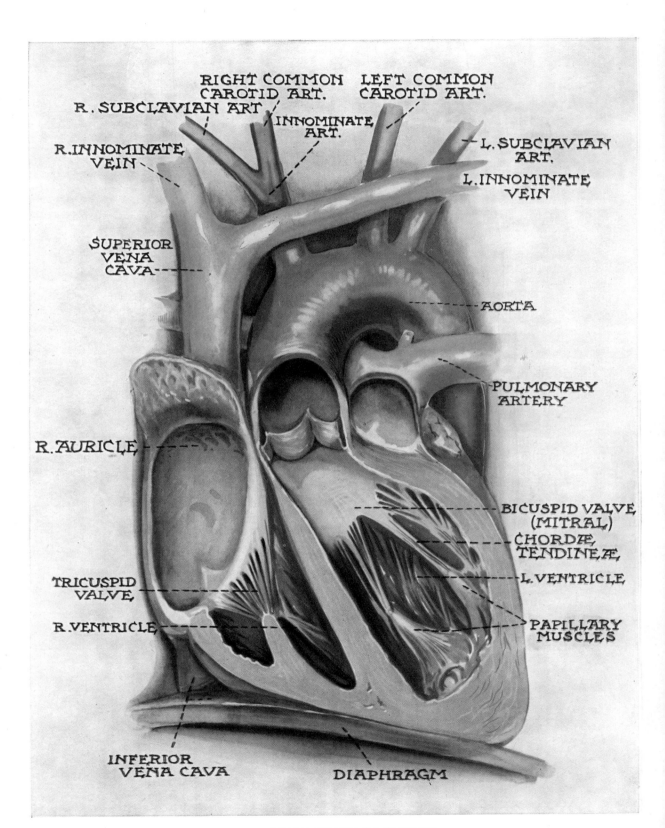

RIGHT COMMON
CAROTID ART.

LEFT COMMON
CAROTID ART.

R. SUBCLAVIAN ART

INNOMINATE
ART.

R. INNOMINATE
VEIN

L. SUBCLAVIAN
ART.

L. INNOMINATE
VEIN

SUPERIOR
VENA
CAVA

AORTA

PULMONARY
ARTERY

R. AURICLE

BICUSPID VALVE
(MITRAL)

CHORDÆ
TENDINEÆ

L. VENTRICLE

TRICUSPID
VALVE

R. VENTRICLE

PAPILLARY
MUSCLES

INFERIOR
VENA CAVA

DIAPHRAGM

THE HUMAN HEART IN SECTION.

X

THE HUMAN MACHINE
THE HEART AND BLOOD-VESSELS

By J. H. BARNARD, O.B.E., M.D., Late Physician to the Victoria Home, Paris.

EVERY tissue in the body requires, for its continued existence, a due supply of food and oxygen, and, in addition, the removal of the waste products formed by it during the performance of its functions. These requirements are satisfied by the blood, whose constant distribution to the tissues is effected by the Vascular or Circulatory System. This consists of a central pump, the heart, and a system of closed tubes called arteries, capillaries, and veins. The heart, with certain assisting forces, drives the blood along the arteries, through the capillaries and veins, and so back again to its starting-point. The interchange of nutritive material and waste products between the tissues and the blood takes place through the delicate walls of the capillaries. The central nervous system regulates the supply of blood according to the ever-varying needs of the tissues by altering the calibre of the vessels conveying the supply.

THE MACHINERY OF THE HEART

The heart is a hollow, muscular organ, of conical shape. It lies between the lungs, and is enclosed in a membranous bag called the pericardium. It is placed obliquely in the chest behind the breast-bone and the adjacent rib cartilages; it occupies more of the left than of the right half of the chest, two-thirds being situated to the left of the middle line and one-third to the right.

Its length from base to point (apex) is about 5 in., its greatest breadth about $3\frac{1}{2}$ in., and its thickness (from front to back) $2\frac{1}{2}$ in. Its weight is from 10 to 12 oz. in man, 8 to 10 oz. in woman; as age advances, it progressively increases in weight, this increase being less marked in women.

The heart is divided into right and left halves, entirely shut off from each other. Each half is subdivided into two cavities, an upper, thin-walled auricle (atrium), and a lower, thick-walled ventricle. As will be seen later, the auricles are receiving, and the ventricles distributing, chambers. Into the right auricle open the superior vena cava, conveying impure blood from the head and the upper limbs, and the inferior vena cava, conveying impure blood from the rest of the body; also the coronary sinus, bringing impure blood from the substance of the heart itself.

The right auricle and the right ventricle form the right half, the left auricle and left ventricle the left half, of the heart; the right half contains dark, venous, or impure de-oxygenated blood; the left half, bright red arterial or pure oxygenated blood. The right auricle opens into the right ventricle by an opening (the auriculo-ventricular opening), guarded by a valve called the tricuspid valve; this is composed of three triangular segments or flaps (cusps), arising from the fibrous junction between the auricle and the ventricle, and hanging down into the ventricle. The flaps consist of connective and elastic tissues; these flaps are so arranged that the blood is allowed passage from the auricle into the ventricle, but denied a flow in the opposite direction. From each flap a number of tendinous threads pass to be attached to muscular projections of the wall of the ventricle, called the papillary muscles.

In addition to the auriculo-ventricular opening, the right ventricle has another opening, that into the pulmonary artery, which conveys impure venous blood to the lungs, to be re-oxygenated and to be rid of its carbonic acid. This opening is guarded by a valve having three semilunar flaps,

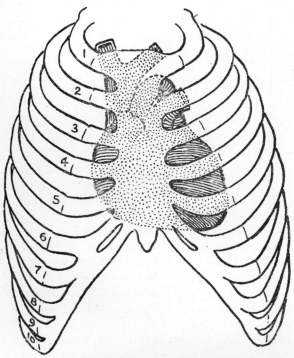

THE POSITION OF THE HEART

The heart lies obliquely in the chest behind the breast-bone, two-thirds of it being on the left side of the middle line.

from the great blood-vessels which arise from it. It looks upwards, backwards, and to the right. The apex is directed downwards, forwards, and to the left, and is overlapped by the left lung and pleura. It lies behind the space between the fifth and sixth ribs, about $3\frac{1}{2}$ in. to the left of the middle line of the breast-bone.

The lower surface of the heart lies on the diaphragm. The right auricle is larger than the left, but its walls are thinner; it is divided into two parts—a principal cavity, situated posteriorly, and an anterior smaller portion, the auricular appendage. This latter is a small, conical muscular pouch; it overlaps the root of the aorta. The left auricula similarly overlaps the root of the pulmonary artery. The right auricle will hold about 2 oz.; the left, rather less.

The right ventricle is triangular in shape, extending from the right auricle to near the apex of the heart. It forms the larger portion of the anterior surface of the heart. Its wall is thinner than that of the left ventricle, the latter being three times thicker. Its cavity, of equal capacity with that of the left ventricle, will hold about 3 oz. of blood.

The left ventricle is longer and more conical in shape than the right ventricle. It forms only a small part of the anterior surface of the heart, but a large part of the diaphragmatic surface. It also enters into the formation of the apex of the heart.

The heart is composed of muscular fibres and of fibrous rings, which give them attachment. It is covered by the Component Tissues. visceral (inner) layer of the pericardium, and its cavities are lined by the endocardium, a fine cellular layer.

The PERICARDIUM is a conical fibro-serous bag, enclosing the heart and the roots of the great blood-vessels. It consists of two bags intimately connected with each other, but differing in structure. The outer sac, the fibrous pericardium, consists of fibrous tissue. The inner sac, the serous pericardium, lies within the fibrous sac, lining its walls. It is a delicate membrane, composed of a single layer of flattened cells resting on loose connective tissue. The heart

composed of strong fibrous and elastic tissue. The centre of the free border of each cusp presents a small fibrous nodule, called the corpus arantii, which strengthens the valve. In the closure of the valve, the flaps come into contact with each other, and, being pressed together, prevent the reflux of the blood into the ventricle.

The circulation is arranged on the same plan in the left chambers. Two pulmonary veins from each lung open into the left auricle. The valve guarding the left auriculo-ventricular opening has only two flaps; from its resemblance to a bishop's mitre it is called the mitral valve. Attached to the flaps are tendinous threads (chordae tendineae) connecting them with the papillary muscles. The left ventricle opens into the aorta, the main artery of the body. This opening is guarded by a valve made up of three semilunar flaps similar in structure to those of the pulmonary valve.

The base of the heart, formed mainly by the left auricle, appears to be suspended

is thus enclosed in a double-fold bag, the space between the folds being merely a chink between the moistened surfaces of the inner fold. In other words, the cavity is a " potential " one, and only becomes real when, in pericarditis, fluid is effused and fills it. The function of the pericardium is to facilitate the incessant movements of the heart.

The ENDOCARDIUM is a thin, smooth, shining membrane ; it lines the inner surfaces of the heart-chambers and their valves, and is continuous with the lining membrane of the larger blood-vessels. It consists of a layer of delicate endothelial cells placed on a layer of connective tissue and elastic fibres.

The HEART MUSCLE, or Myocardium, differs from a voluntary muscle, like the biceps, in the following particulars. Voluntary muscles consist of fibres, each from 1 to 2 in. long, and about as thick as a thread, surrounded by a membranous sheath which isolates it from its fellows, and each with a separate nerve supply. The heart-fibre is not surrounded by a sheath, and an impulse started in one part spreads over the whole, in contrast to a voluntary muscle, where a separate impulse must enter each fibre, the impulse not spreading from one fibre to another. In the heart, the impulse starts in the great veins (the venae cavae and the pulmonary veins), near their junction with the auricles, spreads from cell to cell throughout the auricles and onwards down the ventricles to the apex. The walls of the two auricles and of the two ventricles are con-

tinuous, and this ensures synchronous contraction of auricle with auricle and ventricle with ventricle.

Thus systole (contraction) begins in the cardiac ends of the venae cavae and the four pulmonary veins. When they have emptied their blood into the auricles, they close to prevent reflux. The auricles then contract, and as soon as this contraction attains its height, the wave of contraction reaches the ventricles and the auricles relax. The ventricular contraction runs from base to apex to end in the papillary muscles. After emptying their contents, the ventricles relax, the relaxation beginning at the apex and spreading to the base. Now comes the diastole (pause) during which both auricles and ventricles are quiet. The cycle of movement then recommences, and is repeated about seventy times a minute.

The arteries supplying the heart-muscle are the coronary arteries—branches of the aorta ; they are two in number (right and left). They arise from the aorta immediately above the attached margins of the aortic valves. A free junction between the smallest

Blood Supply of Heart.

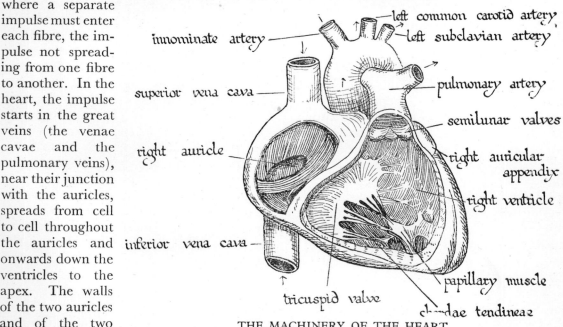

THE MACHINERY OF THE HEART
A section of the heart, showing the interior of right auricle and right ventricle.

branches of these nutrient arteries of the heart exists within its substance.

The sudden blocking of a coronary artery by an embolus, or its gradual obstruction by arterial disease or thrombosis, is a common cause of sudden death in persons beyond middle age (an embolus is a clot or a fragment of a diseased valve carried by the blood into a vessel which it blocks ; a thrombus is a clot of blood formed in the vessel itself). When the obstruction is not complete, an attack of angina pectoris (heart-pang) may ensue. The majority of the veins from the heart-substance empty into the right auricle.

The nerves of the heart are supplied by the pneumogastrics (vagi) and the sympathetic division of the involuntary nervous system. Stimulation of the vagi slows the heart-beats ; stimulation of the sympathetic quickens them. Putting the vagi out of action allows the accelerator nerve, the sympathetic, full scope, and the heart beats very rapidly. In contrast, if the sympathetic nerves are cut, the heart-beats are slowed.

Nerve Supply of Heart.

The average duration of a cardiac cycle (the time between the commencement of one beat and the beginning of the next) is about eight-tenths of a second, contributed in equal proportion by the periods of contraction and of rest. The rhythmical contraction of the heart is of muscular origin ; in other words, the heart-muscle possesses the inherent property of contraction independent of nervous stimulation. The more embryonic (primitive in type) the muscle, the more easily does it initiate the contraction wave. The muscle is most embryonic in its nature at the entrance of the great veins into the auricles ; that is the reason why the normal systole starts at this spot. Between the systole of the auricles and that of the ventricles there is a very slight pause, this being due to the fact that the impulse to contraction is conducted by the auriculo-ventricular bundle (see later), whose rate of conduction is relatively slow. The nerves, although not originating the contractions, are of great import-

ance in regulating their strength and frequency.

Some peculiarities in the circulation in the unborn child which lead to modifications in the anatomy of the heart after birth may here be mentioned.

The Unborn Child.

The principal difference between the circulation in the adult and in the unborn child is the direct communication in the latter between the right and left auricles through an aperture called the oval aperture. With this may be mentioned the large size of the valve of the inferior vena cava which directs its contents, through this opening, into the left auricle.

Other differences are the greater size of the auricles over the ventricles, and the equality in thickness of the walls of the two ventricles. Towards the end of life within the womb, the ventricles become larger than the auricles, and the wall of the left ventricle becomes thicker than that of the right corresponding chamber. Finally, the proportion of the size of the heart to that of the body is at the second month of foetal life as 1 to 50 ; at birth it is as 1 to 120 ; and in adult life as 1 in 160.

The oval aperture which allows direct communication between the two auricles is closed soon after birth. Sometimes the closure is incomplete, and a slit-like opening is left. This condition may last two or three months after birth, and is of no importance unless the deficiency be very pronounced, and is accompanied by other defects, such as obstructive disease of the pulmonary valve and an abnormal communication between the ventricles.

On the arterial side, the heart of the unborn child is peculiar in that the pulmonary artery communicates directly with the aorta through a narrow tube, the ductus arteriosus. This is a short tube, half an inch in length at birth, and as large as a goose-quill. Through this duct the greater part of the blood from the right ventricle is conducted to the aorta. Within fourteen days after birth it is normally obliterated.

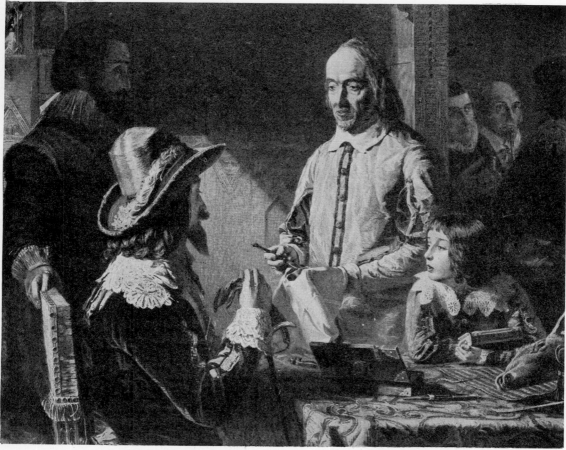

[*After Robert Hannah*

HARVEY DEMONSTRATES THE CIRCULATION OF THE BLOOD TO CHARLES I.
William Harvey's discovery in 1628 was a landmark in the history of medicine. He was the first to show that the blood makes a complete circuit through the body.

Sometimes this obliteration is not effected, but if other cardiac defects do not complicate matters, the child may survive until past middle age.

The infant who is normal begins to breathe at birth. The establishment of respiration brings a much larger supply of blood to the lungs through the pulmonary artery. The circulation through the placenta (afterbirth) is now cut off. The oval aperture is closed by a partition about the tenth day after birth. The ductus arteriosus begins to shrink immediately the infant breathes, and is, or ought to be, closed between the fourth and tenth days after birth. It is converted into an impervious fibrous cord uniting the left pulmonary artery to the arch of the aorta.

THE BLOOD-VESSELS

The blood-vessels are intimately connected with the heart, and their functioning in health and disease is closely inter-related.

The arteries lead from the heart, branching like a tree. Each branch has a smaller diameter than that from which it arises, but the united cross section of the branches is always greater than the section of the parent vessel. The veins lead to the heart, their trunks being larger than their tributaries, and their cross-section is less than that of the vessels which form them. The capillaries are intermediate between the smallest arteries (arterioles) and the smallest veins (venules).

The ARTERIES are thick-walled vessels

389

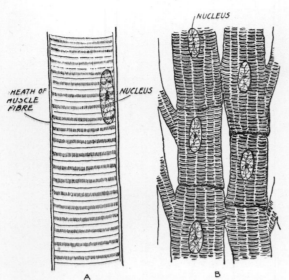

VOLUNTARY AND INVOLUNTARY MUSCLE-FIBRES

The fibres of the heart-muscle (B) are interconnected, and an impulse started at any point spreads gradually over the whole muscle. In a voluntary muscle (e.g. in the arm) each fibre (A) is sheathed from its neighbour, and requires a separate impulse from the brain.

which, when cut across, do not collapse. After death they contract and expel their contents, all the blood in the body being found in the capillaries and veins. The term "artery" or "air-tube" originated prior to the discovery of the circulation of the blood by Harvey in 1628, when, on account of their being empty of blood after death, their contents were supposed to be air.

Arteries have three coats :—

1. Tunica adventitia, the outermost coat, formed of connective tissue. This coat is most developed in the larger arteries, constituting their strongest part.

2. Tunica media, the middle coat, formed partly of yellow elastic tissue and partly of unstriped muscular fibres (called also involuntary, because they are not, like our biceps muscle, under the influence of the will). In the large arteries, the elastic fibres predominate ; in the small arteries, it consists almost entirely of muscle. In moderate-sized arteries, like the radial (the pulse at the wrist), it is muscular, with a certain amount of elastic tissue.

The function of the middle coat is to maintain a continuous pressure on the contained blood and to regulate the supply to each tissue. The maintenance of the pressure is chiefly the work of the elastic constituent of the coat ; the regulation of the supply is the part played by the muscle-fibres. The pressure thus exerted on the blood maintains, with other factors to be mentioned presently, the continuous flow through the capillaries in the intervals between the successive contractions of the heart-muscle.

3. Tunica intima. This, the innermost coat, is composed of elastic tissue (absent in the aorta and in the very smallest arteries), lined by a layer of endothelial cells. The blood, when in contact with this layer, does not clot.

Both arteries and veins are supplied with small nutrient arteries (vasa vasorum), and the muscular fibres of the middle coat are supplied with nerves (nervi vasorum).

The VEINS are thin walled, and collapse when cut across. The aggregate capacity of the veins is three times that of the arteries.

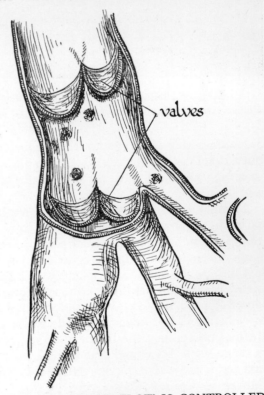

HOW THE BLOOD FLOW IS CONTROLLED

A section of a vein, showing the valves which prevent the blood from flowing in the wrong direction.

Like the arteries, they have three coats—the outer and inner very similar, but the middle containing less muscle and a larger proportion of fibrous tissue. Veins are stronger and tougher than arteries. The medium-sized veins, especially those of the lower extremities, contain valves, which, by preventing reflux, favour the flow of blood towards the heart. The venae cavae, the pulmonary veins, and the vertebral veins, have no valves. When veins become lengthened, dilated, and twisted, and the valves shrunken and useless, a state of varicosity is described. The veins not only convey the impure, dark, venous blood back to the heart, but are capable of great dilatation (especially the systemic veins) ; they thus contain a reserve of blood ready to be drawn upon when wanted elsewhere in the body. In the dead body, they accommodate not only their own normal quantity of blood, but that of the arteries as well.

The CAPILLARIES have walls consisting only of a single layer of endothelial cells, with sinuous margins joined together by a cement substance. This wall is continuous with the inner endothelial lining of the arteries and veins. The capillaries form a network in the various tissues, and there maintain a uniform diameter. Exchanges take place between the blood and the tissues, through the walls of the capillaries, of oxygen, carbonic acid, and nutrient material. The white corpuscles of the blood (leucocytes) are able to pass through their walls and through those of the smallest veins— especially in inflammation. The leucocytes constitute the police force of the body, always on the look out for foreign bodies, especially micro-organisms or disease germs, which may gain entrance into the tissues, and which they attack and endeavour to eat and digest. This process is called phagocytosis (cell eating), and the leucocytes, thus engaged, are called phagocytes.

THE ARTERIAL AND VENOUS SYSTEMS

Some knowledge of the large and important blood-vessels is necessary to understand the circulation of the blood.

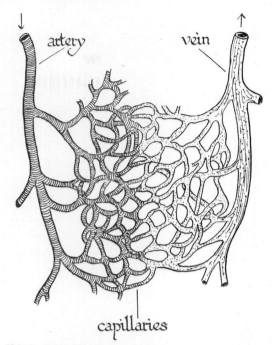

HOW THE BLOOD REACHES THE TISSUES

The veins and arteries divide up into a network of fine capillaries through the thin walls of which oxygen and nutrient material are supplied to the tissues by the arterial blood, and carbon-dioxide and waste products pass into the veins.

The arterial system begins at the left ventricle of the heart with the aorta. This is the chief artery of the body. At its commencement it gives off two branches, the coronary arteries, which supply the heart-muscle. The aorta passes first to the right, then it arches backwards and to the left, and passes down behind the left lung, in close relation to the gullet and backbone. It pierces the diaphragm, enters the abdomen, and ends about the level of the umbilicus by dividing into two branches, the common iliac arteries.

The Aorta.

From the arch of the aorta arise three large arterial trunks, namely, the innominate artery, which, after a short course, immediately divides into the right common carotid and the right subclavian arteries ; the left common carotid and the left subclavian arteries.

The common carotid arteries run up each side of the neck in an oblique line from the junction of the breast and collar bones to the angle of the jaw. They divide into

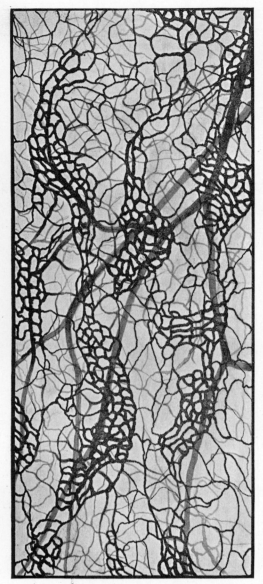

THE NETWORK OF CAPILLARIES

The mesentery, the thin membrane which anchors the bowel of the rabbit, magnified 100 times.

branches to supply the shoulder regions. The axillary arteries are continued in the arms as the brachial arteries which, in the region of the elbow, divide into the radial and ulnar arteries. These pass down the forearms and unite again across the palms of the hands to form arches which give numerous branches to the fingers.

The terminal branches of the aorta, the right and left common iliac arteries, after a short course divide into the in-

Lower Limbs. ternal and external iliac arteries. The former supply the pelvic organs and the latter emerge from the pelvis in the groins as the femoral arteries which pass downwards and inwards in the thighs deep amongst the muscles, until behind the knees they become known as the popliteal arteries. Below the knees the popliteal arteries divide into the anterior tibial arteries which lie alongside the tibiae, and the posterior tibial arteries which pass down under the calf muscles. The latter passes behind the inner ankles to the soles, where they form arches similar to those in the palms of the hands, and supply the feet and toes with branches.

The four pulmonary veins, two from each lung, open into the left auricle of the heart.

The Chief Veins. The superior and inferior venae cavae open into the right auricle. The superior vena cava is formed by the union of the two innominate veins, which result from the junction at the root of the neck of the subclavian vein from the arms and the jugular vein from the neck. The superior vena cava thus receives blood from the head, neck, and upper limbs. The inferior vena cava commences in the abdominal cavity about the level of the umbilicus by the union of the two common iliac veins. It collects the blood from the lower limbs and the abdomen. One of the largest tributaries of the inferior vena cava is the hepatic vein : this conveys the blood which has reached the liver by the hepatic arteries and also the blood conveyed from the digestive organs *via* the portal vein. The superficial veins of the legs, the saphenous veins, are of special interest,

internal carotid arteries, which penetrate the skull to supply the brain, and

Head and Neck. the external carotid arteries, which divide into numerous branches to supply the face and scalp.

The subclavian arteries arch under the middle of the clavicles over the first ribs, on which they may be compressed,

Upper Limbs. and pass into the axillae or armpits, where they are known as the axillary arteries. These arteries give off

because of their liability to become " varicose."

THE CIRCULATION

The blood, as it leaves the heart, makes a double circuit. The venous, impure blood, brought into the right auricle by the superior vena cava, which drains the head and the upper limbs, and the inferior vena cava, which drains the rest of the body, passes into the right ventricle, and thence, by the pulmonary artery, into the lungs. There the blood gets rid of its carbonic acid and acquires a stock of oxygen, being changed from a dark to a bright red colour by this gaseous interchange in the lungs, and is returned by the four pulmonary veins into the left auricle. From this chamber it passes into the left ventricle, which pumps it into the aorta, the main artery of the body, whence it passes throughout the whole of the body *via* the arteries and capillaries. The tissues abstract the necessary nutriment from the circulating blood, which eventually passes into the small veins that unite to form the venae cavae, and these return the blood into the right auricle, thus completing the circuit. There is thus a minor or pulmonary circulation from the heart to the lungs and back again, and a general circulation from the heart to the rest of the body and back again to the heart.

A subsidiary, but highly important circulation, the portal circulation, must be mentioned. The veins collecting the blood from the stomach, pancreas, spleen, and the intestines (excepting the lower part of the rectum) join to form the portal vein. This ramifies through the liver like an artery, its branches ending in capillaries called sinusoids. From these the blood is returned to the inferior vena cava (and, through this, to the general circulation) by the hepatic veins. During this circuit through the liver, important work is done by the liver cells. From the blood circulating amongst them, two products are elaborated, namely, glycogen and urea. Glycogen is a product arising from carbohydrate digestion, and is doled out through the hepatic veins as sugar to undergo combustion in the tissues, and so maintain the body-heat and energy supply. Urea is formed by the liver-cells from the amino-acids, which are the end-products of protein digestion. It is passed into the circulation and eventually excreted in the urine by the kidneys. Urea is a harmless by-product of organ activity.

By introducing into the central end (that nearer the heart) of a severed jugular vein in the neck a coloured solution (methy-

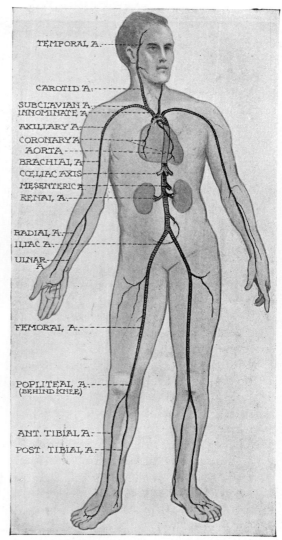

THE ARTERIAL SYSTEM

Indicating the chief arteries of the body by name. There are corresponding veins in every limb to convey the blood back to the heart.

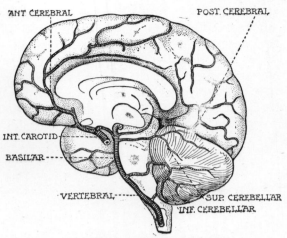

HOW THE BRAIN IS FED

Arteries run up each side of the neck and penetrate the skull to provide the brain with its rich blood supply.

lene-blue or ferrocyanide of sodium), observation of the time it takes to appear at the other end of the cut vein tells us the circulation time. That time is half a minute. In this short time the solution has traversed in succession the right heart, the lungs, the left heart, the arteries, capillaries, and veins of the head. Allowing for a longer journey, such as a visit to the feet and back again, we may reckon one minute to one and a half minutes as the average time. Some corpuscles take longer than others to cover the distance. The blood is apt to flow sluggishly in the veins of the liver and other abdominal organs. Usually one-half of the blood is contained in these veins. The usefulness of these reservoirs may be seen when blood is suddenly wanted elsewhere. A man runs to catch a train; this attracts to his limbs about two-thirds of the whole stock of blood in his body. In this case, the reservoir is depleted to meet the emergency. This resource will not meet the requirements of the brain, whose supply of blood

The Blood Stream.

is dependent on the general blood-pressure. In shock, however, the brain is rendered bloodless by the great accumulation of the blood in these reservoirs, which have received the name of the splanchnic pool.

The principal agent in diminishing blood-pressure is a sensory nerve of the heart called the depressor nerve. It ascends from the heart in company with the vagus, or one of its branches, to the vaso-constrictor centre in the medulla oblongata, carrying a message of distress, in answer to which the splanchnic vessels are dilated and the heart is relieved. When the blood-pressure is too high, the heart is in distress as in heart-pang (angina pectoris). This effort of nature often requires to be assisted. This is effected by administering nitrite of amyl as an inhalation, which dilates all the arteries of the body, and often affords instantaneous relief.

The contraction of the heart-muscle, in its task of causing the blood to circulate,

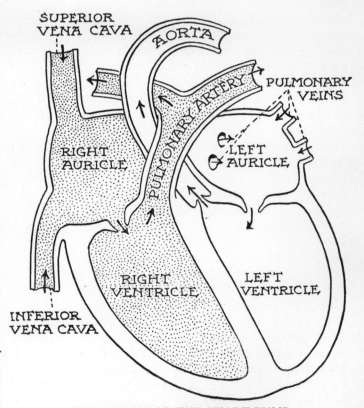

THE ACTION OF THE HEART-PUMP

Showing the course of the blood through the heart. The shaded portions contain the impure, venous blood.

is aided in two ways. One is the pressure on the veins of the muscles in action. This drives on the blood towards the heart. A man engaged in sedentary work should change his posture occasionally. This removes the weight of his body from certain veins that it is compressing. The other powerful force which aids the systole is the suction exercised by the chest in inspiration. This sucks blood into the great veins and is effective in encouraging the flow of blood. Everybody feels better after a good yawn, because the brain then receives an extra supply of blood. From the physical point of view the circulation of the blood is caused by the difference in pressure in the great vessels which first contain it as it leaves the heart, and that in the veins, which return it to the heart. The pressure in the main artery of the body, the aorta, is 200 millimetres of mercury; in the venae cavae, the pressure is nil or negative.

Causes of Circulation.

The auriculo-ventricular openings are very wide—so wide that the contents of the auricles can be emptied almost instantaneously into the ventricles. The tricuspid valve guarding the right auriculo-ventricular opening

The Heart Valves.

has three flaps, while the mitral valve guarding the left auriculo-ventricular opening has only two flaps. These flaps are tough, but thin. Their margins are festooned. The tendinous cords attached to them have been likened to the stay-ropes of a tent. At the other end these thread-line tendons are attached to the small papillary muscles. Each bunch of tendons is inserted into the contiguous margins of two flaps. When the auricle contracts, the flaps do not hang back against the sides of the ventricles. These sides are not flat, but are raised in pillars by muscular projections (columnae carneae—fleshy columns). Between these columns the blood finds its way, and floats the flaps. When the ventricle contracts, the valve balloons, the flaps meet together, not by the free edges, but fold to fold, the free edges being held down towards the ventricle by the tendons. The valve is prevented from bulging into the auricle by the papillary muscles. The flaps of the aortic and pulmonary valves form a half-cup, and behind each is a recess. This arrangement prevents the flaps from being pressed against the sides of the vessel as the blood is forced in.

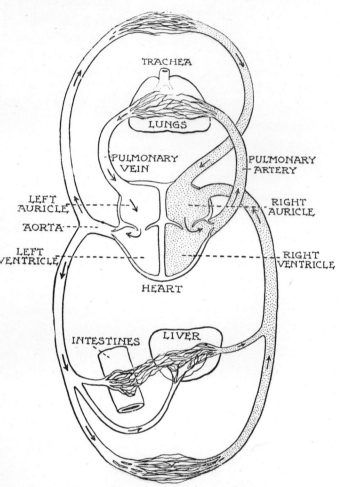

THE COURSE OF THE BLOOD STREAM

A simplified diagram (from the back of the body), showing the path taken by the blood during its circuit. The impure, returning blood is shaded.

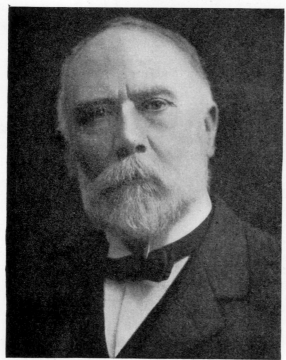

[Central Press

SIR JAMES MACKENZIE
A famous pioneer in the study of heart disease.

The power of rhythmical contraction is inherent in the heart-muscle. The excised heart of a small mammal can be **Nerve Control of Heart.** kept beating a long time when a warm solution containing a lime salt, a potassium salt, and a sodium salt is passed through the coronary vessels—the nutrient vessels of the heart. The rhythm or regularity of beats is controlled by impulses reaching the heart through the pneumogastric (vagus) and the sympathetic nerves. When the branches supplied by the vagus nerve are stimulated, the rhythm is slowed, the amplitude of each beat lessened, or the heart stops. This shows that the vagus (pneumogastric) is always sending impulses to the heart, tending to slow the beats. The cardio-inhibitory centre, whence these impulses flow, is situated in the medulla oblongata (at the top of the spinal cord, between it and the brain). When the sympathetic branches are stimulated, acceleration and augmentation of the beat occurs.

The vasomotor nerves supply the blood-vessels, and like the nerves supplied to the heart, they are of two kinds. Those which correspond to the accelerator fibres of the cardiac nerves and increase the tone or grip of the unstriped muscle in the vessel-walls (especially of the smallest arteries) are vaso-constrictor, *i.e.*, their stimulation narrows the arteries ; those which correspond to the vagus branches in the heart and inhibit the tone of the vessel-walls are vaso-dilators, *i.e.*, their stimulation widens the arteries.

The vaso-constrictor fibres (those which tend to narrow the vessel) come from the sympathetic, and are connected with a vaso-constrictor centre in the medulla oblongata. There are no vaso-constrictor nerves in the coats of the coronary arteries, of the pulmonary vessels, and of the vessels of the brain.

Thus the tone of an artery—a very important factor in the circulation—is maintained, along with the automatic action

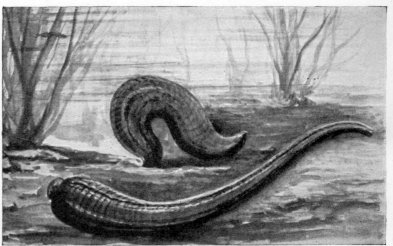

[James's Press Agency

MEDICINAL LEECHES
A panacea of the Middle Ages, when blood-letting was a universal remedy.
Leeches are still applied to reduce certain types of inflammation.

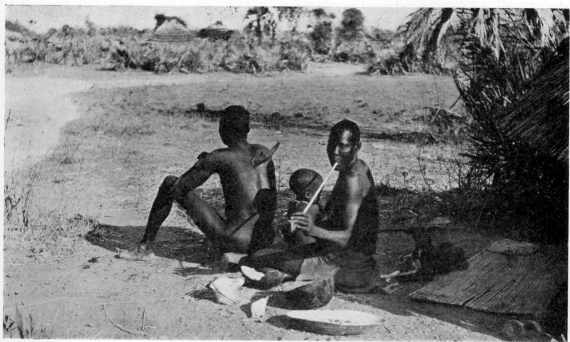

A PRIMITIVE FORM OF " CUPPING "

This African woman doctor is applying a treatment essentially the same as the modern method of "cupping,"
in which blood is drawn to the surface by a vacuum, to relieve a congested organ.

from the pressure inside the artery, acting as a stimulus or spur to the muscle-fibres of its middle coat, by the give-and-take of the vasomotor nerves. From every part of the body impulses or messages ascend every moment to the vasomotor centre in the medulla oblongata, urging it to keep up or relax the blood-pressure.

The importance of the self-adjustment of the blood-vessels to circumstances is shown by their behaviour in different positions of the body. When we are standing, the feet and the brain are adequately supplied with blood ; the latter, notwithstanding its disadvantageous position, not being kept short of blood. Spend some weeks in bed ; when you first get out of bed, your feet will perhaps swell from too much blood, whereas your brain is so badly supplied that you feel dizzy or even faint.

A small loss of blood over an engorged organ procured by the application of a leech produces a beneficial effect. Similarly, cupping (the drawing of blood to the surface by a vacuum) over the kidneys lessens the congestion of those organs. It is to this vasomotor action that we owe the occasional beneficial action of a mustard leaf or a blistering fluid.

The consideration of the heart-beat has been postponed in order to allow the reader an opportunity of familiarising himself first with the physiology of the heart as it was known up to about twenty years ago. At that epoch the discovery in the heart-substance of a structure peculiar to the heart, enables us to explain the mystery of the possession by that organ of an inherent power of prolonging its beats independently of nervous influence. The discoverer (Tawara) called this structure the conducting system ; the late Sir James MacKenzie, who has done so much to elucidate arrhythmia (disorders of the heart-beat), renamed it the genetic system. This system possesses the power of generating and discharging impulses which bring about the contraction of the heart-chambers.

The Heart-beat.

At an early stage in its development the heart is a simple tube made up of muscle-cells. These cells generate impulses which cause contraction, the impulse being passed on from cell to cell. As development proceeds, pouches—the future auricles and ventricles—are formed on the sides of the tube. This primitive tube loses some of its attributes, but becomes highly specialised for its future functions. The contractile function nearly disappears, leaving that task to the newly developed pouches (auricles and ventricles) ; the impulse production and the power of conduction, as well as those of regulation and control, are retained by the relic of the primitive tube. In the human heart, the remains of this primitive tube have been called the sino-auricular node, the auriculo-ventricular node, and the auriculo-ventricular bundle (bundle of His). The cells of this bundle can still contract slightly, but the contraction of the heart-chambers is now left to the recently developed muscle-cells of the auricles and ventricles, which respond only to impulses conveyed by their master, the genetic system, *i.e.* the two nodes and the bundle. This means that the heart-muscle cannot contract unless it receives an impulse or prod from this relic of the primitive tube, and that any disease of this structure results in alterations in the heart-beats, which are often of serious import.

The sino-auricular node, called also the heart's " pacemaker," is a small structure composed of striated and spindle-shaped nucleated cells, embedded in connective tissue, in which are found nerve-fibres from the vagus and sympathetic nerves. It is placed at the spot where the superior vena cava joins the right auricle.

The auriculo-ventricular node has the same structure ; it is situated in the wall of the right auricle, near the partition separating it from the ventricle. Fibres from the vagus and sympathetic nerves are supplied to it.

The auriculo-ventricular bundle, leaving the auriculo-ventricular node, passes over the partition and divides into two branches, which are distributed to the two ventricles. It is made of cells larger than the ordinary muscle-fibres, and less markedly striped. The different fibres are connected with each other so that each fibre is continuous from start to finish. In the ventricles the fibres break up into numerous interlacing branches, which end in the muscle-fibres of the ventricle.

The auriculo-ventricular bundle thus runs from the superior node (the sino-auricular) to the inferior node (the auriculo-ventricular) and, passing beyond, splits into two branches, which, further dividing, supply the heart-muscle of the ventricles, including the papillary muscles already mentioned. The bundle is, in short, a direct communication between the auricles and the ventricles. The significance of this bundle, and of the nodes, will transpire when arrhythmia (abnormalities of the heart's action) are under consideration.

THE CARE OF THE HEART

By G. A. SUTHERLAND, C.B.E., A.M., M.D., F.R.C.P., M.R.C.S., Physician to Paddington Green Children's Hospital ; Consulting Physician to the Royal National Orthopædic Hospital, etc. ; Author of " Modern Aspects of Heart Disease."

THE man in the street knows a good deal about the engine of his motor-car. He is aware that it must be carefully watched, that it is apt to go wrong at times and play curious tricks if it is not attended to, that even with good usage there is a time limit to its efficiency, and that with bad usage this time limit is much reduced. In his own person he possesses a mechanism—the heart—very similar to the engine of his car. The human heart is an engine designed to run, under favourable conditions night and day without intermission for seventy or more years. It is an automatic engine which, under normal conditions, requires no starting, no resting, no handling, and which works silently. When, however, it is disturbed, usually through the fault of the owner, it can back fire and make noises, and become irregular in its action. It has marvellous powers of recovery and of accommodating itself to strains and disturbances of various kinds, but it has always to work single-handed—there is no spare engine available in time of trouble. It is popularly supposed that the doctor can repair any damages to this engine, but, as a matter of fact, he feels himself rather helpless in dealing with a heart that has lost its power of doing its own work. The prevention of engine trouble will always be the best means of avoiding the risk of heart disease.

There is with many a great dread that they have a weakness about the heart or are suffering from heart disease. **Dread of Heart Disease.** No question is more frequently heard in the consulting-room than, " Is my heart all right, doctor ? " Behind that simple question the doctor knows that there often lies a pent-up feeling of fear which has not before found expression. As the public generally is singularly ignorant about the heart and its functions, it is curious that this dread of heart disease should be so common. The origin probably lies in the mystery attaching to some cases of sudden death, often much talked about, and the fact that it is the unknown which possesses terror for all of us.

Certain popular beliefs tend to encourage this dread. One is that a person with any form of heart trouble is apt to fall dead at any moment. If a patient is told that there is a valvular murmur, or some dilatation about the heart, at once arises the vision of dropping dead in the street as the natural sequel. Even if the statement is made that the heart is a little weak, at once precautions are taken to ward off this danger of sudden death, and a healthy individual may be turned into a worrying invalid for life. It is not that there is any real danger of it, but because the individual becomes obsessed with this idea of sudden death. Clearly the only line of treatment is a straight talk with a doctor in whom the doubting and dreading one has confidence. He will probably point out that sudden death is by no means a common thing in connection with heart disease, and that it is the last thing to be expected in the case of the healthy person consulting him.

There are others who suffer from the dread that they are the victims of heart disease because of certain symptoms they have noted in themselves, and which are popularly supposed to be connected with the heart. An attack of breathlessness, or palpitation, or faintness, or loss of consciousness, may be sufficient to rouse this dread. Such a symptom, or symptoms, coming on in one previously free from heart disease will usually be due to some passing disturbance in some other organ of the body. Most frequently these symptoms are due to stomach disorder, an attack of indigestion, or flatulent distension of the stomach. This may not produce any local pain or discomfort, and so the anxious mind settles on the heart as being the source of the trouble. Disturbances of the nervous system, produced by emotion or shock of some kind, are apt to induce similar symptoms. The feeling of palpitation or discomfort about the heart, which may accompany these nervous disturbances, seems to the sufferer to confirm his view that the heart is affected, but there is no real ground for this assumption.

Another word of terrible significance to many is " angina." They have heard of some one dying of angina, and so **Angina Pectoris.** to them the terms " death " and " angina " come to be synonymous. The term " angina " simply means a sense of choking or suffocation, and its fuller description, " angina pectoris," means pain about the chest, or breast pain. While pain in this region may be associated with serious forms of heart disease, it is by no means necessarily or most frequently so. Pain in this region may be induced by over-exertion of any kind and by many forms of indigestion. It is frequently due to poisoning or an exhausted state of the nervous system. It is one of the many manifestations of rheumatism when the muscles of the chest wall are affected.

Hence the person who has " a pain about the heart," and only a slight knowledge of what angina means, should not needlessly alarm himself. It is a curious fact that those who suffer from the serious and cardiac form of angina usually refer their symptoms to the stomach, and do not consider the heart as being involved. Those, on the other hand, who are alarmed by the fear of angina from the symptoms they experience are usually found to be suffering from some form of stomach trouble.

THE HEART AND ATHLETIC SPORTS

The subject of the heart and athletics is a very important one. We are an athletic nation ; we have developed athletics and spread them over the civilised globe, and we believe in their beneficial effect in the production of a healthy race. There is, however, a very general belief that heart strain is a risk associated with all the more strenuous games and sports, and that an " athlete's heart " is a very real complaint. It is more especially in connection with football, running races, and rowing, that

this danger is supposed to exist. Naturally the element of competition, when team is opposed to team, or man to man, adds to the strenuousness of the exertion, and to the risk, if risk there be, to the heart.

It may be stated generally that delicate boys or girls, or youths, should not be allowed to play in the more strenuous forms of games, or in competitions. Quite apart from the question of any danger to the heart, there is the fact that while exercise in moderation will do nothing but good, a definite risk of injury to the body generally follows the strain of strenuous physical exertion. It is also advisable that an athlete at the time of strenuous exercise should himself be in a fit condition physically. The first stage of an illness, such as tonsillitis or influenza, is not the time when the athlete will do the best for his reputation or his body. After any illness the athlete will do well to allow a sufficient convalescent

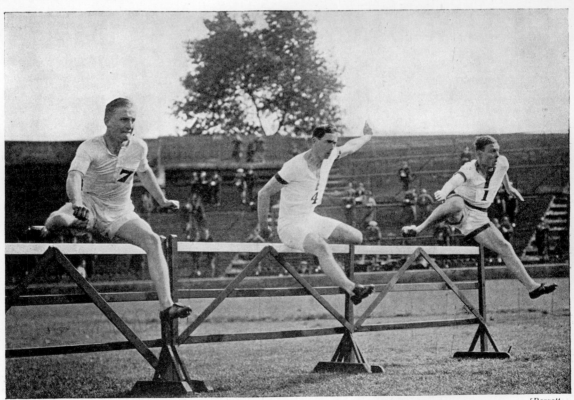

[Barratt

DO STRENUOUS SPORTS INJURE THE HEART ?

Although delicate people should not compete in the more strenuous sports, there is a tendency to overestimate the danger of heart " strain " to normal individuals, since a healthy heart is usually well able to look after itself.

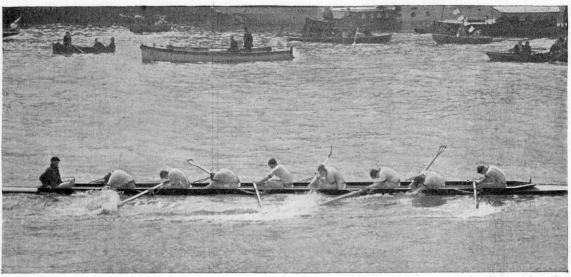

"DOWN AND OUT"

[Sport and General

The end of the centenary Boat Race, showing the losing crew completely exhausted. Such collapse, due to strenuous exercise, is usually a precautionary measure on the part of the heart, to prevent serious damage from overstrain.

stage to make him thoroughly fit before resuming active operations.

Many of the public and some of the doctors have a firm belief in the existence of "a strained heart," or "a strained muscle of the heart," or "a dilated heart," as the result of some active sport. They are familiar with strains and sprains of muscles and joints in the football and cricket fields, and they assume that the heart is equally liable. The usual sequence of events in connection with "a strained heart" would appear to be as follows. After some more than usually severe game or other exertion, a boy has fainted, or complained of severe pain in the left side of his chest, or fallen down completely exhausted. Some one says he has strained his heart, and the mischief is done. As a matter of fact, the heart has been looking after itself all the time, and knows quite well when stress has fallen upon it, and how to prevent itself from being strained. Nature has so arranged things that the heart is very well able to protect itself, and to make its own adjustments to meet conditions of physical stress. When it has had enough it produces in its owner sensations which compel him to pull up. These may take

"Strained Heart."

the form of breathlessness, or pain in the chest, or fainting, or a sensation of complete exhaustion.

The warning and compelling note comes from the heart, and when the athlete is "down and out," the heart gets its opportunity of resuming its normal action. When an athlete strains a muscle in his thigh, it is so painful that the rest which is needed becomes a necessity. If the athlete did in very deed strain his heart, then rest would be essential—but rest is impossible. The human heart is constructed to go on working night and day without a rest for threescore years and ten. The only form of comparative rest is by a lessening of the exertion put forth by the heart, and that is achieved by putting the owner at rest, temporarily. The poor, "strained" heart must carry on—and, curiously enough, it seems to be able to do so.

A well-known athlete once told me that he broke down from exhaustion while running a race, and was "down and out" for some time. This seemed to indicate if not a strain, at least a danger of exhaustion of the heart. The following day he ran the same distance, improved on all his previous records, and was free from discomfort at the end of the run. I have spent a good deal of time in trying to find examples of the strained and damaged hearts due to athletics, and so far have failed to find one. In a recent work by two famous athletes, H. M. Abrahams and Dr. A. Abrahams,* there is the following reference to athletic hearts : " We do not believe that in a healthy person even the most violent exercise can produce strain or disease of the heart, but we are more inclined to regard any strain as something affecting the whole organism." Another statement they make is : " It is the opinion of a physician, who is perhaps the greatest living authority on the subject, that in man even the most intense exertion is incapable of producing any harmful effect on the human heart. The reserve of the heart is enormous ; when the call is excessive other factors fail (and so fatigue results), but not the heart."

There are many individuals going about idle and lazy and leading invalid lives because they had in youth suffered from a " strained heart," and were supposed to be suffering from it still. Their whole life has been occupied in trying to prevent any additional strain of the heart, and thus they have been cut off from any possibility of a useful career. They live under the shadow of an imaginary injury in the past and in the constant dread of imaginary perils in the present and future. Their case is a particularly sad one, but we do not think that a healthy youth with a sound heart need have any fear of a similar fate overtaking him. He is to be encouraged in the pursuit of strenuous athletic exercises. On the other hand, the youth with a heart already damaged by disease should have his exercises strictly limited and controlled, so as not to produce any of those sensations of cardiac distress. If he goes beyond those limits, not only will the accompanying distress be more persistent, but the heart may be still further damaged.

SOME SYMPTOMS SUGGESTING HEART DISEASE

There are certain symptoms which are apt to excite alarm in the family circle,

* *Training for Athletes* (1928), pp. 16, 48.

because they are supposed to indicate a weak heart or even heart disease. One of them is faintness or a fainting turn. The subject is usually a boy or girl of school age, and most commonly at the time period between ten and fifteen years. Very often the fainting attack has occurred when the young person rose in the morning, or had been standing for some time, or had been in a hot, stuffy atmosphere. Now, while it is quite right and proper to take the youngster to see a doctor, it is by no means necessary to impress the doctor with the home diagnosis that heart disease is the cause of the trouble. The doctor will probably point out that the pallor of the face observed during the attack was due to the blood leaving it because the blood had gone elsewhere.

The tendency to faint as a result of heart disease usually shows itself during some active exertion, whereas these children show it when standing still or changing from a recumbent to an erect posture. The blood accumulates in the abdominal veins and lower extremities, and does not reach the brain in sufficient amount, and so the child faints or loses consciousness. This is not due so much to a weakness of the heart as to a weakness in the tone of the blood-vessels, and more especially the arteries. Children with heart disease seldom faint, while in a certain type of child, although the heart is quite sound, fainting is common.

This type of child is popularly described as having " a poor circulation." Other symptoms are commonly present, "Poor Circulations." such as cold, blue extremities, with a tendency to chilblains in winter, sudden flushing of the face, rapid action of the heart on slight exertion or excitement, attacks of palpitation, and a liability to exhaustion on slight physical exertion. These children have no staying power. The symptoms as a whole point clearly to some weakness of the nervous system, and more especially that part which controls the circulation. It is really a condition associated with the development of the nervous system and nervous control in the young, and indicates that there has been a lagging

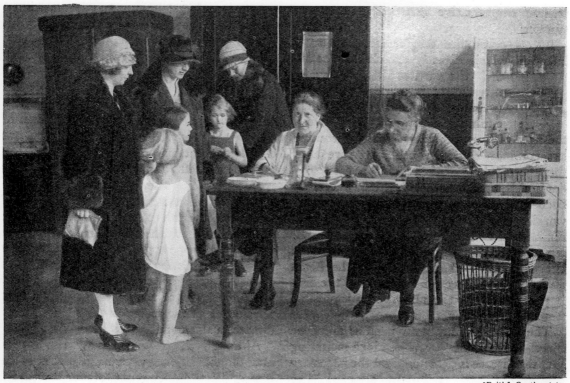

[*British Continental*

MEDICAL EXAMINATION IN A SCHOOL

In rheumatic infection, one of the most fertile sources of heart disease in children, the symptoms are often so slight as to be revealed only by regular medical examination.

behind in certain parts in this development. Every part of a child does not continue developing at the same rate and at the same time. In most cases, Nature will restore the balance if she is not interfered with unduly. The anxious parent may be reassured as to the future of the child's heart. The treatment for this type of child is not to regard him or her as an invalid, but to let him lead as normal a life as possible. He is not to be overworked whether at school lessons or school games ; he is to have an ordinary full diet ; and he is to have plenty of sleep at night.

THE DANGER OF HEART DISEASE

In this country a great number of people die every year of heart disease. The progress of civilisation may be said to be marked by an increasing number of deaths from heart trouble in the community. All classes of society share in this tendency, although different forms of disease may prevail in the various strata. The diseases and the strain of life in large towns are apt to develop different forms of heart disease from those incidental to a life spent in the country and open air.

There are two chief causes of heart disease as commonly met with. The first is an attack, or repeated attacks, of acute disease, which pick out the tissues of the heart, and leave permanent changes there. This is most common during childhood and early adult life. The second is the result of degenerative changes taking place in the heart, weakening its working power, and ultimately bringing on heart failure. This is a slow process, and commences usually after the prime of life has passed. It is intimately associated with those degenerative changes in the blood-vessels, to which reference is made in another section.* This may be

* See " Arterio-sclerosis."

termed degenerative heart disease of advancing life.

In early life the danger is some acute infection which directly attacks the heart, and the outstanding disease of this nature is acute rheumatism (rheumatic fever). It is extremely common in boys and girls between the ages of five and fifteen years, becoming less common during youth, and rare after the age of twenty-five years. The tragedy lies in this, that although the heart may have been seriously affected in childhood, its working power is not necessarily much diminished at this time, and it is not until ten or twenty or thirty years later that the effects manifest themselves, and the heart gives out. Consequently, it is of the first importance to protect all children if possible from rheumatic infection.

Acute Rheumatism.

The infection may show itself as an acute illness—rheumatic fever—so incapacitating that the disease is detected, and the necessary precautions and treatment adopted. In many ways this onset with acute illness is preferable, because under careful treatment the heart usually does not suffer to a great extent. Unfortunately one attack is apt to be followed at some interval by another, and each fresh relapse tends to an increase of the heart disease.

The most dangerous form of rheumatic infection is that in which the symptoms are so slight as not to excite alarm or to confine the patient to bed. Some of them are so common that they have come to be regarded as the usual accompaniments of childhood. Every child is supposed to suffer at times from " growing pains," and many parents regard them as due to growth and development, yet they are invariably a clear indication that the child is the subject of rheumatic infection. Other complaints which should always arouse suspicion of a rheumatic origin are recurring sore throats, a stiff neck, fleeting pains about the limbs, chest, or back, and tenderness or swelling of the larger joints, such as the ankles, knees, or elbows. Every parent should recognise that these com-

" Growing Pains."

paratively slight ailments may be associated with direct involvement of the heart, with progressive heart disease, and with heart trouble which may ultimately, possibly after many years, prove fatal.

Naturally the only time for successful treatment of such heart disease is during childhood and youth, and the chief form of treatment is preventive. It is pointed out elsewhere that parents are often unnecessarily alarmed about their children by symptoms which they erroneously refer to a heart which is quite healthy. In the case of rheumatism, on the other hand, they are not alarmed, because the symptoms complained of do not appear to them to have any possible connection with the heart. It is only by attention to the early symptoms, however slight, of rheumatic infection, that the danger of the most serious form of heart disease in this country can be averted.

Although these facts have been known and taught for many years, it seems to be impossible to get parents to accept and act on them. The medical examination of school children is now doing much good in the recognition of those early signs of rheumatic infection, and great benefit may be expected to follow in the way of diminishing the incidence of serious heart disease in the population generally.

A very difficult problem often arises in the case of a young person who has had an attack of rheumatism in which the heart has been affected. The danger which will present itself to the minds of the relatives is that of cardiac weakness in the future. The regulation of the patient's life under such conditions of the heart will come up for discussion, and the questions of diet, exercises, games, and school life will have to be settled. Unfortunately these questions are often decided not in accordance with the best interests of the patient, but according to the personal feelings of the parents and the doctor.

The parents with a dread of sudden death for the boy, or of some fatal result from school life, will impress their fears on the doctor, and will want to know exactly

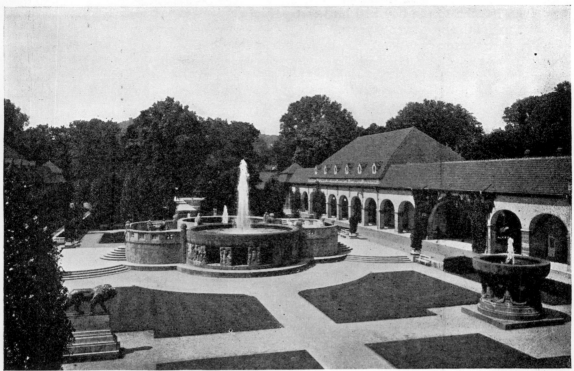

[British Continental

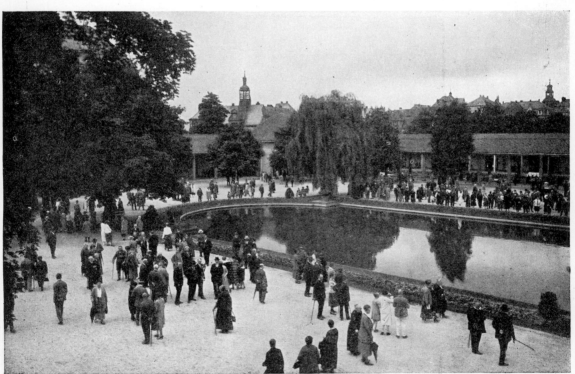

[German State Railways

A FAMOUS GERMAN SPA
Two views of the thermal establishment at Bad Nauheim, near Frankfort, which is celebrated for the treatment of heart disease.

405

what is to happen to the boy and his heart in the course of the next twenty years. This, of course, the doctor does not know, but he knows only too well that if anything goes wrong in the course of following out his advice the result will be ascribed to him, and him alone. He may think that the real injury to the heart is so small in extent that the less interference there is with the ordinary pursuits of life the better for the patient. He knows as a matter of practical experience that a child suffering from real cardiac weakness will not exert himself in an injurious way, provided that he is not placed in competitive surroundings. He knows that there is nothing to be lost and much to be gained in such a case as he is dealing with by allowing the patient to resume his ordinary habits. He is aware that no young heart can develop to its full power if the owner is, so to speak, wrapped in cotton wool.

Those terrible worrying parents, however, want to tie him down to a definite statement as to an unknown future, and they want him to tie himself up with the responsibility for everything that is to happen. It is asking too much of a family doctor to take this burden on his own shoulders. What is required is, that there should be a consultation with another doctor. The responsibility for the future course of action will be shared by the two doctors, and the parents' fears will be much relieved. Thus only will the interests of the one most concerned, namely the patient, be best served.

As regards acute diseases other than rheumatism, and their effect on the heart,

Other Acute Diseases. it may be stated that the effect is usually only temporary. The heart shares the debilitating effect of an acute illness with all the other organs of the body, and recovers with them during the period of convalescence. Scarlet fever and diphtheria are often put down as the starting-point of chronic heart disease, but in the absence of any rheumatic complication it is very rare to find any permanent heart mischief. In the case of acute pneumonia, one often finds that the chief danger lies in the risk of heart failure, but this applies only in the case of elderly people, or those debilitated by previous illness. Healthy children and young adults stand an attack of pneumonia well, and the heart is not usually a cause of alarm. One other disease may be referred to as a precursor of heart trouble, namely, syphilis. This infection is apt to hang about in the system, and after many years to bring about serious changes in the tissues and blood-vessels of the heart. Many cases of unsuspected heart disease are to be traced to this source, and, as in many untreated or imperfectly treated ailments, the condition has gone beyond curative treatment before its gravity is realised by the patient.

The second large variety of heart disease is that associated with degeneration of the heart muscle, the result of ad-

Muscle Degeneration. vancing years. When a man has passed the age of fifty he feels, or ought to feel, that he is not so fit for strenuous exercises, for running upstairs, or for climbing mountains, as he used to be. Expressed in other words, this means that the reserve power of his heart is not so good as it was in his prime. The reserve power of the heart is that called forth when any extra exertion is thrown on that organ. Amongst the other changes with advancing years are certain alterations in the heart muscle which diminish the reserve power. The heart goes on working quite satisfactorily as regards the ordinary exercises and pursuits of life, but it resents any over-exertion. Some have these facts impressed on them by a sudden experience, as when running hard to catch a train they are pulled up by an intense breathlessness or acute pain in the chest. They are fortunate in such an experience if it leads them to recognise the fact that the heart cannot work as it used to do, and learn the lesson that such over-exertion must not be repeated. Others are not so fortunate in that they have no such sudden pull up, and persevere with all their former active pursuits. The result is that the normal changes in the heart as the years advance, the hardening of the muscle and the diminution of the reserve power, go on more quickly than if the heart had not been tried so hard or so long.

He who thinks as the years pass by that he can fight successfully against a tendency to increased shortness of breath or tiredness on exertion is waging a losing battle so far as his own heart is concerned. These risks are greater in people of a stout build, for the extra fat is apt to be deposited in and around the heart, and still further to diminish its working power. The fatty tissue which is scattered in excess throughout the body is also an added strain on the heart, which has to pump the blood through a dense mass of oily tissue. In the matter of preserving a good working heart with advancing years the thin person scores over the stout one every time.

It is not to be assumed from the above that the work of the heart is to be reduced to the minimum in later years, and that a sedentary life is conducive to longevity. The heart is designed to be a working organ. The circulation of the blood and the nutrition of the tissues can only be maintained by a strong action of the heart. This action is much improved by exercise, only that exercise must be reasonable and suited to the powers of the individual. From want of exercise and from want of active functioning, the heart tends to become flabby and lose the power it would naturally have. The circulation is not efficiently carried on, and the different vital organs tend to become sluggish and overloaded with stagnant blood.

Healthy exercise will drive the blood more quickly through all the tissues and organs of the body to their great benefit. Sound sleep at night gives the heart a resting period, when it stores up fresh energy for the activities of the day. These facts are thoroughly accepted in connection with the periods of youth and early manhood, but they also hold good in the case of the seniors. The vital point is that the exertions of advancing years are not to be based on those of adult life, and that each individual must learn for himself the curtailments necessary to preserve an efficiently acting heart.

There is no system of diet which can add years of working power to a man's heart. Undoubtedly a mixed dietary, suited to his digestive powers and his mode of life, is advisable. Some articles of diet have been at times suggested as heart-foods. Sugar at one time had this reputation, at another time it was chocolate, and some hopeful if not helpful spirits have advised the consumption of bullocks' hearts. These suggestions have not stood the test of experience. A healthy heart in old age will, in the absence of previous disease, be the reward of a well-spent life.

THE HEART IN DISEASE

By J. H. BARNARD, O.B.E., M.D., late Physician to the Victoria Home, Paris.

THE diseases to which the heart is subject include those affecting the endocardium (the lining membrane of the chambers and valves), the myocardium (the heart-muscle), and the pericardium (the fibro-serous bag enclosing the heart).

Endocarditis is an inflammation affecting the lining membrane of the valves. There are two varieties : (1) Acute, which may be (*a*) Simple, or (*b*) Malignant ; and (2) Chronic. The distinction between (*a*) and (*b*) is

Endo-carditis.

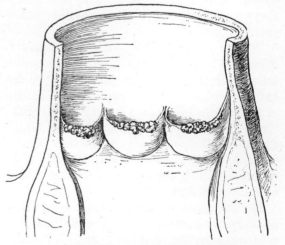

A LEGACY OF RHEUMATISM

Endocarditis of the aortic valves of the heart. Warty outgrowths, called vegetations, form on the valves, most often as a result of some rheumatic affection.

generally well marked, the course of each, and also the outcome, differing greatly. In the simple type (*a*), the symptoms are cardiac, or caused by the damage done to the heart. In the infective (*b*), the symptoms are generalised. This type is, really, a form of blood-poisoning.

ACUTE SIMPLE ENDOCARDITIS is always due to infections, the principal of which are : 1. Acute Rheumatic Fever ; 2. Chorea (St. Vitus' Dance) ; 3. Tonsillitis. All these are related to one another and are included under the " rheumatic " affections. They are the chief causes of simple acute endocarditis. Less common causes are : 4. Fevers, especially scarlet fever ; 5. Pneumonia ; 6. Consumption.

Taking cases of the chief cause, acute rheumatic fever, endocarditis occurs in from one-third to one-half of all cases, especially in those under twenty. The heart is as likely to be affected in a mild as in a severe attack. The endocarditis shows itself early in the attack, usually by the second week. The most common valve affected is the mitral valve. Simple acute endocarditis is very apt to engraft itself on the chronic form, *i.e.* persons suffering from chronic valvular disease are liable to attacks of acute endocarditis.

It is common in childhood, especially young adults. After forty, it is rare. It is also rare in infants, in whom pericarditis is more frequent.

In the vast majority, the left heart is affected, and the mitral valve is most usually selected. On the valves, outgrowths, called vegetations, are formed which consist of fibrin (the solid part of a clot), and white blood corpuscles deposited from the blood. Later this becomes organised into fibrous or scar tissue. Micro-organisms are commonly found in the fibrin or on the surface of the vegetations.

In most cases, the heart-muscle is inflamed in varying degree. The vegetations may subsequently be absorbed and the valve become normal. The occurrence of this, however, is doubtful. The more likely event is thickening and deformity of the valve and adherence of the flaps to each other ; also shortening of the tendinous cords and papillary muscles. This constitutes chronic endocarditis.

There are no characteristic symptoms, but fever and rapidity of pulse may be present. Usually no pain is felt, unless the heart-muscle be involved. Acute simple endocarditis is often a silent disease. In those cases where infective endocarditis supervenes, or where the acute simple form is grafted on a chronic case, there is often a prolonged disturbance of temperature.

The patient may get apparently well, without recurrence, or he may recover with only the doctor knowing that the valves remain affected. He may, in this case, remain well for years, but usually, after a variable interval, there are recurrent attacks of heart failure. The outlook for the future is, as a rule, grave for children. It is serious when the aortic valve is affected alone, and more serious still if both it and the mitral valve are involved.

In treatment, prolonged rest in bed is of prime importance. From three to six months of this rest is not too much, especially if the patient be a child. Parents should warmly second the efforts of the doctor to obtain this most necessary desideratum, for in rheumatic fever the administration of the salicylates or aspirin alone will not preserve the heart valves from infection.

MALIGNANT ENDOCARDITIS (or ulcerative) is a variety of blood-poisoning (septicæmia), the originating focus being in the heart. It is a serious condition characterised by (1) symptoms of general blood-poisoning ; (2) emboli, *i.e.* fragments of valve, or fibrin deposited on a valve, or a clot detached and carried to a distant vessel by the blood current. They either render the area supplied by the blocked vessel bloodless or lead to pus formation ; (3) there may be ulceration of a valve in the heart. Organisms may be found in the blood.

It is almost always secondary to previous endocarditis, which has left damaged valves, or to pneumonia, infective suppuration in bones (osteo-myelitis), or abscess of the middle ear, or infection after childbirth. It is rare after rheumatic fever or chorea.

The symptoms are high fever, profuse sweats, weakness, delirium, enlargement of spleen, purple rashes on the skin, and diarrhœa. There may be rapid or irregular pulse, and signs of heart-failure. Emboli may be numerous in the spleen, kidney, or brain, revealed by paralysis, loss of speech, impairment of sight, diarrhœa or obstruction, and in blood spitting. A fatal termination is inevitable.

When persons are said to be suffering Chronic Valvular Disease. from "heart-disease," it means, in the majority of cases, that they have valvular disease.

Valvular disease is by no means synonymous with chronic endocarditis. Acute simple endocarditis, caused most commonly by rheumatic fever or St. Vitus' dance, generally leaves its imprint on the valves attacked (most commonly the mitral). This constitutes chronic simple endocarditis. Consideration of chronic valvular disease as it affects the mitral valve, shows that pains, miscalled by parents "growing pains," but really rheumatic in their nature, are fre-quently the precursors of the chronic valvular mischief seen in young people. There are, however, other causes that bring about chronic valvular disease. For instance, when leakage of the aortic valve shows itself in middle age, the commonest cause is syphilis. When the same valve is so deformed as to constitute an obstruction to the passage of blood from the ventricle to the aorta, the commonest cause is advanced arterial degenerative changes in old men.

1. AORTIC INCOMPETENCE (LEAKAGE).— This may be the result of either disease of the valve or enlargement of the aortic orifice. Aortic leakage is commoner in males, more especially strong middle-aged men. When occurring in children or young adults the cause is rheumatic endocarditis. Here there is often obstruction of the opening as well, and concomitant mitral valve affection. In middle age, the commonest cause is syphilitic aortitis. When met with later in life, the cause is often arteriosclerosis (thickening of the arteries of the body). At all ages, rupture from sudden strain of a flap of the valve may be the cause, although, with a healthy valve, this is very

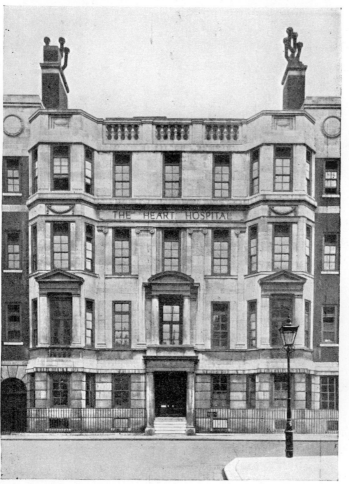

[James's Press Agency

THE HEART HOSPITAL

The national hospital for diseases of the heart, in Westmoreland Street, London.

rare. The remaining cause, enlargement of the aortic orifice, is uncommon.

The blood leaking back into the ventricle makes for deficient supply of blood in the arteries of the body and to overfilling of the left ventricle. Nature meets these defects by what is called compensation. The left ventricle dilates, and then the wall of the ventricles thickens, as a hammerman's biceps enlarges. The overfilling is thus corrected by the dilatation, and the deficient blood supply by the thickening of hypertrophy. Once compensation is established, the symptoms are slight ; the reserve power to meet extra exertion is, however, diminished.

When the cause is arterio-sclerosis, there is narrowing of the coronary arteries, leading to degeneration of the heart-muscle.

The heart may, and often does, increase in weight from the normal, 10 to 12 oz., to 20, 30, or 40 oz. (*cor bovinum*, or bullock-heart).

Early in the leakage, there are often warning symptoms, such as throbbing headache, dizziness, faintness on rising, irritability, palpitations, and shortness of breath. There may be severe pain behind the breast-bone and running down the left arm. Should the compensation fail, the shortness of breath is increased, the feet swell, there is difficulty of breathing at night, and the patient must be propped up, the lungs get congested, and bad dreams are frequent.

Sudden death is always to be dreaded in aortic leakage. The appearance of a patient suffering from this disease is distinctive ; the face is pale, drawn, long, and tired, contrasting with mitral disease, where the face is broad and the cheeks congested. It is the most serious of all single-valve diseases. Heart-failure is hastened by degeneration of the heart-muscle, by auricular fibrillation (see p. 416), and disease of the mitral valve. Angina pectoris is often the cause of death.

2. AORTIC STENOSIS (OBSTRUCTION).—This is essentially an old man's disease, and is associated with far-advanced degeneration of the arteries of the body. It is rarely met with at an earlier age. Except when associated with incompetence of the aortic valve it is a relatively rare condition, and is not regarded as one of the grave valvular disorders. In this disease, there is hypertrophy of the left ventricle, but hardly any dilatation.

3. In MITRAL INCOMPETENCE (LEAKAGE) the mitral valve guarding the left auriculo-ventricular opening closes imperfectly so that, when the left ventricle contracts to drive the blood into the aorta, some of the blood is driven back into the left auricle. There are two forms of this disease met with : (*a*) Valvular incompetence ; (*b*) Muscular incompetence.

(*a*) Valvular incompetence is caused by organic changes in the valve-flaps from endocarditis of rheumatic origin (thickening, contraction, deformity, adherence of flaps, shortening of chordae tendineae and their papillary muscles). Some degree of obstruction of the opening is generally present.

(*b*) In muscular incompetence the valve is healthy, but, owing to dilatation of the left ventricle or to weakness of its walls, the valve acts imperfectly. The dilatation of the ventricle is seen in aortic disease, Bright's disease, arterio-sclerosis, adherent pericardium (see p. 422), and fatty heart. Weakness of the heart-muscle occurs in anaemia and in fevers.

The blood being pumped back into the auricle by the contracting ventricle causes the auricle to dilate, and then to hypertrophy (thicken) from increased work in expulsion. The consequence is that an abnormal quantity of blood being forced by the auricle into the left ventricle causes the latter, in its turn, to dilate and hypertrophy. The mechanical effect of the leakage does not end here, for the emptying of the pulmonary veins into the left auricle is impeded, and the back-pressure makes the right ventricle dilate and hypertrophy. Later on, the right auricle dilates and hypertrophies, and so all four chambers are thus affected.

The changes detailed above—dilatation and hypertrophy—bring about a compensation which may be effective for years. If the patient leads a quiet life, the circulation may be adequate for a long time. In muscular incompetence, where the muscle is weak, compensation is less adequate.

The maintenance of an efficient circulation depends upon the maintenance of compensation; this may be upset by a recurrent attack of endocarditis, by a lung affection, or by fevers. As in all valvular disease, auricular fibrillation is liable to ensue.

Heart Failure.

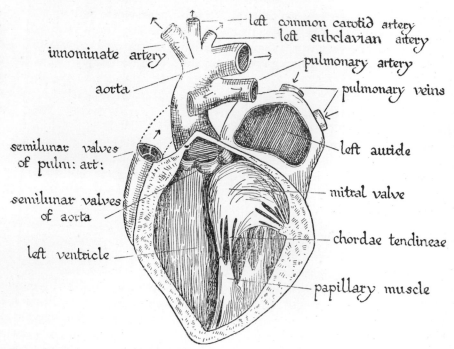

THE STRUCTURE OF THE HEART

" Heart disease " usually means disease of the valves, which form the doors to the heart. Any valve may be affected, but disease of the mitral valve is the most common.

If compensation be adequate, there may be no symptoms excepting shortness of breath on exertion. This is seldom absent. There may be, in addition, palpitations and attacks of bronchitis. The face is broad and ruddy; small dilated veins in the cheeks, and a purplish tinge of lips and ears, are suggestive of leakage. When compensation is failing there will be palpitations, shortness of breath, cough (much phlegm and often spitting of blood), and swelling of the feet. Later, these symptoms become aggravated; the swelling spreads from below upwards to the rest of the body, and there may be an accumulation of fluid in the pleura; the urine becomes scanty and clouded, and the liver swells from congestion. Several attacks of failure of compensation may be recovered from by appropriate treatment, but life is precarious and, eventually, the sufferer is confined to his chair with his body bent forwards in a distressed attitude.

4. MITRAL STENOSIS (OBSTRUCTION).—This is an obstruction to the flow of blood from the left auricle into the left ventricle owing to changes in the mitral valve and the fibrous ring to which it is attached. In some cases there is a history of an attack of acute endocarditis, rheumatic or choreic. In others, no history is forthcoming, though this does not exclude its rheumatic origin. It is commoner in females (2 to 1 male). The symptoms become manifest at all ages, but are most commonly met with in young women of twenty to thirty years of age.

The physical signs of stenosis never show during an attack of rheumatic fever; the development of obstruction being a slow process; it may take from six weeks to several months or years for the signs to manifest themselves. The changes in the diseased valve are, in adults, a button-hole contraction, the aperture being a mere slit; in children, a funnel-shaped contraction. Here the aperture may admit the tip of the little finger; later on, only a pencil.

The left auricle is hypertrophied, and so is the right ventricle. The left ventricle is small. The heart increases in weight from the normal, 8 to 10 oz., up to 12 or 16 oz. In the left auricles are clots; from these clots, emboli are very apt to be carried by the blood-current to distant vessels, which they block.

Besides hypertrophy of the left auricle, followed by hypertrophy and dilatation of the right ventricle (the left ventricle remaining small), there are disturbances of rhythm (auricular fibrillation, heart-block, and paroxysmal tachycardia: see p. 416), because the heart-muscle is frequently involved by the rheumatic process.

Years may elapse before symptoms, except shortness of breath, appear. When compensation fails, there is difficulty of breathing, cough, palpitations, and rapid and irregular pulse. Haemoptysis (blood-spitting) is commoner and more abundant than in incompetence; dropsy (of the abdominal cavity) is more frequent, and so is enlargement and tenderness of the liver. The pulse is very irregular and small, especially when there is auricular fibrillation.

The complications include bronchitis (always serious); recurrent attacks of endocarditis and embolism. (Of this there is special danger in mitral stenosis, because of thrombi in auricles; less frequently, fragments detached from the valve. They are usually carried to the vessels of the brain, causing paralysis and defects of speech; to the spleen, causing pain in left side; to the kidney, causing pain and bloody urine; and to the lungs.) Auricular fibrillation occurs in the majority of cases.

5. DISEASE OF THE TRICUSPID VALVE.—This valve is seldom affected except in consequence of disease of other valves (mitral and aortic), or as a sequel of bronchitis and emphysema. The commonest lesion is incompetence; obstruction is very rare.

6. DISEASE OF THE PULMONARY VALVES.—Acquired disease of this valve is very rare. It is, however, the commonest site of congenital lesions (disease present at birth). In congenital pulmonary stenosis the cusps of the valve are adherent, and often there are coexistent other structural defects.

It is common in rheumatic cases in children to see, existing together, disease of the aortic and mitral valves. It is **Combined Valvular Disease.** also very common to see tricuspid incompetence with organic mitral stenosis, and mitral incompetence with organic aortic disease.

The two types of lesion—obstruction and incompetence—may coexist in the same valve, e.g. mitral incompetence and stenosis.

The outlook depends on the state of the heart-muscle. It should be clear that compensation depends entirely on the condition of the heart-muscle, and hence the prospect is better in cases due to rheumatism than in those due to arterio-sclerosis or syphilis. In the latter, the coronary arteries are always involved, and this causes progressive myocarditis, a condition which leads to failure in compensation. When rheumatism is the cause, the coronary arteries escape. If failure of compensation yields to rest, the prospect is improved. The outlook is bad in children under twelve years. This is due to the proneness of young children

[F. W. Bond, F.Z.S.]

PERICARDITIS IN A LION'S HEART

Inflammation of the pericardium or membranous envelope of the heart. Note the shaggy exudation.

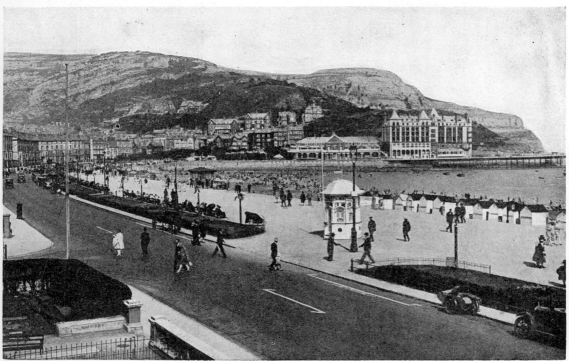

A SPA FOR HEART TROUBLES
A view of Llandudno which, in spring and autumn especially, is beneficial to people with cardiac complaints.

[Photopress

to pericarditis, to affections of several valves, to recurrent attacks of rheumatism, to progressive lesions, and to the strain of puberty.

The outlook is better in females, owing to mitral lesions being commoner than aortic, and to the coronary arteries being less frequently involved (more frequent absence of syphilis and arterio-sclerosis). In aortic incompetence the predominant factor is the state of the coronary arteries. The danger is greatest with syphilis, less with arterio-sclerosis, and least with rheumatism. The blocking of the coronary arteries is important, because it deprives the heart-muscle of its proper blood supply. This starvation is apt to provoke attacks of angina pectoris, which may occasion sudden death. Auricular fibrillation and a coincident leakage of the mitral valve hasten death. Age is important. The duration of life is longest when the disease begins in youth, and most favourable then if the mitral valve be unaffected.

Aortic incompetence is the most serious of all valve lesions. It may exist for years without symptoms if compensation be good, but death is invariably premature and often sudden. In aortic stenosis the prognosis is said to be the best of all. In mitral incompetence the prognosis is improved if a degree of stenosis is present. All hangs upon the condition of the heart-muscle. Adequate compensation may allow a fairly active life for years.

In mitral obstruction, auricular fibrillation is a great danger. The outlook depends upon the response to treatment. If " back-pressure " effects—cough, difficulty of breathing, and signs of venous stagnation—are marked, the outlook is gloomy. Pregnancy should be avoided.

Angina pectoris is a condition characterised by paroxysmal cardiac pain. Frequent references have been made to the importance of the nutrient arteries of the heart—the coronary arteries. In the severer form of angina pectoris

Angina Pectoris.

these arteries are found, after death, hardened and so unable to contract and dilate according to the varying needs of the heart-muscle. Angina pectoris is divided into two groups.

1. Angina major or severe angina. This affects middle-aged or elderly males, and it is due to hardening of the coronary arteries, frequently of syphilitic origin. The pain is usually very pronounced, and sudden death is not infrequent.

2. Angina minor. The patients are usually females. The coronary arteries are not diseased, and sudden death never occurs.

Angina major is rare under the age of thirty years; it is also rare in women. It occurs mainly in men of the professional classes. The onset of the attack is sudden and rapidly reaches its climax. There is a sense of constriction over the heart region, and pain is experienced which starts over the heart, and radiates to the left armpit, the inner aspect of the left arm, and the ring and little fingers. Sometimes the pain is felt on the left side of the lower jaw and the back of the head behind the left ear. There is marked mental anxiety, with a fear of death. If the seizure occurs during a walk the patient invariably comes to a dead stop. The agony is overwhelming. Rigid, and with one hand held over the painful area, with the other he declines assistance. His face is ashy-grey and bedewed with sweat; his breathing is restrained. The attack is short—anything up to two minutes. It commonly ends abruptly, leaving the patient exhausted or, sometimes, none the worse. At the end of the seizure he generally belches " wind " and empties his bladder. The attacks may be repeated. Sudden death is always possible, although the majority of these sufferers do not die in an attack. The common exciting causes of an attack are exertion after meals, especially hearty, mixed meals; a cold wind, especially if a head wind; and violent emotion. The inhalation from a crushed capsule of from three to five drops of nitrite of amyl in many instances puts an end to the seizure, the patient is rapidly relieved. Amyl nitrite should always be available.

In angina minor the attacks are probably due to constriction of the blood-vessels of the extremities, which brings about distension of the ventricle. The pain may resemble that of angina major, but it is commonly less severe. The exciting cause may be excessive smoking or the invasion of such a disease as influenza. The onset is not so abrupt as in the major type. She (the patient is generally a woman) walks about during the attack, and is mentally excited. The seizures are never fatal.

Attacks of angina major, which must be considered as a symptom rather than a disease, are frequent in such conditions as aortic incompetence, where the openings of the coronary arteries are involved.

Of diseases of the heart-muscle (myocardium) there are two varieties, namely, acute and chronic myocarditis.

Diseases of the Heart-muscle. ACUTE MYOCARDITIS, which is an acute inflammation of the heart-muscle, occurs in the acute fevers, more especially diphtheria and typhoid fever. It is seen constantly in the acute endocarditis complicating rheumatic fever, and in acute pericarditis. In the rheumatic forms the auriculo-ventricular bundle (bundle of His) may be involved.

The chief cause of CHRONIC MYOCARDITIS (FIBROID MYOCARDITIS, FIBROID HEART) is a morbid condition of the coronary arteries, which is the outcome of arterio-sclerosis, chronic kidney disease, syphilis, and senility. In this condition the muscle is tough; the muscle-fibres are degenerated, and there is an excess of fibrous tissue. The symptoms are due to inefficiency of the cardiac muscle or to the involvement of the genetic system, producing abnormal rhythms. This degeneration of the heart-muscle may give rise to no particular complaints, although sudden death may occur. Generally there is shortness of breath, sometimes so severe as to be dubbed " cardiac asthma." There may be giddiness, fainting, pain in heart region, and attacks of angina pectoris of varying severity. Implication of the auricular-ventricular bundle may induce the condition of heart-block, in which the ventricle contracts less frequently than the auricle.

FATTY DEGENERATION is a common condition of the heart-muscle. It occurs in wasting diseases and in old age; in pernicious anaemia and in poisoning by phosphorus. It may accompany all forms of myocarditis. In this condition the heart, instead of being firm, is flabby, and, under the microscope, fat is seen to have invaded the muscle-fibres.

FATTY INFILTRATION is always present in very stout people. The muscle-fibres, though not necessarily in a state of fatty degeneration (though the two conditions often co-exist), are pressed upon injuriously by masses of fat, rendering the patient short-winded and the heart-sounds weak. Later this may lead to dilatation and heart-failure.

Stimuli can originate from any part of the primitive cardiac tissue, and these may be blocked partially or completely by disease of the junctional tissues or by meeting muscle in a "refractory" state. These two causes may and often do co-exist.

Contraction Abnormalities.

Abnormalities of contraction are classified as :

1. Variations in Vagus nerve control } Sinus irregularities.

2. Abnormalities of stimuli to contraction } Extra-systoles (premature contractions). Simple paroxysmal tachycardia. Auricular fibrillation. Auricular flutter.

3. Interference with muscular conduction of stimuli } Heart-block.

4. Impairment of muscle contractility } Pulsus alternans.

SINUS IRREGULARITIES are common in children. During inspiration the heart-beats become more frequent, but slow down again during expiration. This condition is of no importance, and children (free from valvular disease) who are the subjects of these irregularities should be encouraged to join in games.

EXTRA-SYSTOLES form one of the com-

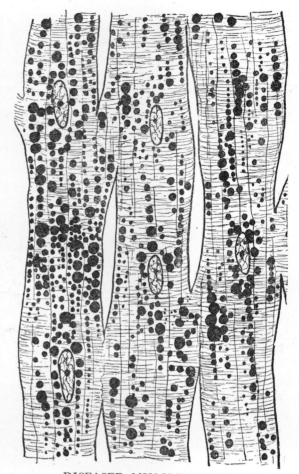

DISEASED MUSCLE-FIBRES
Fatty degeneration of the heart-muscle, a condition common in wasting diseases and in old age.

monest of irregularities of the pulse. They are more often met with in men. Most people who have reached middle age or beyond suffer from these premature beats occasionally. They are met with in those who have heart disease and in those free from it. They disappear when the heart quickens in exercise, and tend to reappear as the heart slows down. The premature beats are caused by impulses started from over-excitable parts of the heart. After the premature beat, there is a pause until the normal rhythm is resumed. This pause frightens the patient; it is ended by a sudden thud in the chest when the normal rhythm starts again. When occurring in persons free from heart disease they are of no importance. Adolescents who smoke numerous cigarettes often have palpitations after a short run, or on getting into bed. Tea, coffee, and alcohol will often have the same effect as nicotine. Even in those cases of extra-systole with valvular disease undue alarm should not be experienced.

In SIMPLE PAROXYSMAL TACHYCARDIA the normal rate gives way, suddenly, to beats varying from over 100 to 200 a minute. This is caused by the temporary abdication of the " pacemaker " (sino - auricular node), its functions being usurped by a new centre in the auricle (the commoner) or the ventricle. They are a kind of extra-systoles. They may occur at any age, being particularly associated with mitral stenosis (obstruction) and myocardial degeneration. There is often found, after death, a fibroid heart and blockage of the coronary arteries. It begins suddenly, and may last from a few seconds to several weeks. The beats are regular, though quick. The end is as sudden as the onset. If the attack lasts some time, it may occasion distress, such as pain in the heart region, exhaustion, and a cold feeling. These, with the exception of the exhaustion, disappear at the termination of the attack.

Patients very rarely die in these attacks, which may be due to nervous influences or dietetic irregularities.

AURICULAR FLUTTER is a form of tachycardia in which the auricle contracts from 200 to 300 times a minute, the ventricle lagging behind with one-quarter or one-half of this rate. It is evident that only a portion of the auricular contractions are conducted to the ventricle.

This, like paroxysmal tachycardia, begins and ends suddenly, but it is more liable to last for a longer period. To diagnose it, an instrument such as the polygraph or the electro-cardiograph is necessary, since a venous pulse tracing must be obtained.

Digitalis (foxglove) has been found efficacious in increasing the resistance to the conduction of impulses along the auriculo-ventricular bundle. Quinidine is another useful drug. On no account should either of these drugs be taken except under the doctor's orders.

The importance of AURICULAR FIBRILLATION may be appreciated when it is stated that more than half the cases admitted into a general hospital for heart-failure are suffering from this form of heart disease.

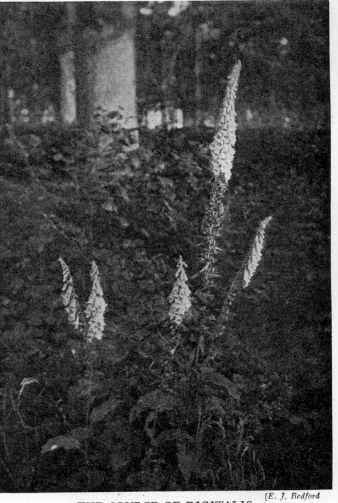

[E. J. Bedford]

THE SOURCE OF DIGITALIS

The Common Foxglove, long used in herbal remedies, provides a drug with a powerful effect on the motion of the heart.

Of these, one-half are cases of mitral obstruction.

In a healthy heart, the sino-auricular node or " pacemaker," the most excitable part of the heart, is the seat of the impulses that excite the contractions of the auricles. This nodal impulse is, in auricular fibrillation, replaced by impulses which start irregular contractions all over the auricles. Otherwise expressed, the proper co-ordinated auricular contractions are suppressed, the auricles being, as it were, delirious. The ventricle has showered upon it a great number of small impulses or stimuli from the delirious auricle, but they do not respond to every one of these impulses ; only a certain number get through.

When the heart beats irregularly and at a greater rate than 120 a minute it is evidence that the auricles are fibrillating. This is confirmed by gentle exercise in bed, which increases the irregularity, contrary to what occurs in extra-systoles or heart-block, in which exercise diminishes the irregularity of the pulse.

Auricular fibrillation, a serious condition, is frequently persistent off and on for the remainder of the patient's life. It means the beginning of the end. Very few survive more than ten years. If the case responds favourably to the action of digitalis or quinidine, and the pulse can be reduced to below 90 a minute, the outlook is more favourable.

Foxglove was introduced into therapeutics by William Withering, a Birmingham physician, in 1775. He acquired a family receipt from an old Shropshire woman, who, it was said, had worked wonders with it. Over twenty plants were contained in the prescription, and Withering has the merit of recognising the active ingredient in it, namely, digitalis. He noticed the beneficent effect of this plant on the heart-beats (doubtless in cases of auricular fibrillation) when he observed, " It has the power over the motion of the heart to a degree yet unobserved in any other medicine."

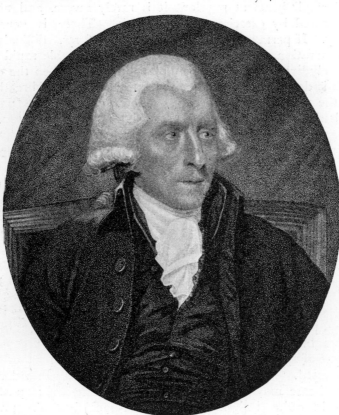

WILLIAM WITHERING, M.D., F.R.S.
The Birmingham physician who first recognised the active ingredient (digitalis) in the foxglove.

HEART-BLOCK is due to an impairment in the conducting powers of any part of the primitive cardiac tissue from the auriculo-ventricular node inclusive to its branches in the ventricles. When temporary, it is due to an infective disease, especially acute rheumatism, and it is also to be guarded against in medication with digitalis. Permanent heart-block occurs in hearts irretrievably damaged by the rheumatic or syphilitic poison and in elderly persons with myocardial degeneration.

In this condition, only a certain number of auricular contractions get through to the ventricles. When the block is complete, the pulse, though regular, is a low one—less than 40 a minute. In some of these cases, fainting, unconsciousness, or convulsions occur. This is called the Adams-Stokes Syndrome. It is due to cerebral anaemia produced suddenly by the blockage, and the convulsions may prove fatal.

In PULSUS ALTERNANS the pulse consists of alternate large and small beats at regular intervals. It is increased by exercise, and it may be temporary. If permanent, there is myocardial degeneration. In marked cases, the patient rarely lives more than two years. The outlook is dark if the condition be observed when the pulse is beating at a slow rate ; not so bad if it only shows itself when the pulse is rapid.

Inflammation of the fibro-serous envelope of the heart is almost always secondary to other diseases, which include :—
Pericarditis. 1. Rheumatic fever ; 2. Pneumonia ; 3. Septicaemia (as in inflammation of a bone and puerperal fever) ; 4. Chronic kidney disease, diabetes ; 5. Acute specific fevers (especially scarlet fever).

In RHEUMATIC PERICARDITIS, if any fluid be effused, it does not become purulent. It is most common between 5 and 20 years. Almost all cases of pericarditis occurring between these years belong to this class. It is rare after the age of 25 years. The two sexes are equally affected.

In children, the disease may exist when the joint-affection is quite insignificant. It may occur with tonsillitis only, or with St. Vitus' dance. In adults, the joints are usually severely involved. Generally endocarditis is coexistent ; in children, we may say, always. In children it usually appears as a late complication.

PNEUMONIC PERICARDITIS is the commonest form in children under five, the lung trouble being lobar pneumonia, broncho-pneumonia, or pus in the pleural cavity. The effusion usually becomes purulent, and the disease is nearly always fatal.

With TERMINAL PERICARDITIS (in chronic kidney disease, diabetes) the effusion is usually not abundant, and does not become purulent.

SEPTICAEMIC PERICARDITIS is always fatal.

In pericarditis, the serous, inner part of the bag becomes shaggy and dull. There may be no effusion, and the two parts of the bag (outer and inner) may adhere together ; this is most common in children. In severe cases the myocardium is inflamed.

The symptoms are often slight. Pain is often absent, especially in young children ; it is rarely severe, and not aggravated by pressure. There is generally fever. In rheumatic fever, difficulty of breathing, pallor, and a feeble rapid pulse suggest the complication. When the effusion is abundant, the difficulty of breathing may become pronounced, and the pain marked, and associated with tenderness. Vomiting may be severe.

The most serious aftermath in cases that recover is adherence of the pericardium. This may occur between the two bags, or, what is more serious, between the pericardium and the surrounding structures, especially the inner surface of the breast-bone ; also to the lungs or midriff (diaphragm). This causes great hypertrophy of the heart-walls, and also dilatation ; the weight may go up to more than 40 oz.

The prognosis is very bad ; young folks generally die, not being able to cope with the strain of puberty. Surgeons now, in selected cases, remove a part of the fourth, fifth, and sixth left ribs in order to free the heart from its adhesions ; part of the sternum (breast-bone) is also removed.

THE DANGERS OF ACUTE RHEUMATISM

By F. JOHN POYNTON, M.D., F.R.C.P., Physician to University College Hospital and to the Hospital for Sick Children, Great Ormond Street.

THERE can be no question that the medical profession is making a great forward step in the close attention it is giving to the problem of acute rheumatism in childhood. It is a disease of great national importance, and to those who have been deeply interested in the subject it has been a cause of regret that the problem has not been approached in real earnest many years ago, but tuberculosis, cancer, and other diseases, together with the Great War, have distracted attention.

One result of this has been that the public, naturally associating the word "rheumatism" with the spectacle of an English spa, with many adults crippled by arthritis, have not yet realised how widely different is the acute rheumatism of childhood, or understood its frequency. How many would imagine that this disease reaches its maximum of frequency at the early age of 10 years, or that of all the causes of organic heart disease in this country acute

A Cause of Heart Disease.

rheumatism is the main one! When this is realised, then it follows that the age at which such heart disease arises is usually in childhood, and, in brief, during school age.

What an awakening it is to grasp the fact that not only is it the young that are thus injured, but that when the heart is severely damaged, the scars left by the disease are a frequent cause of chronic heart disease in later life !

The exact position of the problem will be the more easily understood if, for a moment, we first consider tuberculosis, a disease now much more generally understood. Tuberculosis may attack most of the organs of the body. All recognise the lung affections, acute or chronic as the case may be ; tuberculosis of the intestines ; tuberculosis of the nervous system, including the deadly tuberculous meningitis ; tuberculosis of the joints, as illustrated by spinal caries, and tuberculous hip joint disease. The same infection may also attack the heart, but here we come upon one of the many curious facts in disease ; this occurrence is comparatively rare.

Now, if we turn to acute rheumatism in childhood, we find also that many organs are attacked. We see rheumatic heart disease taking the prominence that the lung affections do in tuberculosis ; when it attacks the nervous system it produces the important malady chorea (St. Vitus' dance) ; when it attacks the joints and muscles, it causes arthritis and fibrositis. In childhood it is a well-known and interesting fact that the joints, though often attacked, are rarely, as in the adult, damaged severely. On the other hand, in the young, the heart suffers greatly, but the adult heart is less often attacked.

As to the cause of acute rheumatism it is accepted that it is due primarily to an

Acute Rheumatism.

infective agent, but, unfortunately, there is no agreement as to this agent, although the writer believes that he is correct in stating that every year brings more evidence to favour the view originally held by Dr. Alexander Paine and himself that it is a streptococcus. Nevertheless, he would add that in order for this streptococcus to produce the disease there may be secondary causes, and there is often a peculiar constitution.

One path by which this infection invades the system is through the tonsils in an attack of tonsillitis, though it is not to be supposed that this is the only path. Even, however, if it is thought wiser at present to hold the streptococcal view to be as yet unproven, the fact remains that the disease is looked upon as the result of *some* infection, and there at once arises the important question : Can we advance our knowledge of prevention by more inquiry and more care, waiting, meantime, patiently for the actual determination of its exact nature ?

If we can, we are striking at the root of the greatest cause of organic heart disease. There is reason to believe that in London alone there are 10,000 children suffering from rheumatic heart disease. And 2000 of these for whom medical service in the broadest sense is not readily available. In other great cities there is good reason also to believe that there are many children thus damaged, and it can be well understood that the medical profession is faced by a very difficult and a very formidable adversary.

It would only complicate and obscure the question if all these difficulties were enumerated, but some examples will make this point clear. One is this. The heart disease of acute rheumatism, though too often most

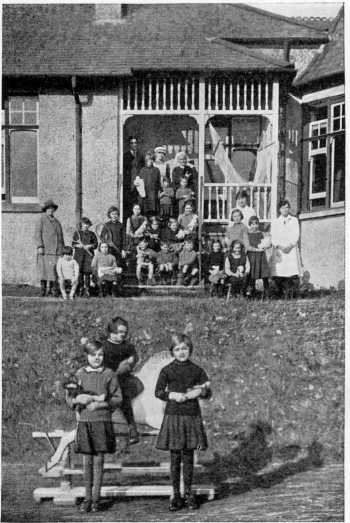

Courtesy]   [Invalid Children's Aid Association

THE RETURN TO HEALTH

A happy group at one of the country homes for children, where accommodation is provided for a thorough convalescence.

after much difference of opinion, must inevitably lead to progress, but time and patience are demanded.

Another difficulty is the result of the frequency and stubbornness of the illness, and its tendency to recur. The hospitals, with urgent cases of all kinds pressing for admission, cannot always keep these cases in their beds a sufficient time to enable the heart to become quite strong, and there is a great need for convalescent accommodation in the country, with special supervision, facilities for education, and open-air treatment. Above all, plenty of time must be available for the heart either to recover completely, or, if damaged, to be trained to the degree of perfection that is available.

Care of Child Patients.

Such an undertaking is not only costly, but, being a progressive step, requires that cautious testing and gathering of experience which are demanded of all pioneer attempts, but there is no doubt that such a step is now generally admitted as one of the definite lines which are justified for trial. Already encouraging results are being obtained, for example, at Kurandai, at Hartfield in Sussex, in an open-air home for forty-eight children, initiated by the Invalid Children's Aid Association. The reader who is intent upon becoming acquainted with the nature of the problem will see that, by freeing the hospitals from the prolonged care of these cases, they will be enabled to give more attention to the earliest developments of the disease, and will thus be in the position to send the children away in a more favourable condition.

The last difficulty to be cited in illustration is occupation, and this requires some com-

serious and obvious, is still more frequently quiet and practically painless in its onset. Parents can easily be deceived, and doctors also, for the disease is amazingly treacherous. No doctor wishes unduly to alarm, or to convert a child into a querulous invalid by prolonged and needless rest. Yet there is no doubt that in the earliest stages of rheumatic heart disease there must often be doubt for some time as to the reality and extent of any suspected heart damage. Increasing knowledge of the disease, laboriously acquired

ments upon the more frequent forms of valvular heart disease and weak hearts left as a result of definite injury during acute attacks of rheumatism in childhood. No one can approach this aspect without long vision. He is compelled to look forward and visualise the future of these children, remembering that the aim must be to obtain for them good, if restricted, lives, when they grow up, and, for the State, citizens who can take their part in some measure in the country's life.

Looking at all aspects, the most important rheumatic valvular damage is probably narrowing of the mitral valve, or mitral stenosis. It is very frequent, and particularly so in females. The result is slowly to unbalance the action of the heart, and the majority of cases die between 35 and 45 years, death being preceded by a varying but often long period of invalidism. For the State, this crippling and loss of life among women in the prime of life means more than appears superficially, for, as a result, we repeatedly find a home desolated by the loss of the mother of a young family, and this, among the working class population, is a particularly grievous disaster.

In many cases, two valves are damaged, the mitral and aortic, and though with care such patients may live useful lives, if they drift into unsuitable occupations they break down rapidly and completely.

The subject of the various occupations in a complex civilisation and their relative **Suitable Occupations.** effects upon the heart is in itself one of great difficulty, and demands much collective experience and knowledge. It is obvious that a man with a weak heart should not become a professional association football player, but there

are many employments not so easy to decide upon, because in all cases of heart disease the nervous strain has to be reckoned with as well as the physical. On the other hand, we know that it is very detrimental, both for children and adults, to be driven to passive rest unless it is absolutely unavoidable, some occupation of body and mind is essential, and the question to be answered is—what is suitable ?

Even if we have a perfect knowledge of the suitable occupations for such cases, there still remains the difficult undertaking of organising for individuals, in a vast population, a mechanism by which they can be duly assigned to their occupations, but there

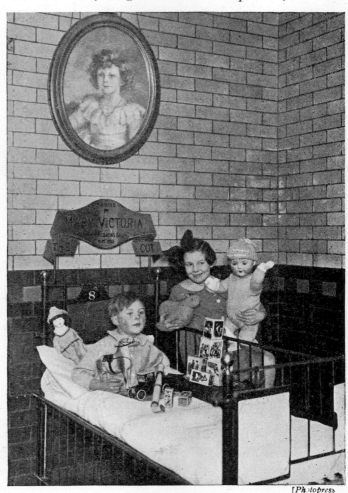

[Photopress

CONVALESCENT

Princess Mary's cot in the Great Ormond Street Hospital, London. Acute rheumatism requires very long convalescence, and accommodation for such patients presents a serious problem.

is no doubt that in this country, unobtrusively and quietly, great progress has been made in this direction in recent years.

Chorea, which is the result of acute rheumatism attacking the brain, is fortunately, in itself, not so serious as heart disease, because at puberty the tendency to it greatly diminishes, and even in childhood, the vast majority recover. But it is a serious condition and an outstanding cause of absence from school, and a child with chorea is suffering from the rheumatic infection, and so is liable to have heart disease also. This, too, is not a rare event, and we repeatedly notice that girls, who are more frequently affected with chorea than boys, after several attacks, begin to develop mitral stenosis.

St. Vitus' Dance.

One great question to be handled is the reason for the frequency of this brain rheumatism. It is by no means settled. The writer's view is that educational strain is a great factor, lowering the vitality of the highly strung child, who is so liable to acute rheumatism, but he is prepared to accept also the additional agents of sitting in damp boots and clothes, and being in contact with other children who may have sore throats. Chorea is very rare in his experience in the private and public schools, and it must be remembered that these children, if they are nervous and out of health, are generally brought to doctors, who advise either a term or half term away from school, or some judicious change in their school routine.

If acute rheumatism in the child began invariably with acute pain and swelling in the joints, the position would be much easier, for then at once and perforce they would be put to bed, and the doctor sent for. Unfortunately vague pains, listlessness, and pallor, a slight sore throat, and a little shortness of breath, are easily misinterpreted or overlooked, and damage is done before alarm has been excited.

More supervision and more beds for the prolonged convalescence of the rheumatic child are urgent needs. In all directions it is to be hoped the public will aid the medical profession to elucidate the disease, to push on the prevention, to improve the opportunities for strengthening the hearts, and to assist in the task of finding suitable employment for those who, though they have some damage to their hearts, are yet able, with some care, to do much good work and lead happy lives.

The writer is convinced, and has been for many years, that when once the medical profession and the public, working hand in hand, determine to improve the health provisions for the rheumatic child, there will be a striking diminution in heart disease in this country, and a great relief to suffering, both for the young and the adult. The great reason for such hopefulness is the fact that heart rheumatism tends to diminish in severity and frequency after puberty, and constitutes the great stimulus for which we are fighting, namely, the rescue of many of the most charming of our English children.

DISEASES OF THE ARTERIES

By GEO. SOMERVILLE, M.D., D.P.M., Deputy Medical Superintendent, West Ham Mental Hospital.

ARTERIO-SCLEROSIS is the term applied to any widespread thickening and hardening of the arterial coats which leads to loss of elasticity and contractility of the arteries. As a rule it is the middle coat which is chiefly affected ; the arteries become tortuous, and their passage becomes narrowed.

Arterio-sclerosis.

The primary cause of arterio-sclerosis is not definitely known, but its constant occurrence in varying degree in the aged suggests it is of the nature of a senile degeneration. It is favoured by any factor which throws excessive strain on the vessel walls, as in the performance of heavy, muscular work ; or by any condition which tends to raise the blood-pressure, as chronic kidney disease, gout, lead poisoning, alcoholism, syphilis ; and probably by excessive secretion of the suprarenal ductless gland.

It should be noted that arterio-sclerosis, high blood-pressure, and chronic kidney

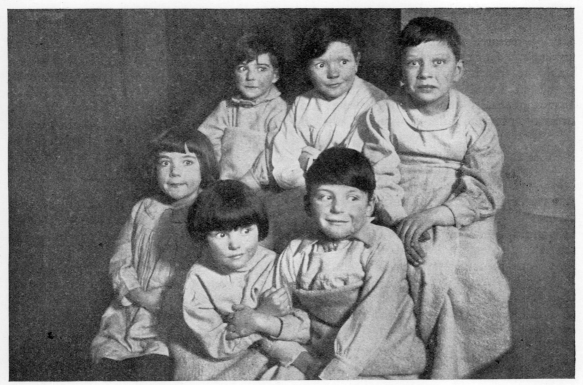

THE DANGER OF CHILDHOOD RHEUMATISM

A group of children at the Hospital for Sick Children, Great Ormond Street. All are sufferers from chorea (St. Vitus' dance), a disease of rheumatic origin which is liable to affect the heart, and four have rheumatic heart disease.

disease are closely related. Arterio-sclerosis, no matter how caused, usually *results* in high blood-pressure and chronic nephritis (kidney disease), and conversely it may be *produced* by high pressure and chronic nephritis.

The disease shows itself in the latter half of life, and is more frequent in men than in women. In certain families, members show a tendency to arterio-sclerosis on reaching a certain age. Loss of vigour, physical and mental, with giddiness, fainting attacks, headache, and attacks of breathlessness, are the earliest symptoms of the disease. Owing to their apparently trivial nature, such symptoms are apt to be disregarded, and consequently the disease is allowed to progress until some dramatic sign such as heart-failure or an apoplexy brings a realisation of the necessity for urgent treatment.

As the arterial thickening advances, the heart becomes increasingly less able to meet the strain, and some degree of cardiac failure becomes manifest. The narrowed blood-vessels deprive the brain of its necessary blood supply, and the mind becomes involved. Clear and connected thought or conversation becomes impossible ; there is a general dulling of the intellectual faculties ; the sufferer is liable to fits of absentmindedness, emotional outburst, and even moral aberrations. All grades of mental disorder are possible, from deficient memory power to complete dementia or mental disintegration.* Epileptiform seizures may occur, and transient paralyses may arise which are ascribed to temporary spasm in narrowed arteries. When the heart is beating forcibly, and the brain arteries are degenerate, a cerebral or brain haemorrhage (shock, apoplexy) is liable to ensue.

The heart-muscle hypertrophies, *i.e.*, increases in size, and the heart eventually becomes dilated ; abnormal rhythms may set in, and attacks of severe cardiac pain (angina pectoris) are of common occurrence. Heart-

* See " Senile Dementia and Old Age."

failure may suddenly arise. Changes in the kidney-vessels result in a form of chronic kidney disease, which may terminate in uraemia. Gangrene of the extremities is liable to result from insufficient or ill-regulated blood supply, and the bodily tissues generally tend to degenerate and are more prone to inflammation and disease. The occurrence of pneumonia or influenza is fraught with great danger to life.

A localised nodular form of arterio-sclerosis is described as " atheroma." In this variety the disease process usually commences in patches of the inner coat. The cells multiply, undergo a fatty degeneration, and often become calcareous, i.e., plates of lime form in the arterial tubes, rendering them very brittle and liable to rupture, or to the occurrence of thrombosis from clotting of the blood on the roughened surface. In the large arteries localised dilatations, aneurisms, are apt to develop. Atheroma is generally widespread, but it nearly always commences and predominates in the big arteries—the aorta and its main branches.

Though nothing can be done to cure or abolish arterial thickening, much can be done to hinder its advance, and to add many years of comparatively useful life. The outlook largely depends on the state of the heart, in other words, upon the power of the heart to compensate and overcome the resistance of the thickened arteries. An irregular and rapid pulse, along with severe breathlessness, are ominous signs.

In treatment, three indications must be kept in mind : (1) No extra strain must be thrown upon the heart or vessels ; (2) the blood-pressure should be kept low ; and (3) the heart must be aided to maintain efficient service. The application of general hygienic measures is the means adopted best to secure these indications, and upon the kind of existence the sufferer can afford to live will depend the actual duration of life. All strain and stress of mind and body must be avoided. Diet should be light and easily digested, highly proteid foods being strictly moderated, and alcohol forbidden. The possibility of **intestinal toxaemia** must be

considered and rectified when necessary. The excretory organs, the bowels, kidneys, and skin, must be made to function at their highest level. Baths and passive exercises, unless the arterial disease is very advanced, are of considerable benefit. High blood-pressure may be reduced by avoiding the causal factors. Any rapid reduction by drugs is not permanent, and may be dangerous if the cause is left untreated. Should signs of cardiac failure appear, urgent treatment is necessary.

Syphilis is a fertile source of arterial disease. In the commonest form the inner coat of the aorta undergoes a patchy degeneration which leads to fibrosis and calcification or deposition of lime salts (aortitis). An aortic aneurism is a frequent complication.

In the smaller arteries an obliterative inflammation, from proliferation of the cells of the inner coat, may lead to choking of the artery and consequently to serious degenerative changes in the tissues supplied. This condition also predisposes to thrombosis or clotting.

An aneurism is a dilatation upon an artery which is caused by weakening of the arterial wall, combined with increase in Aneurism. the arterial pressure due to arterio-sclerosis. The blood-vessels are continually subjected to a considerable pressure, which rises with each heart contraction, but, owing to the natural resilience and elasticity of the arteries, this pressure is more or less equally distributed, and does not give rise to shocks or jars. With advancing years the arteries lose their elasticity, but there is a corresponding diminution of vigour, and consequently the vessels seldom give way. Should, however, degeneration occur in the arteries at a comparatively early age as a result of such diseases as alcoholism, syphilis, and gout, when the heart is still vigorous and hard work is being performed, an artery is liable to become dilated, to give way, that is, to develop an aneurism.

Accordingly aneurism tends to occur in the active period of life, between the ages of thirty and fifty, in men who follow arduous occupations, as navvies and dock labourers, and who suffer from degenerate arteries. Syphilis plays an important part in the production of aneurism, which is seldom seen in women unless they have suffered from this disease.

Aneurisms are classified according to their shape : when the walls dilate uniformly, a " fusiform " or " tubular " aneurism is described (mainly met with in the arch of the aorta) ; when a limited area of the wall is weakened a pouch or sac is formed, and it is called a " sacculated " aneurism (mainly found in medium-sized arteries, and has a tendency to rupture) ; when blood tears its way amongst the coats of an artery it is known as a " dissecting " aneurism, and when a tiny dilatation the size of a millet seed appears on the side of a small artery (often in the brain), it is termed a " miliary " aneurism.

The symptoms of an aneurism naturally vary with its size and position, and may be complicated by other manifestations of arterial disease. The essential feature is the presence in the line of an artery of a globular swelling which pulsates in an expansile manner with each beat of the heart. An aneurism gives rise to symptoms mainly as a result of pressure exerted on surrounding structures which usually become adherent to it. Pain, disturbances of sensation, paralyses, may follow pressure on nerves. The sternum and vertebral column may be eroded from continuous pressure. Adjacent veins may be pressed on and cause congestion and dropsy of the parts beyond. Difficulty in swallowing, breathlessness, and a barking irritating cough may be produced by the pressure on the gullet, wind-pipe, and laryngeal nerve by an aneurism of the thoracic aorta. Other evidences of aneurism include inequality of pupils, differences of pulses, and peculiar murmurs ; these signs can only be detected by the trained observer.

Aneurism must always be regarded as a grave condition. It is liable to progress towards a rupture, when a profuse haemorrhage causes sudden death. The pressure on vital organs is a serious complication,

and it should always be realised that aneurism, in most cases, is evidence of extensive disease of the arteries, so that the outlook is generally unfavourable.

In the treatment of aneurism, the main indication is to imitate the natural method of cure by means of a laminated clot, which gradually increases till it fills the sac, and prevents further growth or rupture.

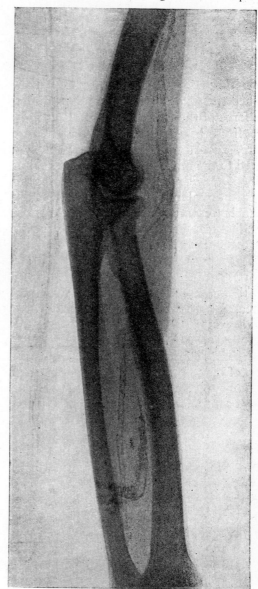

Courtesy]   [" *Manual of Surgery*," *Thomson & Miles* (*O.U.P.*)

A CALCIFIED ARTERY

An X-ray photograph of an arm, showing an artery made hard and brittle by plates of lime formed inside the tube.

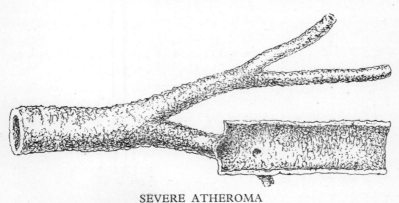

SEVERE ATHEROMA

A diagram showing the appearance of an artery hardened by lime deposits.

painful. Finally, the condition subsides, or in a limited number of cases local gangrene or death of the tissues may ensue, and the tips of the fingers or toes may slough off.

The disease is due to local spasm of the muscular walls of the arteries, followed by a relaxation or partial paralysis. Gangrene is the result of the failure of the circulation to be re-established. The primary cause is unknown. Raynaud's disease tends to occur hereditarily in predisposed persons—most commonly women, and those whose general health is poor. The typical attacks recur with varying frequency ; exposure to cold and excessive fatigue acting as exciting agents.

To this end measures must be taken to reduce the arterial tension and to diminish the force of the heart's action. Rest in bed, free from harass and worry, with a dry, spare, non-stimulating diet, gradually reduced to the minimum necessary to maintain nutrition, with saline purges, are the main constitutional methods of treatment. Failure of such treatment necessitates local surgical interference. Where anatomically possible, the artery may be ligated, usually proximally (*i.e.* at the end of the aneurism nearest the heart), with the object of promoting clotting. In the case of large arteries, such as the aorta, by the insertion of needles which scarify the inner surface of the sac, or by introducing a coil of fine wire through which an electric current can be passed, coagulation of blood or clotting may be obtained.

Non-suppurative inflammation of arteries may occur in children subsequent to infective fevers, such as diphtheria or influenza. Arteritis. It may so soften the arterial wall as to lead to aneurism. Suppuration may occur when an artery is involved in an abscess or where a septic embolus is present. The vessel wall disintegrates, and a dangerous secondary haemorrhage may result.

Raynaud's Disease (Symmetrical Gangrene) is a condition in which the fingers, toes, or extremities of the ears and nose become numb, waxy-looking, Raynaud's Disease. and bloodless—a phase which lasts from minutes to hours, and is then followed by the affected parts becoming livid and

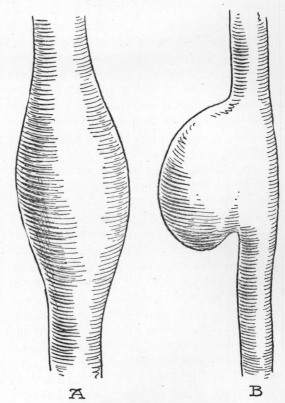

A   **B**

ANEURISM IN AN ARTERY

When the wall of an artery is weakened at any point by disease, it may be distended by the pressure of the blood, forming an aneurism. The diagram shows (A) " tubular," and (B) " sacculated " aneurisms.

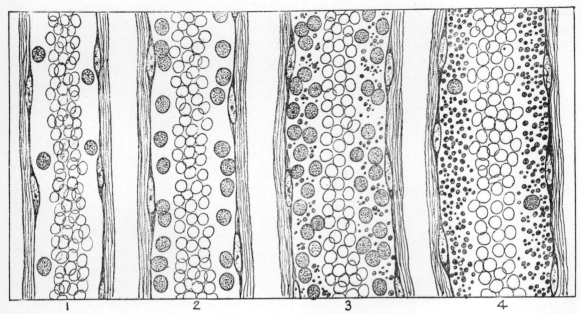

THE CAUSE OF THROMBOSIS

Diagrammatic sections of an artery at successive stages (1 to 4) of the process of thrombosis. Clots of blood form on the inner surface (roughened by lime deposits), retarding, and finally completely obstructing the blood stream.

Treatment is mainly directed to improving the general tone of the system, and to preventing attacks by the use of warm gloves and suitable clothing. Electricity, in the form of galvanism, may be of value in certain cases.

In intermittent claudication of arteries (Intermittent Limp), numbness, tingling, pain, and cramps occur after walking, in the muscles, chiefly of the legs, and lead to a limping gait or complete inability to walk. The arteries of the affected part cease to pulsate, and the foot and leg may become blue and swollen. The disease is always associated with arterio-sclerosis, and is caused by a spasm of the narrowed arteries, depriving the muscles of their blood-supply, which is induced by some disturbance of the arterial nerve control. During an attack, rest, followed by massage, is the best means of obtaining relief. Prevention of attacks is dependent upon the successful control and alleviation of the related arterio-sclerosis.

Intermittent Limp.

DISEASES OF THE VEINS

Inflammation of the walls of a vein tends to occur in rheumatic, gouty, or anaemic subjects, and in those who have been confined to bed for prolonged periods as a result of some operation, or following some febrile disorder, such as typhoid.

The most typical example of phlebitis is met with in the superficial veins of the leg, especially when they are varicose. There is swelling and tenderness along the line of the affected vein, and the skin over it is dull red in colour. In some cases, owing to thrombosis, the swollen vein may be felt as a firm cord. The onset is associated with sudden pain and a rise in temperature. The acute symptoms pass off in a few days, though the swelling and tenderness may persist for many weeks.

If the deep veins of the legs are involved there is great swelling of the whole limb, which becomes pale white in colour, and has an almost wooden consistence. This condition may arise as a complication of childbirth, and is known as " white leg," or " phlegmasia alba dolens."

In treatment, absolute rest in bed—the foot of which should be raised, with the limb immobilised by sandbags—is of first importance. Unnecessary handling of the parts should be avoided, lest a portion of the clot be displaced and embolism occur. Warm fomentations may relieve the pain. When the condition is recovered from, a supporting elastic bandage should be worn.

A more severe inflammation of the veins may occur in relation to some focus of septic infection in the adjacent tissues. The vessel wall is destroyed by suppuration, and the clot within it becomes infected, undergoes softening, and detached portions, entering the circulation, may cause secondary foci of suppuration—pyaemic abscesses. This infective phlebitis most frequently arises in certain veins within the skull as a sequel to chronic suppuration in the middle ear.

Courtesy] [" Manual of Surgery," Thomson & Miles (O.U.P.)

VARICOSE VEINS

The distension is usually due to weakness of the vessel walls and increased pressure of the blood inside the veins.

It is a serious complication, but may be treated surgically by ligating the vein on the cardiac side of the inflamed clot with a view to preventing dissemination of septic emboli.

In the condition known as varicose veins, the veins are so altered that they remain permanently dilated, lengthened, and tortuous. Although any veins in the body may become affected, varicosity is chiefly found in the veins of the legs, in the veins of the spermatic cord (varicocele), and in the veins of the rectum and anal canal (haemorrhoids).

Varicose Veins.

The predominant causal factors appear to be an inherent weakness of the vessel walls, along with a congenital deficiency in the number, size, and efficiency of the valves. Increased pressure within the veins is generally the exciting cause. This may be produced by certain diseases of the heart, lung, and liver, which raise the venous pressure; by the pressure of tumours or the pregnant uterus; by the wearing of tight garters; by muscular straining, and by prolonged standing or walking.

Varicosity of the veins is most commonly met with between puberty and the age of thirty. Men and women suffer equally. In the case of the veins of the leg, the dilated and tortuous vessels can be seen and felt. There are usually one or more bunches of distended veins in the region of the knee, and the small veins of the skin of the ankle and foot often show as fine blue streaks arranged in an arborescent fashion. A good deal of pain and discomfort may be experienced; a sense of weight and fulness in the limb is felt after standing or walking, but this is afforded rapid relief by raising the leg.

Certain complications are apt to arise. A chronic dermatitis or eczema may develop in the skin of the lower part of the leg owing to interference with nutrition. Ulceration of a very chronic nature may follow, and a copious haemorrhage may ensue and prove fatal if the sufferer should be asleep or intoxicated. Phlebitis and thrombosis may prove a dangerous sequel.

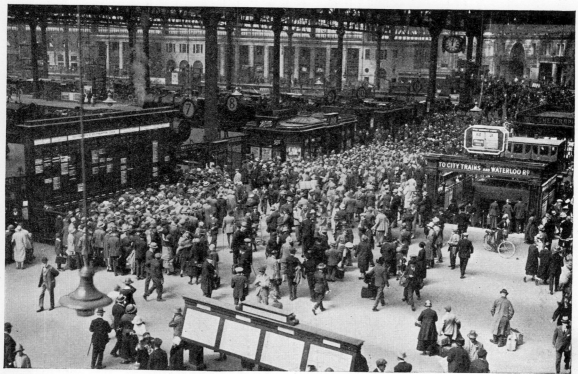

[Photopress

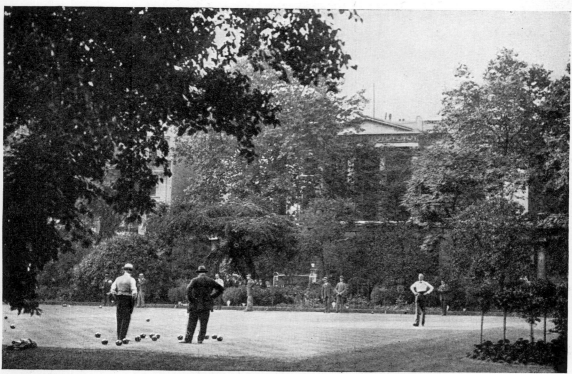

[Topical

A CONTRAST IN CITY LIFE

The worry and strain of present-day life is a prominent cause of degenerating arteries. *Above :* a picture typical of busy city life ; *below :* an antidote for the middle-aged—a game of bowls within the sound of Bow Bells.

As it is quite impossible to restore the veins to their normal structure, all treatment is necessarily palliative.

Any source of pressure on the veins must be removed ; garters should not be worn ; any tumours must be removed ; chronic constipation relieved ; the functions of the liver regulated ; and prolonged standing and walking are to be avoided. A light porous elastic bandage applied as a puttee may be worn to support the distended vessels. Such an appliance should be put on before the sufferer leaves bed in the morning, and should not be removed till he lies down at night.

When severe pain is suffered, and when the occupation or mode of life is markedly interfered with, operative measures are called for. The younger the subject, the clearer is the indication for operation.

The commonest tumour of the blood-vessels is the naevus (mole), a form of capillary angioma. It consists of an aggregation of dilated capillaries in the substance of the skin, and may assume the " port-wine-stain " often seen upon the face. It may be accompanied by overgrowth of the epidermis and of the hairs. The naevus shows little tendency to spontaneous disappearance. It is present from birth, and may tend to increase in size as the child advances in years. The treatment is unsatisfactory owing to the difficulty of removing the naevus without leaving a disfiguring scar. Exposure to radium or electrolysis, in suitable cases, may produce good results.

Tumours of Blood-Vessels.

HIGH BLOOD-PRESSURE

By G. A. SUTHERLAND, C.B.E., A.M., M.D., F.R.C.P., M.R.C.S., Physician to Paddington Green Children's Hospital ; Consulting Physician to the Royal National Orthopædic Hospital ; Author of " Modern Aspects of Heart Disease."

THERE is a subject which is now frequently discussed in clubs and at dinner-tables, and is called blood-pressure. Some people assert that they are suffering from blood-pressure, as if that were a disease instead of being a necessary factor in maintaining the circulation. Others are more precise, and say they possess a high blood-pressure or a low blood-pressure, the former being the more common and popular. This subject of a high blood-pressure has interested the medical profession during the past few years, chiefly because of the precise instruments introduced for its measurement and also because it raises many puzzling questions not yet solved. The problem why one person should have a high blood-pressure and another a low tends to become as absorbing and as insoluble as the old trouble as to why one person is fat and another thin.

Certain facts have to be recognised. As the years advance, say after the age of forty, the larger blood-vessels (arteries) tend to lose their fine elasticity and softness, which help to facilitate the flow of blood through the body. There comes on a gradual process of hardening in the soft walls of the arteries, and these previously distensible tubes become more rigid. The result is that the blood does not flow through them so easily. Consequently more force is required in pumping the blood, and with this increase comes a rise in the pressure of the blood in the arteries. In fact, if the circulation is to be carried on satisfactorily through these more rigid tubes, the only method of securing this is by means of a higher blood-pressure. If symptoms of local or general ill health arise, they are not really the result of higher blood-pressure, which is beneficial, but of the hardening and degeneration of the arteries.

Hardening of the Arteries.

Into this subject we do not go further here, because our object is to discuss the prevention of such hardening of the arteries. It must be recognised that in the majority of people this tendency to hardening of the arteries is merely a sign of advancing years, just as baldness, or failing sight, or deafness, or stiffening of the muscles is. To some it comes sooner, to others later, and to all its extent will depend very greatly on their previous habits of life.

Some unknown poet has probably had hardening of the arteries in mind when he put up the following prayer :

" Give me a good digestion, Lord,
  And also something to digest.
  Give me a healthy body, Lord,
  With sense to keep it at its best.
  Give me a mind that is not bored,
  That does not whimper, whine, or sigh.
  Don't let me worry overmuch
  About the fussy thing called " I."
  Give me a sense of humour, Lord,
  Give me the grace to see a joke ;
  To get some happiness in life
  And pass it on to other folk."

Here we have a very good summary of the preventive treatment of hardened arteries.

Prevention. The digestion is most important, but sometimes a good digestion leads one into the error of thinking that one can eat and drink as much as one likes. Unfortunately appetite and digestion are not the same thing. There is no doubt that over-eating as well as excessive drinking leads to hardening of the arteries by loading the blood with excess of food products, which become irritants. The healthy body prayed for must be maintained by " sense to keep it at its best," and that will be shown by moderation in eating and drinking. The typical example of the hardened sinner with the hardened arteries is seen in the city man who has indulged in excess and for years in the pleasures of the table, and has taken little exercise.

Our poet considers the frame of mind to be of some importance, and he is right. A life of stress and strain from business, or professional occupation, does seem to be an important factor. Some take life lightly, and perhaps do not suffer, but it is more especially the worrying type of individual whose arteries tend to be affected. Care-free people are to be envied in many ways, and they score also in the matter of their blood-vessels. Those on the other hand who have had great business losses, or family troubles, or worries which have engrossed their lives for long periods, are apt to show early the signs of degenerating arteries. All

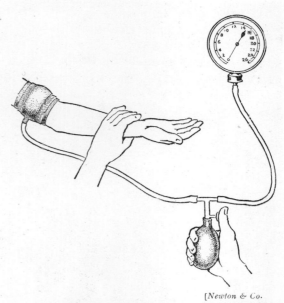

[Newton & Co.

HOW BLOOD-PRESSURE IS RECORDED

Air is pumped into a rubber sleeve placed round the upper arm until the pressure is sufficient to block the arm artery. The clock-like instrument registers this pressure.

the more reason is there for those who would have a healthy old age not to " worry overmuch " about themselves or anything else.

There is something very insidious about the onset of high blood-pressure and thickening of the arteries, because the subject of it often feels in particularly good health and spirits, up to a certain stage. This means that the heart has responded well to the additional strain thrown upon it, and maintains a good circulation through the brain and other organs of the body. Those who at this stage have a warning note in the form of a severe attack of nose bleeding, or a giddy feeling, or noises in the ears, are fortunate because attention may thus be directed to the progressive changes which are going on, and preventive treatment adopted. If, on the other hand, there is no such warning, the degenerative changes in the arteries go on, and the strain on the heart leads to changes there which in time weaken its working power. Another special risk lies in connection with the kidneys, in which the blood-vessels may degenerate to such an

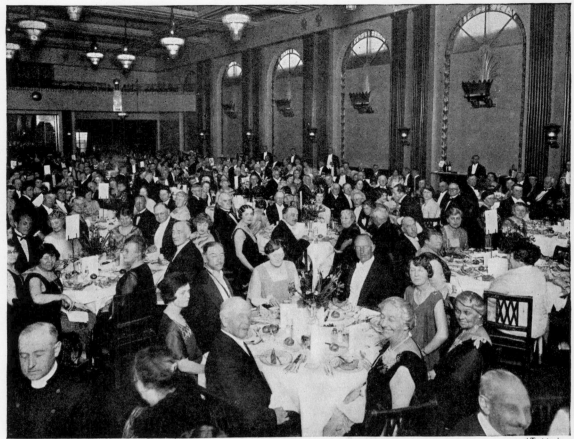

[Topical

THE PLEASURES OF THE TABLE

City life presents many temptations to depart from the golden rule of moderation in diet—one of the first rules for avoiding the hardened arteries of middle age.

extent that their normal function is seriously interfered with and the blood-pressure rises higher.

There is nothing special about the preventive treatment of high blood-pressure and degenerated arteries. As already stated, there is a normal change in this direction with advancing years, and many people with a moderately high blood-pressure live to a good old age. The seeds of it are usually laid during the period of adult life, and the chief causes are the habits of the individual and sometimes, although less frequently, a severe or prolonged illness. The preventive treatment may be summed up as healthy living. It is not a question of a special dietary, but of moderation in eating. Wholesome food of all kinds, alcoholic beverages in strict moderation, exercise sufficient to keep the muscles supple and strong, sound sleep, plenty of water drunk between meals, and an absence of worrying, represent the general indication. The " worrying " part must be stressed : there is a large class of the population which makes its own worries without any real foundation, simply from the possession of a worrying disposition. They should remember that therein lies a great danger of the development later on of high blood-pressure. The normal pressure of a healthy adult is about 120 : that is to say, it requires a pressure of 120 millimetres of mercury to overcome the pressure produced by the heart and blood-vessels. A high blood-pressure signifies that the blood in the heart and blood-vessels may be under a pressure of 180, 200, or even as high as 220.

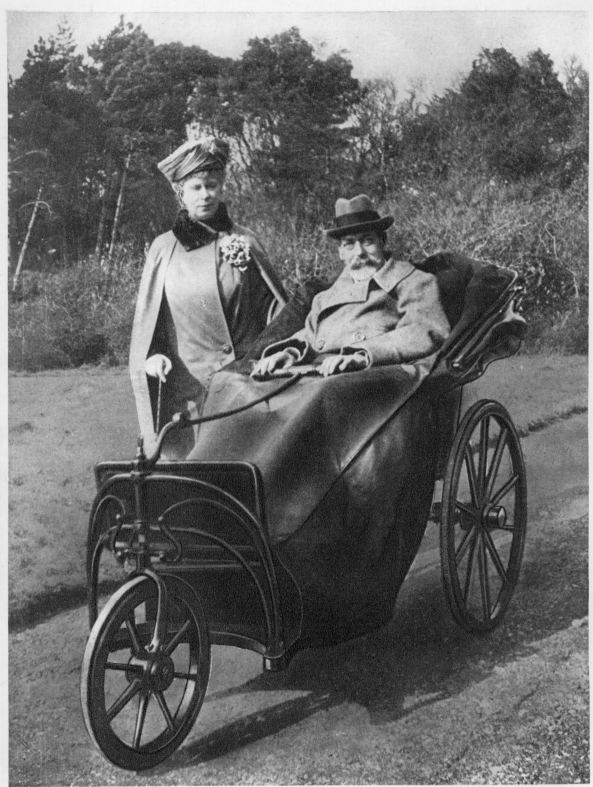

[*Central News*

CONVALESCENT.
The famous first picture taken of His Majesty The King after his remarkable recovery from serious lung trouble.

THE BLOOD IN HEALTH AND DISEASE

By GEORGE SOMERVILLE, M.D., D.P.M., Deputy Medical Superintendent at the West Ham Mental Hospital.

THE BLOOD AND ITS WORK

THE blood is the medium through which all the active cells and tissues of the body are kept in intimate relationship. Nutritive substances, including oxygen, pass from the blood to the tissues : waste materials, including carbonic acid, pass from the tissues to the blood. This constant interchange furnishes the tissues with a source of energy and the means of repairing loss of substance : it allows materials which are of no further use to the body to be carried to the excretory organs. It is by means of the blood that the secretions of certain ductless glands are carried to the various tissues which they are destined to influence. As the blood flows through the muscles and glands it is warmed, for these are heat-producing organs ; when it traverses the capillaries of the skin it is cooled. Hence the circulating blood serves to equalise the temperature of the different parts of the body.

The BLOOD is a red, viscid, opaque fluid, alkaline in reaction and with a faint but characteristic odour. It consists of a pale yellowish transparent liquid, called the plasma or liquor sanguinis, in which are suspended enormous numbers of minute bodies, the red and white blood-corpuscles and the blood-platelets.

The RED BLOOD-CORPUSCLES are circular bi-concave discs without a nucleus, yellow in colour when seen singly but red when massed together. There are on an average roughly 5,000,000 to the cubic millimetre of blood. These hollow envelopes contain in solution hæmoglobin, an iron compound, which has an affinity for oxygen. It is in virtue of this power of the hæmoglobin to combine with and give up oxygen, that the red cells act as carriers of oxygen from the lungs to the tissues. In post-natal life the red corpuscles originate from nucleated cells in the red marrow of the bones. When there is rapid destruction of the normal cells, such as occurs in pernicious anæmia, these immature nucleated red cells appear in the blood. Each red corpuscle appears to have a definite life history or term of existence. When worn out it is destroyed by the liver or spleen and the resultant colouring matter is excreted by means of the bile.

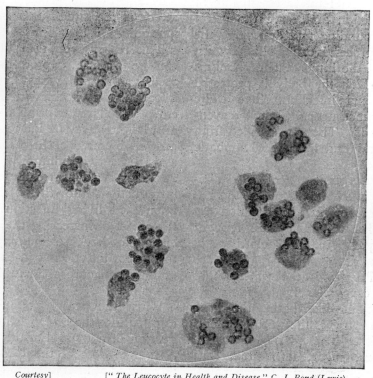

Courtesy]   [*" The Leucocyte in Health and Disease," C. J. Bond (Lewis)*

THE BLOOD'S SCAVENGERS AT WORK

A microphotograph showing white blood-corpuscles engulfing foreign bodies (red blood-corpuscles from a sheep). In this way the white corpuscles help to rid the blood of disease germs.

The White Blood-Corpuscles (leucocytes) are colourless nucleated cells of varying shape and size. They are larger than the red cells but are much less numerous (about 1 in 500). The leucocytes possess the power of amœboid movement and are able to make their way through the capillary cells into the tissue fluids. They are susceptible to the presence of foreign bodies which they are able to engulf and destroy. Invasion by micro-organisms causes a great increase in the number of the white-corpuscles (leucocytosis) which tend to congregate at the site of infection and serve the useful purpose of surrounding and destroying the invaders. This process is called phagocytosis, and it is one of the important mechanisms by means of which the body is protected against organismal infection. The white corpuscles are sometimes called the " scavengers of the blood." They are derived from the bone marrow and from the lymphatic glands.

The Blood-Platelets are colourless disc-shaped bodies, much smaller than the red corpuscles, whose origin and function are not definitely known. They are thought to play a part in the clotting of blood.

The Blood-Plasma is the watery fluid in which the corpuscles float. It is the nourishing solution which bathes the tissue cells and which removes the waste products of their activity. The plasma holds in solution proteins, sugar, fats, urea, salts (notably sodium chloride and bicarbonate), and the gases, oxygen, carbonic acid and nitrogen. One of the proteins of the plasma is called fibrinogen. It is present in solution, but when the blood is shed it is altered by a ferment, believed to be derived from the blood-platelets, and deposited in the form of threads known as fibrin. The corpuscles are entangled in the resulting meshwork and form a clot which at first is soft and jelly-like but later becomes firm and tough. This is the process of blood coagulation and it is the physiological method of sealing an injured blood-vessel and preventing loss of blood.

THE PROTECTIVE POWERS OF THE BLOOD

The normal blood contains substances inimical to bacterial life and is consequently pre-eminent amongst the body defences against disease. It is a commonplace that certain people when exposed to infection do not contract disease. This is due to certain protective qualities of the blood, and such persons are regarded as possessors of a " natural immunity." It is also a familiar fact that one attack of an infectious disease protects against another attack of the same disease. An " acquired immunity " is developed.

Immunity.

This response on the part of the blood can be artificially produced and can be used as a preventive measure against possible infection. By vaccination a mild attack of cowpox (believed to be an attenuated variety of smallpox) may be induced. The natural protective powers of the blood are stimulated and a relative immunity to smallpox is attained. Vaccine treatment is simply the introduction into the body of dead or attenuated living infectious material with the object of increasing the resistive powers of the blood. A vaccine may be used either to prevent infection as in enteric or cholera or to aid in cure as in rabies or catarrhal inflammations.

When the actual poison of bacteria is injected into the body it stimulates the production of a natural antidote or antibody. A minute dose of the toxin of diphtheria introduced at intervals into the blood stream of an animal results in the formation of a considerable quantity of antitoxin. Such an animal is now able to survive a dose of toxin many times larger than that which previously would have killed it. An immunity to the toxin has resulted. The antitoxin neutralises the toxin in much the same way as an acid neutralises an alkali and their mixture in equal quantities is harmless. Blood serum, rich in antitoxin, can be procured by the gradual immunisation of an animal (usually the horse) and this serum—standardised—can be used to combat a toxæmia in human beings. This is known as " passive immunisation " to distinguish it from the " active immunisation " of vaccine inoculation. Passive immunisation by the injection of antitoxin is universally adopted in the treatment of diphtheria and tetanus.

The blood-plasma possesses natural protective powers in the form of " bacteriolysins," substances antagonistic to organismal life. Also, invasion by bacteria stimulates the " agglutinating power " of the plasma. The invaders are rendered immobile and are clumped together so that their activities are hindered.

It is the function of the phagocytes (white blood cells) to eat up invading organisms, but they appear unable to do so unless there are present in the plasma substances called " opsonins " which prepare the organisms for destruction. The activities of the phagocytes, upon which the power of resistance depends, varies with the quantity of opsonins, *i.e.* the opsonic index.

The means of combating bacterial foes are many. They may be killed by bacteriolysins ; rendered immobile by agglutinins ; eaten up by phagocytes aided by opsonins, or the toxins may be neutralised by antitoxins. These are the main methods by which the body is enabled to resist or to recover from diseases of organismal origin.

DISORDERS OF THE BLOOD

The blood is the circulating medium and readily responds to alterations in organic functioning. The constitution of the plasma is altered in metabolic disorder such as diabetes and gout. Poisons either from within as in chronic constipation or from without as in organismal infections not only have a deleterious effect on the tissues generally but also gravely impair the quality of the blood. Diseases of the blood are characteristically revealed in certain changes in the corpuscular elements and in the quantity of hæmoglobin.

Anæmia. Anæmia is the comprehensive term which signifies deficiency in certain of the elements of the blood. There may be a decrease in the total amount of blood, in the red corpuscles, or in the

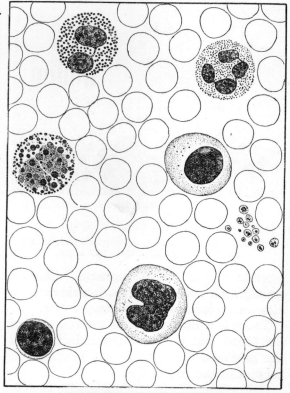

NORMAL BLOOD CELLS

The circles represent red blood-corpuscles ; the larger white corpuscles have been shaded to show the different types with their nuclei ; the small bodies on the right are blood-platelets—all greatly enlarged.

hæmoglobin. It results either from defective blood formation or excessive blood destruction. Impoverished blood impairs the vitality of all the tissues : vicious circles are set up. The lungs suffer from want of oxygen : the heart muscle loses its tone : disordered stomach and bowel functions cause dyspepsia and constipation : malnutrition of the brain causes headaches and mental irritability. Morbid changes in the quantity or quality of the blood lower the level of healthy functioning throughout the whole body.

" Green Sickness." " Green Sickness " (Chlorosis) is almost entirely confined to young women. It is mainly dependent upon want of fresh air, unsuitable diet, or deficient exercise and insanitary surroundings. It occurs at the phase of life when the girl is being moulded into the woman—the time which demands the best

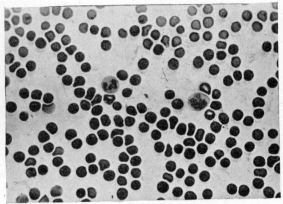

[Frank Harrison, M.R.C.S., L.D.S.]

UNDER THE MICROSCOPE

Red and white corpuscles, floating in a transparent fluid, are here magnified 750 times.

possible hygienic environment. Chronic constipation with its auto-intoxication is also an important contributory factor.

There is a diminution of the red cells of the blood, but the most marked change is the profound decrease of the hæmoglobin content of the corpuscles.

Girls who suffer from chlorosis are usually plump but have a waxy-looking complexion which often assumes a greenish tinge. They are breathless on the slightest exertion and their capacities for physical or mental work are greatly reduced. Loss of appetite and persistent constipation are invariably present. Mental irritability, capriciousness and hysterical outbursts occur at times.

A condition similar to chlorosis may occur in early tuberculosis and the possibility of this renders careful medical examination necessary in all cases.

This disease is not dangerous to life and under treatment rapid recovery takes place in the majority of cases in about two months. The essence of treatment is to improve the hygiene of the surroundings and of the self. Diet should be simple and nutritious : fresh air and sunshine are vital ; saline laxatives are necessary for the bowels and, if there is any heart strain, rest is imperative. Iron is the outstanding remedy for chlorosis. It may be administered in the form of Blaud's Pills. These should be taken after meals and the mouth and teeth should always be

cleansed afterwards. Any definite causal factor must be eliminated and it is essential that the hygienic life should be maintained, otherwise relapses are inevitable.

Pernicious Anæmia is a form of anæmia showing marked diminution in the number of red blood-corpuscles. It is a **Pernicious Anæmia.** disease of middle life and is probably due to some poison which destroys the blood cells. The actual nature and source of the toxin is at present unknown, but by many it is believed to originate from oral or intestinal sepsis.

Most cases commence gradually. There is severe pallor of the lips, gums, and conjunctivæ. The skin assumes a lemon-yellow tint and as a rule the body fat is not diminished so that sufferers often exhibit a fairly well nourished appearance. There is progressive debility : breathlessness results from the slightest exertion ; the heart dilates and the pulse becomes rapid and feeble. Dyspepsia, vomiting, and diarrhœa occur as the disease advances. Sleeplessness and mental peculiarities result from starvation of the brain,

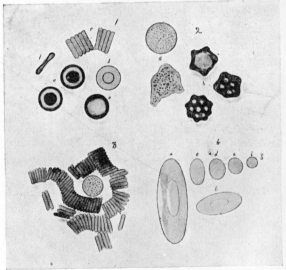

[Newton & Co.]

THE COMPOSITION OF THE BLOOD

Group 1 shows different views of the biconcave red corpuscles. Group 2 represents the varying shapes of white corpuscles, and two mulberry-shaped globules sometimes present in unhealthy blood. Group 3 is coagulated blood ; and 4 shows corpuscles of different animals as follows : (a) proteus ; (b) frog ; (c) lizard ; (d) birds ; (e) fishes ; (f) man ; and (g) musk-deer, which has the smallest blood-corpuscle known.

and there may be degenerative changes in the spinal cord. The signs of pernicious anæmia appear to be produced not only by the morbid state of the blood but also by the poisons which originate the disease. Pernicious anæmia may progress uniformly towards a fatal termination, but more frequently the disease is subject to fluctuations, and there are remissions and relapses which extend over a number of years.

and intestinal tract may not be the fundamental cause, undoubtedly it is an aggravating factor and its alleviation promotes the general well-being and hinders the rapid progress of the disease. The administration of iron is useless in pernicious anæmia ; arsenic appears to be the only drug which has any beneficial effect. Transfusion of blood has been tried, but any subsequent improvement is only transitory. Although

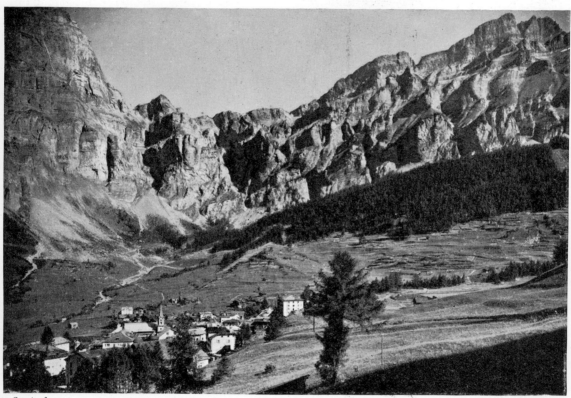

Courtesy] [Swiss Federal Rlys.

A HEALTH RESORT FOR THE ANÆMIC
Loèche-les-Bains, a spa among the mountains of Valais, Switzerland, which undertakes the cure of anæmia.

In treatment, which unfortunately can only be palliative so long as the primary cause or causes are unknown, it is important to place the patient under healthy conditions with regard to food, air, and rest. Diet should be restricted to milk, fruit, and vegetable foods as the feeble gastric secretions are unable to digest meat proteins. Rest in bed improves the body functions generally and relieves the heart. Hill air appears to be specially beneficial in these cases. Though sepsis of the mouth, teeth,

radical treatment must remain impossible until the nature of the toxin and its source are discovered, recently an effective remedy has been discovered. It consists of feeding the sufferers on a diet rich in animal liver. The mechanism of the cure is unknown At present the treatment remains more empirical than rational, nevertheless accumulated scientific evidence reveals that liver-feeding is apparently a specific agent in obtaining remissions in cases of pernicious anæmia.

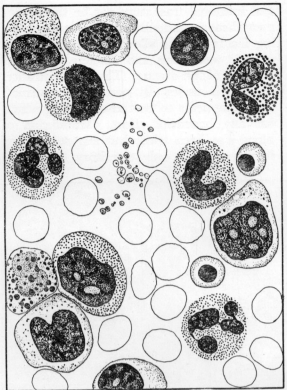

BLOOD IN LEUKÆMIA
In this disease the white blood-corpuscles greatly increase in number. They are shaded in these diagrams to show the different types.

Anæmias which are subsequent to any known cause are termed "secondary anæmias." The simplest variety results from loss of blood either from internal or external bleeding. Repeated small hæmorrhages from the nose, kidneys, womb, congested piles, or in relation to such diseases as scurvy or hæmophilia lead to severe forms of chronic anæmia. The large hæmorrhages from ulceration of vessels in phthisis, gastric or duodenal ulcer, injury or childbirth lead to relatively acute anæmias. Albuminuria in nephritis, prolonged suppuration, inanition from deprivation of nourishment, over-lactation and chronic poisoning by means of lead, mercury, or arsenic, reduce the capacities of the blood forming tissues and are productive of anæmias of varying intensity. Anæmias are an accompaniment and a consequence of acute fevers such as typhoid, and of chronic wasting diseases such as phthisis, cancer, malaria, and syphilis.

Secondary Anæmia.

In secondary anæmias the red cells are diminished in number and are poor in quality; the hæmoglobin may be diminished; the white cells, especially in septic conditions, usually show considerable increase.

Pallor of the skin, lips, and conjunctivæ is the most obvious sign. Languor, loss of mental and physical energy, giddiness and faintness are complained of. Appetite is fickle and digestion is impaired. The heart may dilate and its action become feeble and irregular. Swelling about the ankles from dropsy results from the enfeebled circulation and the impoverished blood.

Treatment must be directed to the primary cause to which the anæmia is secondary. Unless this can be found and eradicated, permanent cure is impossible.

Leukæmia is a disease in which the white blood-corpuscles are greatly increased in number. It is associated with enlargement of the spleen and lymphatic glands. Leukæmia is due to a morbid over-activity of the bone marrow or the lymphatic tissue. It is a disease of middle-age, insidious in its onset and chronic in its course. Discomfort and breathlessness from swelling of the abdomen are usually the first symptoms. Signs of a secondary anæmia develop. Dropsy may occur as a result of obstruction of the lymphatics from the enlarged glands and spleen. Hæmorrhages are common and there are often slight rises in temperature.

Leukæmia.

Examination of the blood reveals an enormous increase in the white blood-corpuscles: they may be multiplied sixty-fold. Two types of cell increase are found: lymphocytes may predominate or immature white cells (myelocytes) may appear in vast numbers.

As with most blood diseases there are remissions and relapses but each relapse leaves the sufferer in a less satisfactory state and the total duration is seldom more than a few years.

Fresh air, a well balanced diet, and rest are the main indications for treatment. So long as the origin of the disease is unknown treatment cannot be radical.

Hæmophilia is an interesting hereditary disease, almost entirely confined to young males who appear predisposed to the recurrence of hæmorrhages. The actual cause is unknown, but it is believed to be related to a diminished coagulability of the blood due to deficiency of lime salts. The peculiar feature of hæmophilia is its manner of hereditary transmission. Only the males of the family suffer, but it is transmitted by the females.

Hæmophilia.

The disease reveals itself in early life by the occurrence of hæmorrhages from slight injuries. A trivial operation such as the extraction of a tooth may cause an uncontrollable and fatal hæmorrhage. Bleeding may also occur, without previous injury, from the nose, mouth, stomach, bowels, urethra, and lungs. There is a steady oozing from the capillaries and a serious anæmia may follow.

Bleeders should be guarded against any possible injury or operation. The general health should be maintained at its highest level. The ordinary methods for controlling bleeding must be adopted. Large doses of calcium lactate are of some value by increasing the coagulability of the blood. To some extent the tendency to bleeding may be overgrown.

HYGIENE OF THE BLOOD

Sunlight and oxygen may be described as tonic blood foods. The rays of the sun increase the oxygen-carrying capacities of the corpuscles; fresh air increases the available quantity of oxygen and hastens the excretion of the toxic carbonic acid. Vigorous exercise is accompanied by deep breathing and the residual air in the lungs is continually refreshed. A well-balanced dietary promotes the general well-being and also nourishes the blood.

Sepsis anywhere in the body causes a constant draining of poison into the blood and reduces the vitality of all the blood cells. Chronic constipation acts in a similar manner. The prevention of hæmophilia is a eugenic problem; the daughters of

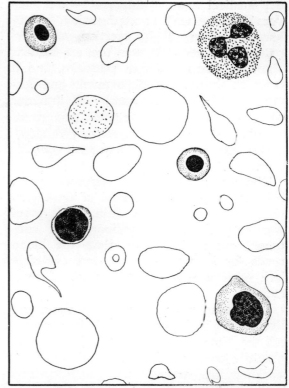

BLOOD IN PERNICIOUS ANÆMIA
The red blood-corpuscles, which in normal blood are about 500 times as numerous as the white, diminish in number and become misshapen and degenerate.

hæmophilic families should be dissuaded from reproduction.

A healthy blood is a *sine qua non* for a healthy mind and body.

BLOODLESSNESS IN GIRLS

By C. W. SALEEBY, M.D., Ch.B., F.R.S.E., F.Z.S., Founder and Chairman of the Sunlight League.

ANÆMIA, or bloodlessness, may be due to many causes. Within recent years we have learnt how to conquer the two most striking and characteristic kinds of anæmia; in both cases the means are extremely simple and the results are glorious. In this article I shall deal with the conquest of primary anæmia, so called, known as "green-sickness" in Shakespeare's time.

The "primary anæmia" of young girls gives their faces a greenish pallor—hence our medical name " chlorosis "—and burdens their lives with a poor digestion, breathlessness on very slight exertion, and perpetual weariness. It was the too-familiar " green-sickness " of past centuries, and it crowded out-patients' departments and doctors' consulting rooms until well into our own. As you walked the street you passed scores of chlorotic girls out of every hundred. Where are they now ? They have gone for ever.

The great remedy was supposed to be iron, for certainly the blood of these girls was pale and poor in iron. Yet proof was easy that their ordinary diet contained more daily iron than the blood needs for its maintenance, and evidently lack of iron was not the cause of their malady.

The cause was the pitifully unnatural lives those girls led—confined indoors nearly all the time, taking very little exercise, absurdly overclothed in long skirts, thick stockings, high-necked blouses, and deprived of the breath and the light of life. Of course they were constipated, and thus their blood was always being poisoned from within and was therefore destroyed more quickly than it could be made without the wonderful blood-forming action of sunlight upon the skin.

Needless to say, these chlorotic girls were easy prey for the germs of tuberculosis—a dread disease which has immensely diminished among young girls since the disappearance of chlorosis.

For it has gone, and doubtless for ever. No collective madness of fashion or half-witted notions of maidenly modesty can ever be permitted to imprison and bleach and blight our young girlhood again as in the past. The formula for safety is very simple—favour the factors which make blood and avoid the factors which destroy it. The physical, social, and spiritual liberation of young womanhood in our time has not been specially designed to meet these needs, but it has done so.

The clock must never be put back. Indeed, some day we must spread the light even into the dark prisons, palaces though they be, of Oriental womanhood: while our own women keep their new heritage of rich, red, running blood, giving their lips and cheeks the colour of life—the only colour worth looking at there—and endowing them with the joy of life which is born and borne in that incomparable stream.

THE LYMPH VESSELS AND GLANDS

By GEORGE SOMERVILLE, M.D., D.P.M., Deputy Medical Superintendent to the West Ham Mental Hospital.

THE LYMPHATIC SYSTEM AND ITS WORK

THE lymphatic system is an accessory circulatory system whereby the lymph, after nourishing the individual cell units in the tissues, is collected and returned to the blood stream.

The lymph is virtually the plasma, or liquid part of the blood, which has passed through the thin walls of the capillaries. It contains oxygen, sugar, salts, emulsified fats and protein which are required by the cells for the performance of their vital functions. The lymph is exuded from the bloodvessels partly as a result of the high pressure within the capillaries and partly owing to the vital action of the cells of the capillary walls. The lymph penetrates the gaps and crevices between the cells and as well as nourishing them receives and carries away the waste products of their activity.

The lymph capillaries take origin in the lymph spaces of the tissues and in the walls of serous cavities (pleuræ : peritoneum), and unite to form fine vessels, " lymphatics," which have a structure similar to that of veins but are more abundantly provided with valves. The lymphatics ramify throughout the whole body. At intervals their course is interrupted by the presence of the lymph glands—pea-like bodies—which act as filters. Ultimately they unite to form the largest lymphatic vessel, the " thoracic duct," which is about the size of a crow quill. It commences just below the diaphragm, runs up the back of the thorax, and enters the left subclavian vein at the root of the neck, thus returning the lymph to the blood stream.

In certain of the lower animals (amphibia and some birds) the movement of the lymph is produced by muscular sacs, named " lymph-hearts " but in man and most of the higher animals such " hearts " do not exist and the lymph circulation is brought about by several agencies. By means of the valvular mechanism all pressure on the exterior of the lymphatics from muscular contraction propels and accelerates the lymph onwards. The respiratory movements greatly favour the current of the lymph through the thoracic duct. A certain contractility in the walls of the vessels also aids in the general propulsion. For the maintenance of a free circulation of lymph— essential for the health of the tissues— regular exercise is obviously of first importance.

The lymphatic glands are round or oval bodies which vary in size from a hemp seed to a large bean. They are interposed in the course of the lymphatics and the lymph is filtered through them before being discharged into the blood-vessels. The lymph glands have a similar structure throughout the body. Externally is a capsule of fibrous tissue which sends inwards partitions and bands to form a fibrous scaffolding. Within the meshes are masses of lymph corpuscles which ultimately form one of the varieties of leucocytes found in the circulating blood. The lymph enters the gland by several afferent vessels (which pierce the capsule) and percolates through it, leaving by efferent vessels which commence in the central portion of the gland.

Lymph glands not only manufacture lymphocytes—but also act as filters. From the circulating lymph they arrest inert substances such as carbon pigment and living elements such as bacteria and cancer cells. The lymph is brought in intimate contact

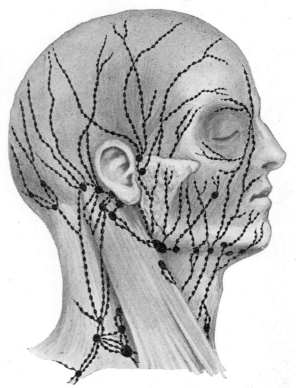

THE NETWORK OF LYMPHATICS
Lymphatic vessels ramify throughout the whole body, and the little globular lymph glands in their course act as filters for waste products.

with the lymphocytes which are inimical to bacterial life and consequently the glands may be regarded as an important line of defence retarding or preventing the passage of organisms and their products into the general circulation.

Lymph glands are arranged in groups or chains, and vary in number and size in different individuals. They increase in number following certain stimuli, as in the case of the axillary glands during lactation. New glands may arise subsequent to their removal by operation. A few glands are situated in the vicinity of the elbow and knee joints, but the main gland barriers of the extremities are found in the armpit and groin. Below the jaw and on both sides of the neck there are chains of glands, familiar to all from the frequency with which they become enlarged and painful. Lymph glands are found in great numbers in the mesentery of the intestines and along the great vessels of the abdomen. Deep in

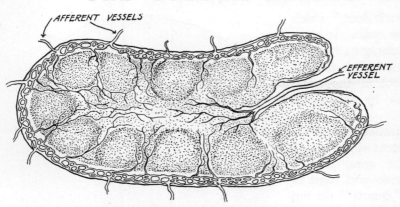

AFFERENT VESSELS

EFFERENT VESSEL

A LYMPH GLAND IN SECTION

The lymph enters the gland by several *afferent* vessels, and returns to the blood by the *efferent* vessels which spring from the centre of the gland.

the thoracic cavity, in relation to the roots of the lungs, lie the " bronchial glands " which receive the lymphatics from the lungs.

DISEASES OF LYMPH VESSELS AND GLANDS.

Inflammation of the surface lymph vessels commonly originates from some focus of

Lymphan-gitis.
infection in the skin such as a wound or a suppurating blister. The inflammation chiefly affects the walls of the vessels and to some extent the surrounding cellular tissue. It is attended by clotting of the lymph.

Lymphangitis is revealed by wavy red lines corresponding to the inflamed vessels which run from the source of infection to the nearest lymph glands. There is a burning pain and tenderness and the glands become swollen and painful.

Provided the primary source of infection is promptly dealt with, the inflammation rapidly subsides. If suppuration occurs, the pus must be allowed to escape by incision. On recovery from the inflammation the limb should be massaged to promote the lymphatic flow and prevent dropsy.

Recurrent attacks of lymphangitis may obliterate the lymph vessels by the formation of connective tissue and a persistent solid dropsy results which eventually culminates in a form of " elephantiasis."

The lymph vessels play an important part in the local spread of tuberculosis and malignant tumours ; they act as channels for the conveyance of organismal infection and frequently transport the migrating cells of cancer.

Owing to their protective function, the lymph glands are peculiarly liable to suffer from inflammation of organismal origin.

Inflammation of lymph glands results from the presence of a bacterial or toxic irritant brought to the glands by the afferent lymph vessels. The glands of the neck, armpit, and groin are those most commonly affected.

Lympha-denitis.
The degree of the inflammation varies. It may be mild and transient as in the glandular enlargement in the neck which often attends tonsillitis or other varieties of sore throat. It may be persistent as exemplified in the enlargements associated with adenoids, carious teeth, ear disease, and scalp eczema. Or, it may exhibit a very acute character and tend to abscess formation as in infected wounds of the fingers, gonorrhœal or soft sore infection, and following the severer forms of sore throat of diphtheria and scarlet fever.

In the treatment of inflamed glands it is obvious that the primary source of infection must first be dealt with. Alleviation of this is rapidly followed by a subsiding of the inflammation. In most cases the glands are best let entirely alone or at most supported by a bandage, but in very acute forms artificial congestion by means of a suction bell, or if suppuration has occurred, incision and drainage are advisable.

Scrofula or tuberculous infection of the lymph glands is exceedingly common and

Scrofula.
of great importance. Though any group of glands may be involved, the disease is most often met with in the cervical or neck glands which are already enlarged as a result of chronic septic irritation following adenoids, tonsillitis,

442

carious teeth, pharyngitis or middle-ear disease.

As a rule the disease affects several glands on one or both sides of the neck. At first the glands are solitary and movable, but later become fixed and matted together from inflammation of the surrounding tissue. The active disease process may be arrested at any stage and the tuberculous glands may become converted into scar tissue or even become calcified. More commonly, however, the gland softens, suppurates, and a " cold abscess " forms. The covering skin is undermined, becomes reddened, and finally the pus ruptures through the skin to form ulcers and sinuses which may persist indefinitely discharging pus or may eventually heal leaving unsightly puckered scars.

Tuberculosis of the glands most often occurs in childhood and in youth : it is rare in advanced life. It chiefly attacks the debilitated and those who exist in unhygienic surroundings, but occasionally it affects the apparently robust and affluent. After lupus it is the least dangerous to life of all forms of tuberculosis, but although many cases may recover completely, others may develop tuberculosis in other organs of the body at any later period of life.

There is considerable variance in opinion regarding the treatment of tuberculous glands. Certain authorities advocate their removal by operation ; others adopt conservative methods endeavouring to promote the general health and to hasten cure by exposure to sunlight or ultra-violet radiations. Treatment must be adapted to the problem of the individual. If the disease remains localised and confined, and there are no signs of its breaking down, constitutional methods should be adopted. The child should be made to spend all his time in the open air—by the seaside if possible. Diet should be generous, after the manner of that which is adopted in other forms of tuberculosis and should contain cod-liver oil and malt extract. Tonics containing iron and arsenic are beneficial. If, however, the disease shows aggressive tendencies, the glands becoming matted together and cold abscesses forming, the mass is best removed by operation, otherwise, should the abscess rupture through the skin, unsightly scars are inevitable. At the same time it should be noted that, owing to the number and deep situation of the glands to be removed and their adherence to surrounding structures, the operation is often by no means an easy one.

In the primary stage of acquired syphilis involvement of the lymph glands in the groin is a prominent feature. A **Syphilitic Disease.** few days after the appearance of the primary sore the glands become swollen and hard—the so-called bullet-bubos. Later in secondary syphilis a general enlargement of the lymphatic glands occurs, while occasionally in tertiary syphilis gummatous disease in the glands may arise.

A primary sarcoma may commence in a lymph gland. It is a rapidly growing **Tumours.** malignant tumour and usually consists of a central enlarged gland with numerous satellites. The

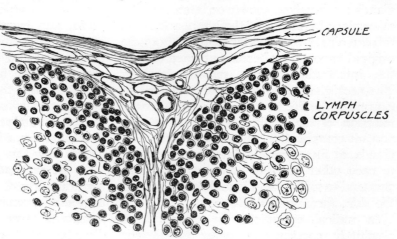

CAPSULE

LYMPH CORPUSCLES

TISSUE OF A LYMPH GLAND

A small section of a lymph gland showing the outer capsule of fibrous tissue and the masses of lymph corpuscles which ultimately form an important contribution to the blood stream.

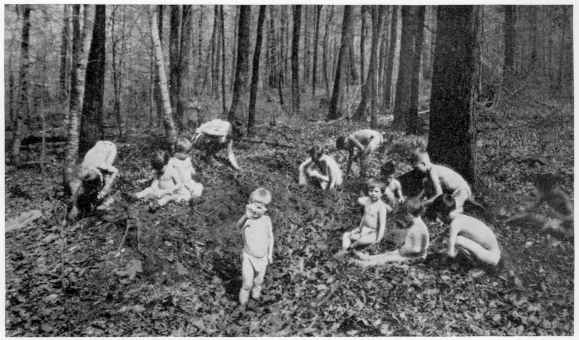

[*Keystone*

THE NATURAL CURE
An open-air life and exposure to sunlight are the best methods of combating tuberculous lymph glands.

outlook is very grave. Early incision followed by the use of radium or X-rays is the only method of treatment possible.

Secondary cancers are exceedingly frequent in lymph glands. Next to tuberculosis they are the commonest affection met with in such glands. When any organ or tissue is affected with cancer the neighbouring glands are involved sooner or later. Spread takes place by means of the lymphatics, and this explains how organs far removed from the original cancer may become affected though the intervening tissues remain healthy. The neck glands are commonly involved in cancers of the lip, tongue, tonsils, or throat ; infection of the axillary glands is an important complication of breast cancer. The glands, at first movable, later become fixed to each other and the adjacent structures, and tend to soften, liquify, and burst through the skin, forming foul ulcers.

In radical operations for cancer it is absolutely necessary in order to prevent recurrence that all the glands which drain the organ or tissue affected should be eradicated.

In the comparatively rare disease, known as Lymphadenoma (Hodgkin's Disease), the origin of which is at present unknown, there is a gradually progressive enlargement of the lymphatic glands throughout the body.

Hodgkin's Disease.

Hodgkin's disease is chiefly met with in young subjects. Glandular masses develop first in the neck, then in the arm-pit and groin, and eventually in the thoracic and abdominal cavities. The glands are firm in consistence and at first discrete and freely movable, but later they become matted together and, from pressure, cause serious interference with important structures such as the windpipe, gullet, and great veins. Breathlessness, difficulty in swallowing, and dropsy may thus ensue.

In the early stages of the disease there is a gradual loss of strength accompanied by a degree of anæmia. There is a tendency to attacks of fever and some gastro-intestinal disorder is of common occurrence. The disease is fatal, and usually extends over a period of several years, the affected person becoming progressively weaker and exhibiting signs as a result of pressure. There is an acute form in which the glandular enlargement is rapidly disseminated and results in early death.

Treatment in both forms is of little avail. Arsenic has been found beneficial in some cases and exposure to radium may temporarily diminish the glandular enlargement.

Surgical operation may be necessary to give relief when important structures are pressed upon, for example, tracheotomy is indicated if there is danger to life from asphyxia.

Enlargement of lymphatic glands is also found in the blood disease called "leukæmia." (See section on Disorders of the Blood.)

THE RESPIRATORY SYSTEM

THE PROCESS OF BREATHING

By MARY G. ADAMS, M.Sc. (Cantab.), Tutor in Biology to the Cambridge University Board of Extra-Mural Studies.

BREATHING in animals and plants, the rusting of iron, or the burning of fuel, are all forms of combustion or oxidation. Fuel and air are supplied, and the fire burns ; food and oxygen are transported by the blood, and the various organs of the body do their work. Work done means that energy has been liberated and heat evolved. Chemically this result is effected by the union of oxygen with the food in the tissues, or perhaps with the tissues themselves. A plentiful supply of oxygen is therefore essential to life (although there are certain bacteria which can, apparently, live without oxygen). In lower animals living in a moist environment, oxygen simply soaks through the skin and diffuses into the blood capillaries of the skin. Higher animals require a more elaborate mechanism for securing a constant oxygen supply.

Lungs, bronchial tubes, trachea, larynx, mouth and nose constitute the respiratory system in man.

Breathing consists essentially of the exposure of a large surface of blood in the capillaries of the lungs to a large volume **Nature of Breathing.** of air. It is extremely desirable that air should enter the lungs through the nostrils. For, in passing through the chamber of the nose, the air is warmed,

moistened if necessary, and cleansed of dust or bacteria by a filter of hairs. Even if bacteria get past the hairs they tend to get entrapped by the sticky mucus which is constantly being poured out over the surface of the passages.

Air is drawn into the lungs through the windpipe mainly by the muscular movements of the chest and diaphragm. The value of the chest as a breathing agency depends, however, not on its size, but on its mobility. Small chests are often more mobile than large ones. The lungs themselves are like

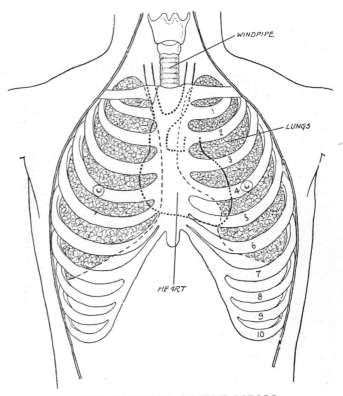

WINDPIPE

LUNGS

HEART

THE POSITION OF THE LUNGS
The lungs lie behind the ribs on either side of the heart, and are surrounded by a smooth membrane called the pleura.

445

elastic bags of spongy material consisting of an immense number of tiny air cavities opening into tubes called bronchi, which finally unite into the single windpipe. All the bigger bronchial tubes are lined with hairs whose constant rhythmical motion works back towards the throat any foreign particles which may have trespassed so far. Moreover, if the tubes become infected with certain injurious bacteria, *e.g.* bacteria of the common cold, glands in the tubes pour out quantities of mucus in an endeavour to remove the cause of irritation. This mucus is coughed up or blown out during the progress of a " cold."

The lung chambers contrive to expose a surface to the air a hundred times as great as the surface of the whole body. Their walls are as thin as soap-bubbles, and pressed against them are the thin walls of the blood capillaries. Through this delicate permeable partition oxygen passes in and is absorbed by the red corpuscles of the blood. In this way revitalised blood passes back to the left chamber of the heart, and, after pursuing its devious course through the body, returns again via the heart to the lungs with a load of carbon-dioxide which it will there expel.

A good deal of water and heat is lost in breathing ; a pint of water may be exhaled every twenty-four hours. In order, therefore, to sustain the temperature of the body more oxygen is required for burning in the tissues. But an abundant supply of oxygen is useless unless the blood is rich in the oxygen-collecting red corpuscles. When there is not a plentiful supply of oxygen the red corpuscles may increase in number, thus improving the oxygen-capturing power of the blood ; or the number of heart-beats per minute may be increased. This happens in the blood of people living at high altitudes. But naturally there is a limit to the power of adjustment, and at great heights unconsciousness is followed by death. Oxygen deficiency can be made good to a certain extent by inhaling pure oxygen. It might therefore be expected that oxygen might be administered to the body during times of special demand. It is true oxygen may be given in pneumonia, or bronchitis, or to athletes before racing, but its usefulness depends on the ability of the heart to transport it to the tissues when it is required. In normal circumstances, however, there is an excess of oxygen in the lungs. Air which is breathed out still contains 17 per cent. oxygen as against 21 per cent. in that which is breathed in. So that only in exceptional cases can more oxygen be utilised.

Few people use their lungs to their fullest capacity, a habit which is reflected in the pale faces and flat chests of sedentary workers. Deep-breathing exercises ought to be the daily practice of those who are denied the stimulus of open-air activity.

The mechanism by which breathing is automatically controlled is very ingenious. There is a nerve-centre in the medulla oblongata of the brain, sensitive to the amount of carbon-dioxide in the blood, from which messages are sent to the muscles of the chest and the diaphragm, bringing about expansion and contraction. Any increase of carbon-dioxide in the blood causes messages to be sent speeding up the breathing—panting is the response.

THE MOVEMENT OF BREATHING

A diagrammatic section through the body showing how the chest expands during inspiration (*left*) and subsides, with the diaphragm drawn up, during expiration (*right*).

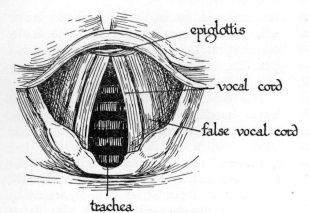

epiglottis

vocal cord

false vocal cord

trachea

THE ORGANS OF SPEECH
Interior of the larynx or voice box, showing the vocal cords and the epiglottis, a trap-door which prevents food and drink from entering the trachea during swallowing.

THE BREATHING APPARATUS

By W. H. HORNIBROOK, F.R.C.S., L.R.C.P., D.P.H. (Irel.), late Medical Officer of Health to Mackenzie County, New Zealand.

THE respiratory apparatus includes the larynx, trachea, bronchi, lungs and pleuræ.

The prominence in the front of the neck, known as Adam's Apple, marks the front of the thyroid cartilage. This is the hard wall of the hollow cavity—the larynx—which contains the vocal cords. It is a long piece of hard cartilage bent round on itself so as to enclose a somewhat triangular space; the apex of the triangle being in front, while the back, or the base of the triangle, is left open. The open space at the back is completed by muscles and ligaments. Each side of the cartilage is roughly square, but prolonged in front above to form the prominence of the apple, and at the back extends into two horns at its upper and lower corners. If the finger be pressed on the top of the prominence of the apple a shallow notch will be felt on the middle line. Immediately below this and inside, the " epiglottis " is hinged. This is a leaf-shaped piece of cartilage that stands up behind and below the base of the tongue, which is supported as in an arm-chair by the hyoid bone. At the moment of swallowing it shuts down like a trap-door on the top of the larynx which it covers tightly until the food has reached the gullet. This is the mechanism which prevents food and drink from entering the windpipe and lungs. Below the lower border of the thyroid cartilage a narrow space may be felt which divides it from the round front of the " cricoid " cartilage. This latter is a ring of cartilage somewhat like a signet ring in shape, the seal being at the back, where the two lower horns of the thyroid cartilage are hinged to it. On the upper edge of the back part rest the two arytenoid cartilages, small solid pyramids having the minute cartilages of Wrisberg and Santorini in relation with their upper pointed ends.

The vocal cords are attached behind to the arytenoid and in front to the thyroid cartilage just below the epiglottis. These are thin bands of elastic tissue stretched tightly across the larynx, having an opening, the " rima," between them through which air enters and leaves the chest. The size and shape of this opening are constantly varying. It is divided into an anterior, or vocal part,

ŒSOPHAGUS

EPIGLOTTIS

TONGUE

HYOID BONE

LARYNX

THYREOID CARTILAGE

VOCAL CORD

CRICOID CARTILAGE

TRACHEA

INSIDE THE ADAM'S APPLE
A section through the neck showing the position of the larynx and vocal cords, which lie behind the Adam's apple.

447

and a posterior, or respiratory part. When at rest, that is to say, during quiet respiration, it is a narrow triangle seven-eighths of an inch long, with the apex in front, and a somewhat bulging base line at the back. It is the narrowest part of the upper respiratory tract. During forced inspiration the orifice is lozenge-shaped, while during spasm and at the moment preceding the explosive effort of coughing, it is tightly closed. The varying tones of the voice are produced by muscular action altering the position and tension of the vocal cords, while they are vibrating in the air current driven between them from the lungs, the higher the note the closer together and tenser are the cords. Above the true vocal cords are two folds of membrane called the false vocal cords. The modifications of the sounds which constitute speech are brought about by muscular action in the pharynx and mouth in conjunction with the tongue, teeth, and lips. Until the age of puberty there is practically no difference in size between the male and female larynx ; but afterwards the male larynx enlarges considerably. The marked alteration in boys' voices at this period is evidence of the changes taking place. The cartilages of the larynx are covered with muscles and fasciæ, and are lined inside with mucous membrane. All these tissues are continuous with, and form part of, the pharynx. The whole of this region is richly supplied with blood vessels and nerves.

THE WINDPIPE, or Trachea, begins at the under border of the cricoid cartilage and extends downwards for four and a quarter inches, when it divides into the two " bronchi." It is a nearly circular tube about one inch in diameter, lying behind the breast bone, from which it is separated by the great blood-vessels, which also lie at both sides of it. Behind, it lies on the gullet. It is composed of fibrous, muscular, and mucous tissues, in which is embedded a series of from sixteen to twenty hoops of cartilage that pass round the front of the tube, leaving the back flattened and smooth where it rests on the gullet. If the hoops were complete rings they might interfere with the swelling of the gullet during the swallowing act, and consequently hinder the easy descent of the food.

THE BRONCHI pass outwards and downwards to the lungs, the right being wider and shorter than the left. The ridge standing up within the end of the trachea marking the angle of its division into the bronchi is placed rather to the left side, which explains why foreign bodies accidentally drawn into the trachea are oftener found in the right bronchus. The bronchi are composed of elements similar in all respects to those of the trachea. The mucous membrane in the trachea, the bronchi and their subdivisons is covered with ciliated cells. Each cell has one, or more, little

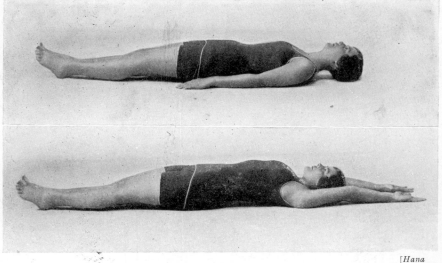

[Hana

AN EXERCISE FOR THE LUNGS

Beginning in the first position, inhale through the nostrils slowly and deeply, expanding the lower part of the chest first, until the arms, with elbows stiff, are brought behind the head, as in second position. Exhale fully through the mouth while returning the arms slowly to the first position.

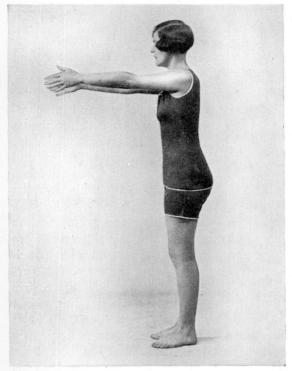
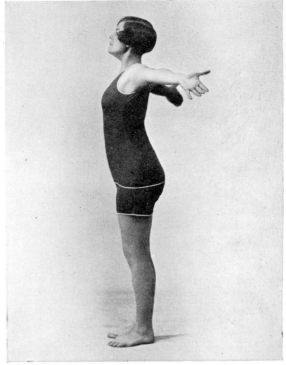

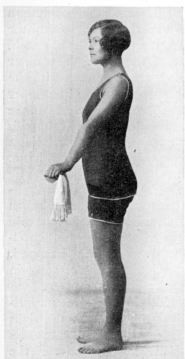
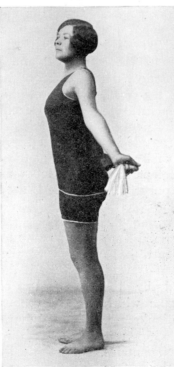
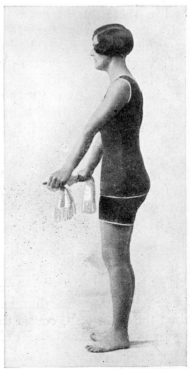

[*Hana*

TWO BREATHING EXERCISES FOR DAILY USE

Above—Stand in first position, inhale through the nostrils slowly and deeply, expanding the chest from below upwards while bringing the arms back to second position; bring arms straight back to first position, exhaling fully through the mouth and letting the chest walls collapse. *Below*—Hold a towel in front of the body; inhale as before, bringing arms upwards and backwards, with elbows stiff, to second position. Exhale slowly, ending in third position. Repeat exercises six times, pausing between each.

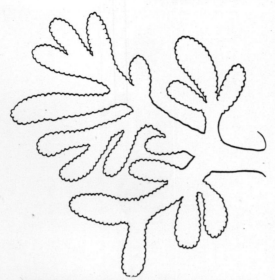

WHERE OXYGEN REACHES THE BLOOD
The smallest divisions of the lung are tiny
air-cells called alveoli. In these the air comes
into contact with the blood in the surrounding
capillaries.

reed-like projections, which are possessed
of movement. The combined movement
is like that seen in a field of corn over
which a breeze passes. In the lungs the
movement is towards the trachea. The
object of this arrangement is to move
onwards the mucus which is secreted by the
membrane. When the mucus is increased,
as in bronchitis, etc., this movement alone
will not be able to expel it ; but it brushes it
along to the trachea where its presence sets
up coughing, and it is got rid of by that
means. Therefore a cough, although perhaps
distressing, serves a very useful purpose at
times.

The two lungs are placed within the
cavity of the chest and are separated from
The Lungs. each other by the heart, large
blood vessels, windpipe, and gullet.
They are surrounded by the
pleura, a thin, smooth membrane which
lines the chest wall, covers the diaphragm,
and passes back to the root of the lung ; it
covers the sac (pericardium) which contains
the heart and then passes on to the surface
of the lung to which it is intimately adherent,
and dips down into the divisions between
the lungs. From this it will be seen that the
pleura is really a closed bag empty except

for a little lubricating fluid between
surfaces which are everywhere in contact.
It acts in the same manner as the lining of
a joint, and enables the lung to move easily
during its expansion and contraction.

The lungs are of a light spongy texture,
dark grey, or black in colour, and are composed of tissue representing the ultimate
divisions of the bronchi, through which are
interspersed the pulmonary arteries and
veins, the lymphatics, and nerve structures.

The blood vessels and bronchi enter the
lungs together, forming its " root." The
right lung weighs about 156 grammes, the
left 142 grammes. In males, the lungs are
larger and heavier than in females. Each
lung consists of a base, an apex, two surfaces, and three borders. The apex rises
into the root of the neck extending about
one inch above the collar bone. This is
the part of the lung which is most frequently
first affected in pulmonary tuberculosis.
The base, which is hollow and wide, rests
upon the upper surface of the diaphragm
which separates the right lung from the
liver, and the left lung from the stomach,
spleen, and part of the liver. The outer
surfaces of the lungs are in contact with the
inside of the chest wall, while the inner
surfaces enclose a space which contains the
heart and great vessels. The left lung is
divided into two lobes, an upper and a
lower ; the right lung into three lobes.
The lobes are made up of lobules. The
lobule is the final termination of the bronchus, which is expanded into a little bunch
of air cells called alveoli. These have a thin
cellular wall around which the finest capillaries of the blood-vessels are wrapped.
Here it is that the interchange of gases in
the process of respiration takes place.

The venous blood, charged with impurities, is pumped into the lungs by the right
ventricle through the pulmonary arteries
whose final sub-divisions constitute the
capillaries, which are also the commencement of the pulmonary veins. These latter
conduct the purified blood back to the left
auricle of the heart. The process of respiration is dependent upon natural phenomena.

If gases of different densities be admitted into a common chamber they will become intimately mixed in time if no chemical action takes place between them. This is known as diffusion. The air taken into the lungs by the inspiratory act contains more oxygen and less carbonic acid gas than the air already in the lungs. The venous blood contains an excess of carbonic acid gas. When this venous blood is exposed in the capillaries to the fresher air which has been inspired, and which contains carbonic acid gas at a less tension than it is held in the blood, the blood parts with its gas, that is to say, the gas escapes from the blood through the walls of the capillaries into the air in the alveoli. Oxygen is absorbed from the air in the alveoli into the blood through the capillary walls. The absorption of oxygen is dependent upon a peculiar property of a substance (hæmoglobin) contained in the red blood-cells. It is by means of these oxygen-charged cells that the vital gas is brought to the various tissues of the body, there to be given up in exchange for carbonic acid gas which represents one of the products of combustion, in other words, of the vital processes that have taken place in the body.

DISEASES OF THE RESPIRATORY SYSTEM

By J. H. CUTHBERT, M.B., Ch.B., D.P.M., Medical Superintendent, West Ham Mental Hospital.

THE whole respiratory system is prone to diseases which include some of the commonest, some of the most trivial, and some of the most serious which afflict mankind. Many may be attributed to our faulty habits of life—social and personal.

ACUTE CORYZA, "CATARRH," OR "COLD IN THE HEAD" is often epidemic and is of microbic origin. In some cases there is a hereditary predisposition. Exciting causes are exposure to cold, wet feet, "stuffy" atmospheres, and irritating vapours.

The Common Cold.

The delicate lining of the nasal passages becomes engorged and swollen while the secretory glands which at first cease to

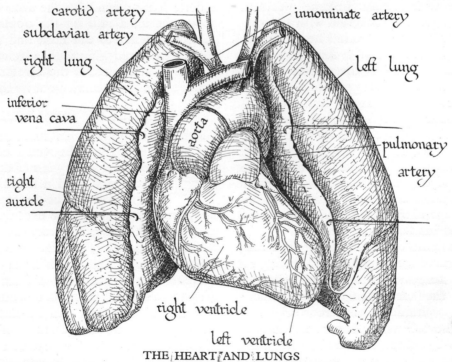

carotid artery
subclavian artery
right lung
inferior vena cava
right auricle
innominate artery
left lung
aorta
pulmonary artery
right ventricle
left ventricle

THE HEART AND LUNGS
Showing the intimate connection between the lungs which purify the blood and the pump which keeps it in motion.

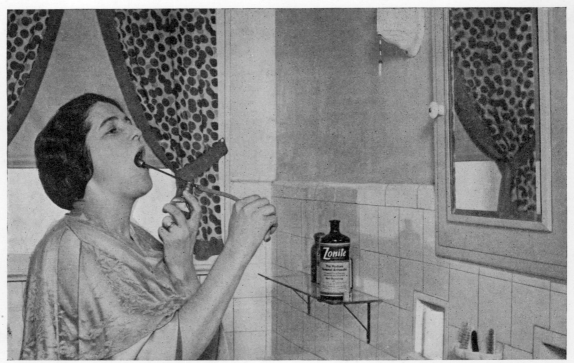

[Topical

A PRECAUTION AGAINST COLDS
Spraying the throat and mouth with an antiseptic to destroy cold germs.

secrete, later manufacture a copious clear discharge which may become purulent. These changes are associated with sneezing, loss of sense of smell, frontal headache and slight fever which last a few days. The catarrh may spread to the middle ear and produce deafness and suppuration or extend downwards to the larynx and bronchial tubes, producing laryngitis and bronchitis.

The tendency to coryza may be largely averted by keeping up the general health and by the use of vaccines. In acute cases an attempt may be made to cut short the attack by a hot bath, bed, a hot drink, and a Dover's powder, together with local nasal sprays and inhalations.

The symptom of nose-bleeding (epistaxis) may be due to local conditions affecting the

Nose Bleeding. nose such as adenoids, polypi, or the ulcerations of tuberculous, syphilitic or cancerous origin. It may, however, arise from constitutional causes as in chronic heart, kidney, and blood diseases. In certain individuals there is a hereditary tendency to epistaxis. In most cases the situation is met by the sufferer lying down with the arms extended above the head and by the application of cold compresses to the neck and nose. In severer cases plugging with adrenalin (1 in a 1000) usually arrests the bleeding. This minor operation is carried out by the doctor.

DISEASES OF THE LARYNX

Acute Laryngitis is an inflammation of the larynx involving the vocal cords and resulting in dryness of the throat,
Acute Laryngitis. hoarseness, and a tickling cough. It is usually due to exposure to cold, irritating vapours or excessive use of the voice. Usually, recovery takes place, but there is a risk of œdema or swelling of the vocal cords, and death from asphyxia. Absolute rest of the voice is essential, and the patient should remain in one atmosphere —in bed if necessary. An inhalation consisting of menthol and tincture of benzoin is often soothing and efficacious. A teaspoonful of the mixture is added to a jug of steaming water and the vapour is

452

inspired. Cough sedatives and medicines to stimulate the excretory organs should be given, and a wet compress applied locally.

Chronic inflammation of the larynx may be due to excessive use of the voice or to excess in alcohol and tobacco. If **Chronic Laryngitis.** the condition does not respond to ordinary remedies the possibility of tuberculous, syphilitic, or malignant disease, warrants a complete examination by the physician.

DISEASES OF THE BRONCHIAL TUBES

Acute Bronchitis is a catarrhal inflammation of the bronchial tubes and is usually **Acute Bronchitis.** the result of cold and damp or irritating vapours. It also occurs in association with measles, whooping cough, and influenza. There is always a risk of an extension of the inflammation to the lung substance with the production of a broncho-pneumonia. It is a dangerous condition in infancy and old age. Should the individual return to his work too soon he may suffer from repeated attacks each winter until the condition becomes a chronic bronchitis.

The onset is usually gradual and is associated with a feeling of tightness of the chest, " rawness " behind the breast-bone, and slight fever. At first there is a frequent, dry, hard cough and scanty viscid expectoration—occasionally blood-stained. In a few days the expectoration becomes copious, watery, and easily coughed up.

The patient should be kept in bed in an atmosphere of uniform temperature and put on a light diet of milk and milk foods until the temperature is normal. Considerable relief may be obtained from inhalations, the application of linseed or mustard poultices, and the administration of cough medicines such as ipecacuanha wine. Later, stimulant cough mixtures and iron tonics may be given.

This condition is predisposed to by such diseases as chronic rheumatism, Bright's disease, heart disease, and chronic **Chronic Bronchitis.** alcoholism. The exciting causes are frequently cold and exposure. The coats of the tubes become thinned and less muscular and dilate under the strain of the constant coughing. Portions of the tubes

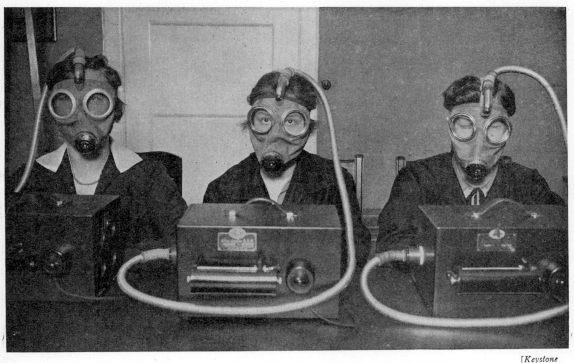

[*Keystone*

A MODERN METHOD OF TREATMENT FOR ASTHMA
Masks and inhaling apparatus which are being used in Germany to relieve asthmatic attacks.

may bulge and produce the condition called "bronchiectasis" with stagnations of the secretions, or actual areas of the lung tissue may become permanently distended and ineffective for purposes of aeration—this latter condition being called "emphysema." The right side of the heart may become dilated owing to the constant cough and the efforts made to drive the blood through the emphysematous area.

The typical cases occur in old people who, in winter, suffer from persistent cough with copious frothy expectoration but no fever. They show marked shortness of breath ; often the chest becomes "barrel-shaped," and evidence of cardiac failure manifests itself. During the more acute phases the treatment is similar to that for acute bronchitis, but of the greatest importance is the question of climate—warm and dry resorts being necessary.

Asthma is characterised by recurrent paroxysmal attacks of severe dyspnœa (difficulty in breathing), the inspiration
Asthma.   being short and the expiration prolonged and wheezing. These attacks are produced by a spasm of the smaller bronchial tubes in which there is usually an associated catarrhal condition. Recently asthma has come to be regarded by many as a manifestation of anaphylaxis—a train of symptoms produced through the reaction of the body to a foreign protein. This protein may have its origin in the food or in some area of infection on the body.

The attacks frequently occur at night, and are commonly associated with chronic bronchitis. The patient remains quite well between the paroxysms. A neurotic herity is an important predisposing factor while exciting causes are to be found in dust and irritating particles, pollen, nasal conditions such as polypi, adenoids, and dietetic errors. During the attacks various remedies may be tried such as tincture of lobelia, hyoscyamus, or burning stramonium or nitre paper. An injection of five drops of adrenalin (1-1000) may arrest an attack or the nose may be sprayed with the solution. All exciting causes must be removed, and the diet should be restricted—no heavy meals being taken at bedtime.

DISEASES OF THE PLEURÆ AND LUNGS

Pleurisy may be of two varieties : (1) Dry pleurisy, where the two layers of the pleura
Pleurisy. are in contact and are inflamed and roughened ; (2) Pleurisy with effusion, where the surfaces are separated by a watery fluid or actual pus—the latter condition being called "empyema." Dry pleurisy is usually due to a chill, or may be of rheumatic origin. It is the "robust" type. Where there is effusion—the "unhealthy" type—the condition is usually of a tubercular nature. Pleurisy may also be secondary to such conditions as pneumonia, abscess of the lung or phthisis.

Sharp stabbing pains on one side, increased on deep inspiration, and associated with moderate fever and slight cough are suggestive of the dry type. If there is effusion the pain is a less marked feature, but the difficulty in breathing becomes more evident. If the effusion is on the left side the heart is often displaced, thus increasing the dyspnœa or breathlessness.

In the early stages strapping the affected side or the application of a linseed poultice will afford relief. Painting with tincture of iodine is often beneficial. The diet should be restricted and measures to stimulate the bowels adopted. Anti-rheumatic and cough remedies should be used. When effusion is present, if this does not respond in two or three weeks to medicinal treatment, tapping the chest may be resorted to by the physician. Whenever pus is suspected (empyema), as indicated by the "swinging" temperature and drenching sweats, tapping becomes imperative ; the surgeon may be consulted with a view to rib resection and drainage.

Chronic pleurisy with marked thickening of the pleural layers is usually associated with chronic phthisis.

Hæmorrhage into the pleural sac may
Hæmo-thorax. result from penetrating wounds or a fractured rib. More rarely it occurs in blood-diseases, pulmonary

tuberculosis, or from a ruptured aneurism.

Air or gas in the pleural cavity is usually associated with fluid and this is often purulent. The condition may arise **Pneumothorax.** from wounds of the chest, fractured ribs, or by the ulceration into the sac of cancerous growths from the œsophagus or stomach. In other cases the pneumothorax arises from the rupture of a tuberculous cavity into the sac or from a lung abscess. The complication is indicated by sudden severe pain in the chest with increasing difficulty in respiration, lividity, and a feeble, rapid pulse. The treatment is mainly surgical.

Broncho-pneumonia is an inflammation of the terminal bronchial tubes and their air cells. More or less circum- **Broncho-Pneumonia.** scribed areas throughout the lung are involved. The process may subside or lead to suppuration or gangrene in patches. Usually many varieties of germs are present. It may be a primary disease, but it is more often secondary to bronchitis, influenza, or one of the fevers, especially measles or whooping cough. It is frequently fatal in early childhood and old age.

The disease usually commences with a rigor or shivering fit, and, in children, frequently with convulsions. The temperature rises to 104-5° F., and difficulty in respiration is marked. The patient becomes livid and critically ill. The pulse and respiration rates are markedly increased. The temperature may " swing " for three or four weeks ; as recovery sets in it drops in a gradual manner. Measles, whooping cough, and bronchitis may resemble an early case of broncho-pneumonia, but the rash, " whoop," and comparatively mild constitutional symptoms help to distinguish these from the more serious condition.

Great care should be taken to prevent broncho-pneumonia ensuing in such infective fevers as measles and whooping cough. At the earliest stage of the disease the child should be placed in a steam-tent and small doses of brandy given at frequent intervals. Poultices or liniments may be applied and

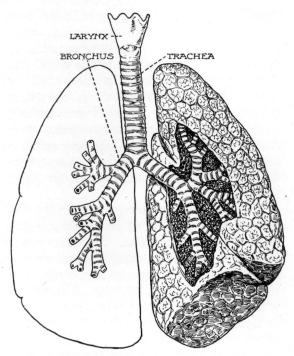

THE BREATHING APPARATUS
Diagram of a normal lung, showing the bronchial tubes and the spongy substance composed of tiny air-cells.

expectorants given to prevent the tubes from being filled up by mucus. An occasional emetic may also be advantageously given with this end in view. To reduce the temperature cold sponging may be necessary. The diet should consist largely of milk and eggs and should be given at short intervals. Every effort should be made to procure sleep by efficient nursing.

Acute lobar pneumonia is now recognised as an infectious disease, and one due to a **Acute Lobar Pneumonia.** specific micro-organism which can be obtained from the sputum, blood, and organs affected. An acute inflammation of the lung tissue results from the infection. The inflammation more frequently commences at the base of the lung and extends upwards to affect a whole lobe or even the whole lung. The other lung may also become involved, or a general blood-poisoning may occur with widespread infection of other organs. The part of the lung affected becomes more or less solid owing to the air-cells being crammed with inflammatory material and respiration thus becomes greatly impeded. The partly solidified area may become gradually looser, partly by the absorption of the inflammatory material by the protective mechanism of the blood and partly by expectoration. In other cases the area becomes dissolved and an abscess or gangrene may result. The disease does not always select the debilitated subject ; quite frequently the robust and healthy adult is attacked. Sometimes it occurs as a secondary and terminal complication to other maladies.

The disease commences suddenly, frequently with a rigor or convulsions, headache, and general malaise. The temperature rises rapidly to 104°F. or higher, and remains high until the seventh to the tenth day, when it falls suddenly by crisis. The patient wears an anxious expression with flushed face, and often a vesicular skin eruption round the lips is present. The skin is dry, the tongue furred, and vomiting may be an early indication of the onset owing to irritation of the nerve which supplies both the lung and the stomach. Pain in the side, a short painful cough at first dry but later attended with a " rusty " coloured sputum, and a pulse-respiration ratio of 2 : 1 instead of the normal 4 : 1 are all significant features of pneumonia. High fever and delirium are danger signs calling for urgent treatment. A pleurisy with effusion may complicate pneumonia, or symptoms may arise from infection of the coverings of the brain, producing a meningitis. Sometimes the joints, the lining of the abdomen, or the heart valves may become infected, and result in an arthritis, peritonitis, or endocarditis.

In the treatment of pneumonia nursing plays an extremely important part. Everything should be done to anticipate the patient's wants, to reserve his strength, and to promote sleep. A fatal termination results usually from cardiac failure. The patient should be clad in a light, loose, armless " pneumonia-jacket " fastened by straps over the shoulders. Light blankets and bed-coverings should be used before the temperature drops, and plenty of fresh air is of great importance. The diet should be fluid at first, and consist of milk, barley-water and broths given frequently along with copious drinks of water. The mouth should be attended to before and after each feed, and the bowels regulated. Should the pain be very prominent local application of ice or a poultice may be resorted to. The high temperature may be a reason for sleeplessness, and should be met by tepid sponging. The insomnia may call for the use of the milder hypnotics such as paraldehyde. Should pain or cough be factors in the sleeplessness, sedative cough mixtures are useful and also aid in the expectoration of inflammatory material. It is important to guard against cardiac failure by giving stimulants such as digitalis or ammonia. When the crisis is due the patient must be watched for sweating. Blankets should be put on ; hot bottles applied to the feet, and hot drinks given. When the sweating ceases the patient should be rubbed down with a hot towel and a warm shirt put on. Oxygen inhalations may be necessary to aid the respiratory difficulty. During convalescence, tonics and respiratory exercises are beneficial.

Pulmonary tuberculosis (phthisis : consumption) is due to a definite micro-organism—the tubercle bacillus. Consumption. The germ usually enters the body by being inhaled, or it may be swallowed in infected meat or milk. If not destroyed by the blood it sets up a process of inflammation and ulceration which may lead to destruction of the lung tissue with cavity formation or severe hæmorrhage. The most frequently affected part of the lung is near its upper end or apex, and this may be due to the normal deficient expansion of this portion of the lung. If the process is not an acute one the infected area heals up and leaves behind a scarred site. This is frequently seen in post-mortem, where the subject has died from some other disease. In some cases the infection is a rapidly advancing one with acute onset, widespread involvement of the lung resembling pneumonia, and a rapidly fatal termination. This type is the so-called " galloping consumption."

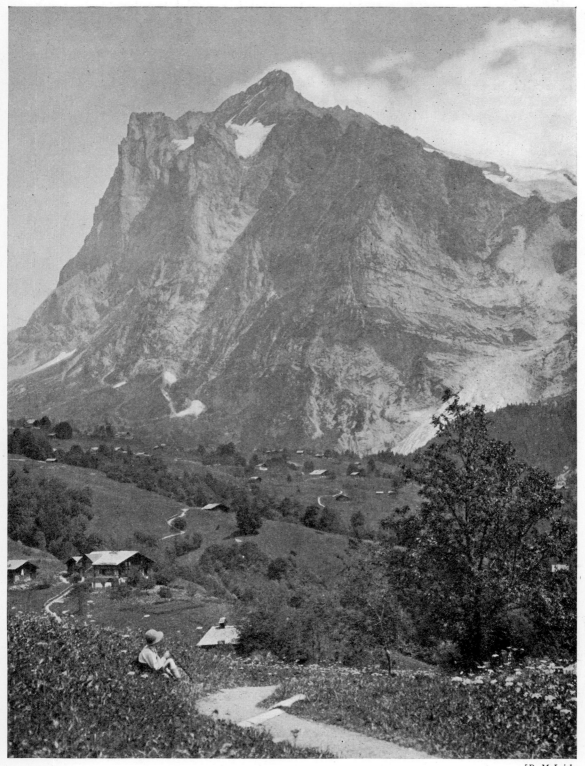

[D. McLeish

THE GRINDELWALD VALLEY, SWITZERLAND
A sunny, sheltered, and mist-free resort where sufferers from respiratory diseases benefit from the pure mountain air.

The disease may occur at any age, but is commonest between the ages of 25-45. Hereditary predisposition is important but is a question of resistive powers in the individual and not a di ect transmission of infection from the pa ents. The habits of the subject as regards excesses and his occupation are also factors. The inhalation of dust, exposure, exhaustion, and malnutrition all help to prepare the ground for the activities of the tubercule bacillus. Bad hygienic conditions as regards climate, damp, overcrowding, and absence of sunlight also play their part, and pulmonary tuberculosis may supervene in the course of many debilitating diseases. A marked characteristic of the germ is its resistance to a dry environment, and the dried sputum of a phthisical patient is a fruitful source of infection to non-sufferers. On the other hand it is more easily killed by direct sunshine than most germs, and on this fact is based most on our prevention and modern treatment of tuberculous conditions.

The disease usually begins insidiously and frequently runs a protracted course. The patient may have felt " run-down " with increasing languor for six months or so, and is often somewhat anæmic or suffers from dyspepsia. There may be a persistent slight cough and gradual loss of weight. As the disease advances the " hacking " cough becomes looser and the sputum becomes thick and purulent ; night sweats are then a marked feature, and the temperature is of the hectic type, i.e., with an evening rise to 101-2° and a morning fall. In the later stages the tendency to hæmorrhage (hæmoptysis) becomes greater—although this may occur at any time. Towards the end diarrhœa may set in from infection of the intestines. The larynx may also become the seat of a tuberculous laryngitis which adds a very distressing complication. Pleurisy, pneumothorax, tuberculous glands, and tuberculous skin are all possible concomitants.

It cannot be too strongly emphasised that this is a disease in which prevention should obviate the necessity for cure. Continuous effort is essential to educate the public to the hygienic procedures which must be understood and applied if this deadly disease is to be combated with a reasonable hope of success. Much has been done by dispensaries in detecting early cases.

As regards actual treatment, if there is fever the patient should be at rest in bed, and he should be placed in the best possible hygienic conditions. This usually means a sanatorium. He will there be under continuous medical supervision and have plenty of fresh pure air and suitable food, both as to quantity and quality. He will there also obtain the requisite rest and have his exercise regulated. Wherever treated, he should live in the open air—in a hut, shelter, or a verandah protected from the worst weather. Feeding is of great importance. The diet should be as liberal as the digestion of the patient permits, and the weight should be recorded regularly. Cod-liver oil alone or combined with malt or an antiseptic such as creosote or guaiacol is usually given. Inhalations of the latter drugs, sometimes with parolein, are of local value.

The complications must receive attention as they arise—hæmorrhage by the application of an ice-bag and injection of morphia ; sweating by atropine ; diarrhœa by bismuth or morphia, and the cough by such mixtures as Brompton's, which contains morphia, hydrocyanic acid with syrup of tolu, and acid infusion of roses. When improvement sets in, increasing exercise and graduated respiratory gymnastics may be carried out. In some cases benefit may be obtained from " tuberculin " injections. This treatment depends on the principle of immunisation. There are various preparations of tuberculin on the market, but the treatment can only be carried out by those who are expert at controlling the dosage of such vaccines. In suitable cases a change to Switzerland, the Riviera, or Egypt may be very beneficial, but sea voyages may do much harm if the sufferer is not strong enough. High altitudes should be avoided if there is a tendency to hæmorrhage.

Fibroid phthisis is most commonly caused

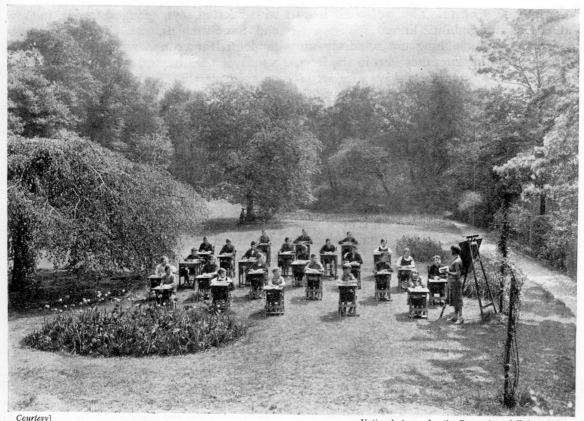

Courtesy]   National Assoc. for the Prevention of Tuberculosis

AN OPEN-AIR CLASS FOR TUBERCULOUS CHILDREN
At the Day Sanatorium, where an open-air life helps to restore diseased lungs to health.

by a pulmonary tuberculosis which runs a chronic course, leading to much scarring and contraction of the lung. It tends to occur in older people. The patient complains of chronic cough, increasing emaciation and shortness of breath. High temperature may be absent. There may be copious purulent expectoration owing to bronchiectasis, and the various symptoms of pulmonary tuberculosis may manifest themselves at some time during the course of the illness. Treatment is largely a matter of relieving the symptoms.

Pneumono-coniosis. Pneumonoconiosis* is the term given to a group of diseases of the lung which arise from the inhalation of irritating particles resulting in coal-miners' lung (anthracosis), stone-mason's lung (silicosis), and steel-grinder's lung (siderosis). The disease produces a fibroid thickening of areas in the lung, the severity of the condition varying with the type of dust inhaled and the duration of exposure to the irritating agent. In some cases there may be inflammation, ulceration, and cavity formation in addition to the fibrous thickening, and the subject is liable to develop pulmonary tuberculosis. Gradual loss of health with persistent cough and expectoration of perhaps black purulent sputum indicate the condition. Treatment is carried out on the lines of that for chronic bronchitis or pulmonary tuberculosis. The adoption of hygienic industrial conditions and preventive measures in factories has lessened the incidence of this disease.

Syphilis of the Lung. Syphilitic disease of the lung is not common. It may occur in congenital cases of syphilis, but the infant does not usually survive. In the third stage of syphilis areas may become involved which may lead to tissue destruction, or a more generalised thickening throughout

* See section on Industrial Diseases.

the lung may occur. The treatment is on the usual anti-syphilitic lines.

Tumours of the lung are relatively uncommon. Sometimes they start in the lung, **Tumours of the Lung.** but frequently they arise secondarily to a growth (cancer) in the breast, stomach, or other organs. Difficulty of breathing, pain, cough, and sometimes hæmorrhage are present. The sputum is described as " prunejuice-like." There is often a pleurisy with effusion. Should this latter condition exist in a patient after middle life, with failure to improve after repeated tappings, and if it is associated with anæmia and emaciation, tumour should be suspected.

Abscess of the lung occurs in such conditions as broncho-pneumonia, lobar-pneumonia, pulmonary tuberculosis **Abscess of the Lung.** and tumours when the organisms of ordinary suppuration are superadded. It may also occur in the course of a general blood-poisoning. The patient becomes more acutely ill with fœtid breath, putrid expectoration and swinging temperature. The treatment is mainly surgical.

Gangrene of the lung may arise from similar conditions to those which lead to abscess, and the symptoms mani- **Gangrene of the Lung.** fested are similar though much more severe. The treatment is directed to maintaining the patient's general condition by stimulants. Antiseptics may be administered or surgical advice sought if the patient's strength warrants it.

THE PREVENTION OF THE COMMON COLD

By *NATHAN MUTCH, M.A., M.D., F.R.C.P., Physician to Guy's Hospital ; Consulting Physician to St. Paul's Hospital ; Lecturer and Examiner in Pharmacology to the University of London ; Examiner in Therapeutics to the University of Cambridge.*

THE common cold is produced by microbes which invade the mucous membranes of the nose and throat of a susceptible person. Spread takes place by coming in contact with infected toys, sponges, towels, pillows, and handkerchiefs, etc. The air is contaminated for a considerable distance around a sufferer who sneezes, coughs, expectorates, or even merely speaks. Germs are passed directly from one victim to the next. Infection is above all from mouth and nose to mouth and nose. Hence when colds are prevalent it is wise to avoid speaking into the mouths and noses of other people—and to hinder them speaking into yours. After all, the ear is the organ of hearing. The sufferer from a cold should realise that he is a serious menace to his fellow-creatures. He should isolate himself as far as possible, and should always sneeze or cough into a handkerchief.

The common cold can be prevented by avoiding the microbes. If circumstances render this impossible then two courses of prevention remain open : firstly—destruction of the microbes ; secondly, raising personal resistance against infection.

Warmth and moisture prolong the life of micro-organisms floating in the air. Therefore the living rooms should be kept cool, dry, and well ventilated. At night the bedroom windows should be wide open, but the bed should be so arranged that a draught does not blow directly on the head and neck. Sunlight kills microbes and also raises our resistance against them, but their health-preserving qualities are lost if the sunlight passes through ordinary glass. Hence let the sunlight stream into the rooms freely through widely-opened windows if colds are to be avoided.

A " responsive " skin is a valuable safeguard against chills, and this responsiveness can be fostered by accustoming the skin to cool air and water as by bathing, cold sponging, cold showers, outdoor exercises in light clothing, and by avoiding scarves, neck wraps, and heavy overcoats. At the same time it is imperative never to rest in a cold place or a draught on coming from a hot room or after severe exercise.

Diet is of considerable importance. Indigestion and constipation seriously weaken the natural resistance of the body and leave it an easy prey to infection. Excess of meat and sugar are to be avoided, but wholemeal bread, raw fruit, raw salads, green vegetables, rye bread, and fresh butter are to be the main constituents of the diet and are to be taken freely.

Finally, breathing through the nose is imperative. "Unless you have something to say or to swallow, the mouth should be shut" is sound advice and cannot be too often emphasised when colds are epidemic. It must be remembered that nose-breathing is the correct or physiological method, and in order that this may be carried out to greatest advantage it is obviously necessary that both

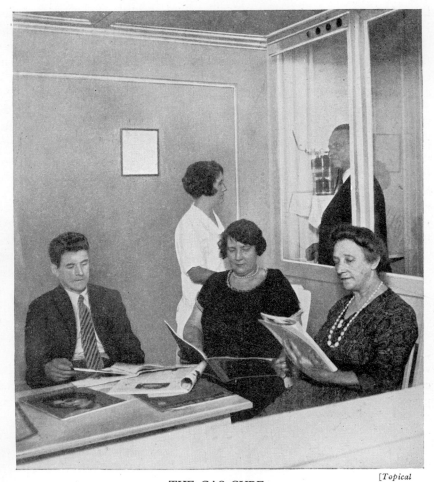

THE GAS CURE

[*Topical*

Patients undergoing treatment in a chlorine gas chamber—a new method for curing colds and other respiratory diseases.

nostrils should be absolutely clear. If this state of affairs does not exist, then consultation with a doctor is indicated. A few simple nose-breathing exercises carried out each morning are invaluable preventive measures. On these occasions it is best to breathe in energetically, making a definite sniffing noise and filling the chest to the utmost capacity and to breathe out slowly and quietly.

Chronic catarrh and colds which recur with great persistency afflict persons who have some defect or ailment in the nose or throat, or in whom some underlying cause of continued low resistance is at work. In such cases, the skill and advice of a medical practioner are required.

The means to prevent the common cold may be summarised thus :—

Avoidance of the microbes.

Destruction of the microbes.

Raising personal resistance against the microbes.

Nose-breathing only.

Above all, let the infected always give due consideration to the non-infected.

CARE OF THE TONSILS AND ADENOIDS

By Sir W. ARBUTHNOT LANE, Bart., C.B., M.S., F.R.C.S.

MANY parents have accepted the frequency of operations for the removal of the enlarged tonsils and adenoids of their progeny as natural events in the course of their young life. Nothing can be more fallacious. The infections of these masses of lymphatic structure represent a lowered vitality on the part of the child and consequently of every tissue in the body. The condition is absolutely unknown amongst natives leading normal lives in their natural surroundings, but it occurs with an appalling frequency among the ill-nourished children of the community whose diet and habits have ceased to resemble the natural habits of the native, and whose vitality has depreciated in a corresponding degree.

Nothing can be more detrimental to the health of the child than the food which is too frequently supplied to it at its home, at its preparatory school, and still more so at the public school, where the diet and sanitation are often deplorably insufficient and incorrect.

Diet in Schools.

Surely the time has arisen when the authorities of some recently established school will have the courage to publish broadcast a correct diet, a sufficient sanitation, and a proper and independent control by medical officers. Numbers of parents would gladly send their sons to such an establishment, and the amount of infection of the throat and ears of the pupils would diminish in a most marked manner.

That regular medical supervision can effect marvels in the prevention of disease of all sorts, even in adult life, is shown by the wonderful success which has resulted from the action of many of the American insurance companies. This is so palpable that some of our insurance associations are following the example set by them, to their great financial advantage. The statistics of the American offices showed that by submitting their clients to regular and systematic examination by expert medical officers, they were able to make more money for their shareholders, to cover the cost of the medical men employed, and also to reduce materially the premiums of those insured with them.

Let us benefit by this experience and see that our children shall be examined periodically by medical men during their life in their homes, in their preparatory schools, and especially in their public schools. It is obvious that if health can be preserved and disease prevented among those adults who insure their lives, an infinitely better result can be secured by looking after the growing youth of the country during a period of their lives when they are developing, and when they can be moulded so that they may become either healthy citizens or permanent invalids.

One cannot too strongly urge on the community that *ill health, disease, and premature death are criminal,* and that those on whom the chief responsibility rests, are the parents, the nurses, the preparatory school masters, and later the authorities in charge of the public schools. If further evidence is desired as to the immense influence which a proper diet can exert upon the health of the individual, it is only necessary to point again to the wonderful work done by Dr. Hindhede in Denmark. He, in one year, besides staving off disaster, starvation, and famine, reduced the mortality of the people of that country to the lowest figure ever published, and, at the same time, improved their resisting power to infections of all sorts in a phenomenal manner. Too much importance cannot be attached to the work that this great man effected so quickly, and in such an extraordinary, simple manner. Yet we still read of statements by interested people advocating the use of white bread and white flour.

It is not merely such cases as require operation for the removal of adenoids and enlarged tonsils, and the frequently associated infections of the ears, but a very much larger number exist in whom the condition is not sufficiently severe or acute to call for operative interference, but which suffer both mechanically and physiologically from the permanent obstruction which results from it. The projecting incisor teeth, the open mouth, the cramped jaws, the hollowed cheeks, the pinched nostrils and the poorly developed chest, are all evidences of neglect early in life, and are all avoidable by proper care and attention.

Let parents realise the great part that the medical profession can play in preventing

Parents' Responsibilities. so much of the degeneration which is consequent on their own ignorance, carelessness and neglect of parents and teachers, and how much it can help them by care and attention to avoid the dreadfully frequent incidence of what are called the minor ailments of young life. While apparently regarded as trivial at the time, they leave results that too often cause the unfortunate individual to possess an enfeebled physique and a limited capacity to perform his share of the duties and to enjoy the pleasures of life. It would appear that the whole arrangement of the diet and habits of our schools wants to be thoroughly overhauled and that the public should be informed of how these changes are being carried into practice. This must all be done openly and in the light of day.

THE CARE OF THE LUNGS

By Sir BRUCE BRUCE-PORTER, K.B.E., C.M.G., M.D., M.R.C.S., L.R.C.P.

PUBLIC Health statistics reveal that on an average half a million of the population die annually as a result of affections of the respiratory organs. Consumption (pulmonary tuberculosis) accounts for a large proportion of these deaths, as also pneumonia which so often forms the terminal phase of other diseases.

Tuberculosis is a highly preventable disease, though it is so widespread that it is quite impossible to avoid risk of picking up the tubercle bacilli. In fact, it seems probable that every child goes through an invasion of tubercle during its early years. Most children escape actual disease but many succumb, and it should be realised that, once tuberculosis has been allowed to obtain a hold in the chest, there are no drugs which of themselves can bring about a cure. The method of combating this terrible scourge is, first and foremost, by a general raising of the health of the body as a whole. The Hippocratic saying that " the body has in it the nature to cure," is as applicable to tuberculosis as to any other disease.

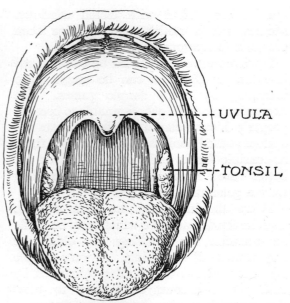

THE POSITION OF THE TONSILS
View inside the mouth with normal tonsils—these, when diseased, may become much enlarged.

A good chest expansion and a good blood supply defy tubercle. To attain these is the object of the hygiene of the respiratory system.

Frequent interchange of air is necessary. The normal rate of breathing is about seventeen times to the minute, and during the same short time the heart beats about seventy-two times. At each beat in the adult it pumps about two ounces of impure blood into the lungs and extracts the same quantity of purified blood. It is obvious that unless the air is changed thoroughly the blood on its way can neither get rid of all its waste material nor collect enough oxygen for the requirements of the body. The act of breathing is an aid to circulation, as can be seen by the way in which the rate quickens on exertion.

In man's natural condition he had fresh air and few clothes to hamper his breathing. The exertion necessary to collect his food caused full movement of the lungs. To-day the picture has changed. Civilisation has increased the wants of the people and industry has resulted in large collections of human beings in confined areas. Most of the working hours are spent in closed rooms, the leisure hours largely in crowded places of amusement, and the sleeping hours in

463

THE GOLDEN HEALTH LIBRARY

small rooms, often with closed windows. Modern men's clothing might have been designed to hamper chest movement.

Hygienic measures should be commenced in infancy. Children can be taught deep breathing by many simple games. The expression of a child who is unable to breathe properly is very characteristic ; the stupid, open-mouthed look is a reproach to those responsible for its early care. Children are better cared for in this respect than they were a generation ago.

There should always be some definite exercise for the purpose which may be made an occasion for teaching the child the importance of breathing. A very simple game is to have two bottles connected by tubing and encourage children to blow the water from one bottle into the other with as few breaths as possible. For this game it is essential that each child has its own glass mouthpiece.

Obstruction of the airway by enlarged tonsils and adenoids is fatal to good breathing, and they must be removed, especially when they have become infected and are thus a source of danger.

Fresh air is of paramount importance. Every effort should be made to ensure a change of air in the rooms occupied whether for rest, work, or play. It is not always an easy matter when the window is on one side only, but, however great the difficulty may be, it must be overcome, as healthy lungs cannot be maintained in a badly overheated room.

Habits of health like those of morality are the results of early training. Teach the child to hold himself or herself correctly and to take some pride in doing so, and we shall start it with a great advantage. We need open-air schools for the fit ; it seems so stupid that we wait till a child breaks down in the ordinary school in a crowded

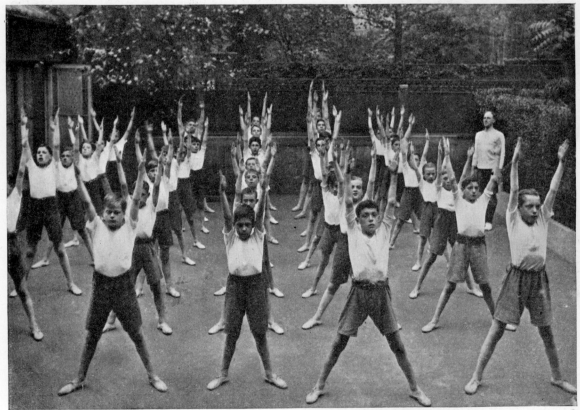

[*Keystone*

VENTILATING THE BODY
Regular breathing exercises in the open air are one of the best preventatives of adenoid trouble.

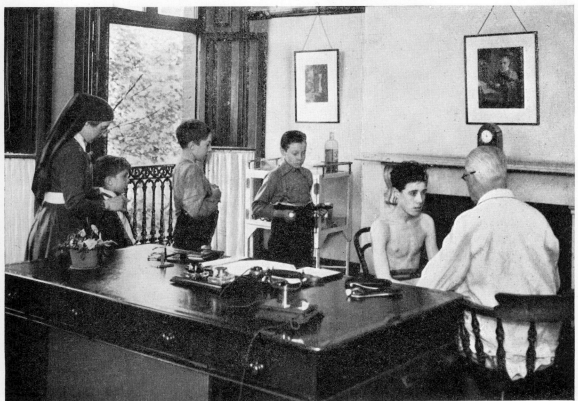

Courtesy]   [*Naticnal Association for the Prevention of Tuberculosis*

A TUBERCULOSIS DISPENSARY
Testing " contacts " with an infected person for the first sign of the disease.

street and then send it to do lessons in the park, instead of sending more fit ones for periods of open-air classes to prevent the breakdown.

The care of the lungs is of vital importance : it repays with a sense of mental and physical fitness. It is advisable to seek medical advice early rather than wait for a breakdown : it is better to have weak tendencies recognised early, even if it means a change of occupation and a readjusting of life.

The doctor of tc-day is in a much better position than his ancestors in the profession. He can use his stethoscope or call in the assistance of X-rays as a means of diagnosis. It is a tragic mistake to allow disease to progress until the tubercle bacilli are found in the sputum as if they were the only evidence of lung disease. Regular examination by the doctor should prevent the disease advancing to this stage unrecognised.

The early signs of weak lungs are loss of energy, loss of appetite, loss of weight, a slight evening rise of temperature, a cough which is more noticeable by the friends than by the sufferer, and later on sweating at night.

For those whose lungs have given way to infection of tubercle, while, in theory, an outdoor life is indicated (patients are often advised to live on a farm or run a chicken farm), the fact must be kept in mind that farm work is not easy, and it is often better to teach a working man a trade, providing his workshop is free of dust and well ventilated.

Early lung trouble is a curable disease in most instances, not by drugs but by hygiene.

THE HYGIENE OF THE BREATHING APPARATUS
By GEORGES ROSENTHAL, M.D. (Paris), D.Sc., ex-Chef de Clinique of the Faculty of Medicine of Paris ; Laureate of the Institute and of the Academy of Medicine.

WHETHER we have to deal with a machine or with an organism, it is the normal working that determines the minimum wear and tear. But while the machine, be it a locomotive engine, the motor of an airship, the mechanism of a watch or of a bicycle, maintains its integrity by the smoothness of its action, the living organism through its regular round of existence and activity becomes, in conformity with natural laws, stronger and more vigorous. This is the law of physical exercise ; it is this law that should serve as a guide to the hygienist in the rules he observes in training.

The first or essential consideration for the specialist of the respiratory tract is to see that the lungs perform their work in accordance with the rigid laws of human physiology ; it is this principle that has guided us in all our researches during the past twenty-five years into respiratory gymnastics.

We must not wander beyond this guiding idea and not overpass the goal we desire to reach. The problem is how, without imitating records difficult of attainment, to adapt oneself to rules that it would be as hurtful to go beyond as to ignore. We shall recur to this point. The conditions of existence in civilised communities due to the aggregation of individuals, the necessary conditions of work and such difficulties as physical failings, result in the respiratory apparatus becoming the prey of feverish ailment recognised, since Pasteur's discoveries, to be of microbic origin. The organism, rendered stronger, thanks to the physiological workings of its organs, should be capable of resisting the invasion of germs. Even if actually invaded, the organism should find its way to recovery and to the attainment of the strength necessary to avoid further attacks.

It should, however, not be overlooked that the human organism constitutes a unity, the various organs of which are so interdependent in their functions and the performance thereof that a diseased organ exercises a deteriorating influence on the rest of the human body. In the same way, what we call our general health, which is (largely) due to the integrity of our muscles, is far from being an indifferent factor in the equilibrium of the breathing apparatus.

(1) On the birth of an infant, a physiological event of the utmost importance *The Process of Breathing.* takes place. While enclosed in the womb, the fœtus is supplied with oxygen by the oxygenated maternal blood ; no sooner is the child born than it begins to breathe. It is the contact of the external air with the skin that, through what is called a bulbar reflex, makes the breathing muscles contract and relax alternately. A nervous message is sent to the bulb (medulla oblongata) situated in the upper part of the spinal cord ; thence a return message is sent to the breathing muscles which are thus stimulated. The rhythmic contraction of these muscles at the rate of about fifteen a minute introduces air into the lungs and thus supplies the oxygen necessary for existence. From the moment of birth, the contact of air with the skin, thanks to the sensibility of the latter, sets up a reflex action, *i.e.*, a nervous message travels to the bulb, where it is reflected along the motor nerves to the muscles whose contraction expands the chest.

The important spot in the bulb that receives and re-transmits the nervous message bears the name of the respiratory " knot of Flourens " (after its discoverer).

Let us then first grasp the fact that the starting point of the respiratory act is the skin surface, the stimulator of the chest movements. It follows that, in a fainting attack, in all threatenings of or actual stoppages of the breathing, we have in the skin a natural and often efficacious resource for inducing a return of the breathing. Be it a case of suspended animation of a child after difficult labour, one of shock in a workman's accident or a fall from a horse, rubbing the skin surface is a useful expedient.

But, *a fortiori*, in the healthy man and especially in the youth, let us not forget the importance of the skin, that member of what may be called the breathing staff. The contact of the air with the skin should be fostered, the neck should be free, the hands ungloved, the sleeves wide, the drawers also wide and not closely stuck to the legs. Daily morning ablutions of the

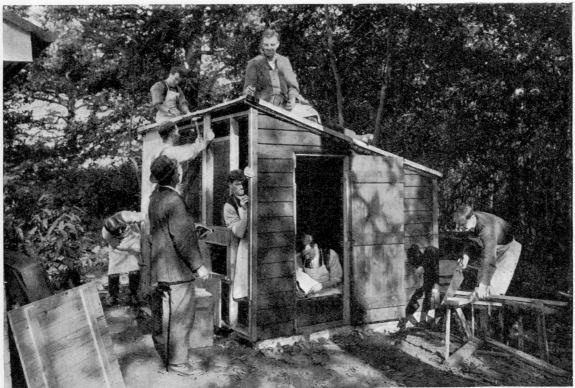

National Assoc. for Prevention of Tuberculosis

THE CARPENTERS AT BURROW HILL, FRIMLEY
A colony for tuberculous patients, where an important part of the curriculum consisted in teaching suitable trades to convalescents.

entire body in cool water, even cold water, if the doctor approves, should be varied by frequent shower-baths. In the foregoing we have a few prescriptions of easy application.

The precious effect of the stimulation of the skin on the respiration enables us to understand the benefits accruing from helio-therapy, that is, the methodically arranged exposure of the cutaneous surface to sun-rays at mountain stations. Sunshine is the best respiratory tonic. Artificial helio-therapy replaces the forces of nature, and, in their absence, acts, though less powerfully, in such a manner that the dosage is more under control.

Dr. Mathias Duval used in bygone days to dwell upon an accident met with in old-fashioned breweries. A superficial extensive burn, the result of a fall into a vat, had the effect of suppressing the reflex working, through the skin, of the respiration. The unfortunate sufferer, compelled to breathe by voluntary effort, soon succumbed to exhaustion : so true is it that the skin is the primordial organ of normal, automatic, and reflex respiration.

(2) Originating in the skin surface, the nervous message travels along the nerves of common sensation to the bulb, where the respiratory " knot of Flourens " deflects it to the chest muscles in co-ordinated and rhythmic waves. The second point in our hygienic activities should be the control of bulbar action. This is, however, a singularly difficult task. The tenacity of asthma is a proof that the application of general prin-ciples does not suffice. Fortunately, the bulb, an essential part of the organism, retains, most frequently, a normal physiological working power.

(3) From the bulb there starts the true respiratory impulse ; it is a synergy or an associated action by means of which the chest muscles raise the ribs while the

diaphragm, in its descent, increases the height of the thoracic cage or cavity. The lung is thus compelled to expand and thus it absorbs the air, taking possession of the oxygen in it ; this is genuine respiration.

Breathing is, then, a synergy, *i.e.*, it is due to an associated muscular action. In order that it should take place, it is consequently necessary that the chest muscles and the diaphragm be healthy ; it is, however, not necessary that these muscles have acquired an athletic development. Compare dancing, swimming, and violin-playing. The dancer, the swimmer, and the violinist require good muscles, more especially educated and trained muscles. The old-fashioned wrestler, endowed with huge masses of muscle, would, in the water, sink like a stone. Thus, for satisfactory breathing, we must know how to make use of normally developed muscles.

(4) Thanks to cutaneous stimulation, to the bulbar reflex, and to the synergetic contraction of the inspiratory muscles of the chest, the lung expands and unfolds to receive the outer air, these being the conditions necessary for the penetration of the air into the lungs.

The breathed air enters by the nostrils, follows the course of the nasal passages, the back of the nose, the aerodigestive space, that is, the place where the naso-laryngeal gangway crosses the mouth and gullet gangway, the voice-box, the windpipe, the bronchial tubes as far as the air-cells of the lungs. No anatomical obstruction should be encountered on this route ; unfortunately, this free passage is not always present. In some cases, the patency of the nostrils is imperfect, the turbinated bones (inside the nostrils) are enlarged, the gristly partition between the two nostrils is deviated ; polypi obstruct and call for treatment. More especially is the obstruction due to adenoid growths. This, with the commonly associated enlargement of the tonsils, is of considerable importance.

Not only do these adenoid vegetations prove in the child a source of inexhaustible infection of the middle ear (causing ear discharges) and of descending bronchitis, but more especially do they constitute an obstacle to the penetration of the breathed air ; this brings about the shrunken chests so favourable to the breaking out of pulmonary consumption.

No hesitation is possible. The inflamed adenoid growth is of no use ; it is hurtful both mechanically and as a source of infection ; it is the cause of the narrow chest with concave walls and prominent shoulders. It should be removed. In the lad, who, though afflicted with this growth, may appear fairly normal—measure the transverse diameter of the chest ; it will be found to be superior to the transverse diameter of the pelvis. In the healthy male child these diameters should be equal or the pelvic diameter should be the greater. Have these growths removed without delay, and, with them, the enlarged tonsils.

For a long time we have all believed that nasal and adenoid obstructions constituted the only mechanical obstacles to healthy breathing. But recently we have become familiar with the trouble caused in respiration by the fall of the base of the tongue into the aerodigestive space. This glossoptosis or mal-placed tongue can be corrected by a dental apparatus, which is well borne by children.

(5) It is also necessary that the air available for breathing purposes be pure. That is a social problem that London has solved by separating the business centres from the inhabited districts ; it is hoped that Paris will follow this example. Rearing children in a dusty atmosphere and amidst the noisome emanations of motor vehicles is an outrage to common sense. The urbanism of the future should remedy this state of things.

(6) It is not sufficient that the air-passages be free and that the air be pure. Even if the healthy and groomed skin make a call on the breathing process, it is necessary to avoid the establishment in the lungs of inert zones (" dead points "), where the germs infesting the air can find a culture ground for their development. For this reason, breathing exercises should be controlled in their three stages.

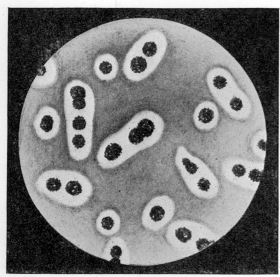

[*James's Press Agency*

A CAUSE OF PNEUMONIA

A microphotograph of Bacilli Pneumococci, one of the types of organisms responsible for pneumonia.

The first step is what my colleagues call the " educative phase of Georges Rosenthal." It consists in giving the growing child, duly rid of his adenoid growths or with his glossoptosis remedied, a series of physiological breathing exercises. These are breathings executed to the word of command given under the direction of the doctor and following a cadenced and normal rhythm in various attitudes or with ordinary movements such as the separation of the arms, for instance. These respirations are exclusively nasal, that is, the air penetrates and is expelled through the nose. This is the only method for obtaining unconscious and automatic breathing—qualities that all organic functions should possess.

This favours the development of the chest in all diameters and corrects the inertia too often shown by the diaphragm. The importance of this inertia was shown in 1904 by the writer in the columns of the *Presse Medicale*. The above-mentioned technique can also be regulated by the will of the breather.

The second step in qualitative training consists of exercises with the aid of the spirometer (spirometers of Dupont Brucker, Blum, or the very practical instrument of Pescher).

The third stage for the subject, now become expert in the art of breathing, brings this knowledge into operation in sports. We give the preference to sports conducted in the open air, as these favour the development of good muscles, good lungs, and a healthily-acting heart. Such are, for men, bicycling, football, races in the open air ; for the young woman, lawn tennis ; for all, swimming.

(7) The lung tissue does not escape the results of wear and tear. If the liver and the kidney become hard and fibrous, the lung, on its part, may find its elastic tissue becoming altered, thinned, and even ruptured. The rupture of the elastic tissue spells emphysema, either diffuse or localised.

However careful one has been to superintend, maintain, or re-establish the normal play of the breathing apparatus, one must reckon with negligence, impossibility and wavering, as well as with unknown factors that bring disease in their train.

The majority of diseases of the respiratory tract are due to infections, the most serious of these being pulmonary tuberculosis (consumption), of which the responsible germ is Koch's bacillus. Therapeutic hopes have been awakened in

Prevention and Cure.

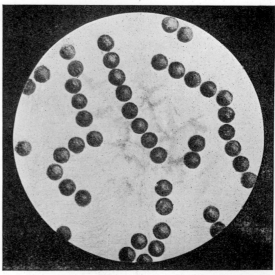

[*James's Press Agency*

A CAUSE OF INFLAMMATORY DISEASES

A microphotograph of Streptococci. These germs occur in strings and may produce severe inflammation.

PONS

MEDULLA
OBLONGATA

SPINAL
CORD

**HOW THE SKIN
CONTROLS
BREATHING**
Showing the con-
nection of the
medulla oblongata
with the spinal
cord.

recent years by the induce-
ment of artificial pneumothorax, that is, the admission
of air or nitrogen into the
pleural cavity ; and vac-
cination at birth with the
bacillus of Calmette and
Guérin.

Two factors above all
propagate this terrible disease : contagion through
the dried expectoration of
the patient, and the weakening of the powers of
resistance by overwork,
debauchery, insanitary
dwellings, alcoholism, insufficient sleep, and poor
feeding. Professor Hayem
used to say that consump-
tion was picked up from
the zinc counters of inferior
wine-shops.

The ordinary diseases of
the respiratory tract were,
before Pasteur's era, attributed to the action of cold
(chills). Now it is known
that they are the outcomes
of the activities of such
germs as the staphylococcus
of Pasteur, the streptococcus
of Fehleisen, the pneumo-
coccus of Talamon and Frankel, and the
enterococcus that Thiercelin described after
researches by him and the writer.

A satisfactory, reasonable care of the
general health, moderation in food and
drink, the avoidance of fermented beverages
are the bases of preventive measures against
these ailments.

But, frequently, the breathing apparatus
is the victim of epidemic diseases or of accidental contamination by germs. Every one
is familiar with the ravages of influenza,
limiting that appellation to undoubted
epidemics such as that of 1918, which proved
a disastrous plague. Who does not remember
how hundreds of young men, returned un-
scathed from the World War, died in a few

days from the complication of massive pulmonary congestion ?

Rare germs such as the anærobic (growing
in an unoxygenated medium) bacillus of
pulmonary gangrene (lung mortification),
the destructive power of which is probably
prepared by the spirochætes of Etchegoin
and Bezancon, are the cause of broncho-
pneumonia of a special type, happily
relatively rare.

Despite the tendency of modern medicine
to make separate studies of affections of the
great systems (respiratory, circulatory, etc.),
we should not lose sight of the fact that the
organism is an entity, and that the functions
of one organ are intimately connected with
those of its fellow-organs. It thus happens
that every disease, every failure of the heart-
muscle will inevitably excite or aggravate
troubles of the pulmonary circulation, and
thereby favour infection. An uninterrupted
chain links the simple congestion of the
bases of the lungs so commonly present in
heart disease to broncho-pneumonia, to
which the patient succumbs because of the
easy development of the devastating microbes
in congested tissues. Fat and gouty subjects
are victims of their defective nutrition and
of the bad condition of their hearts. Without
following, even on broad lines, the cycle of
respiratory pathology, we cannot ignore the
fact that patients who have undergone an
operation on the stomach or on the intestines
not infrequently fall victims to broncho-
pneumonia.

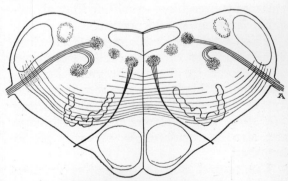

THE BREATHING CONTROL
A section through the medulla oblongata, the bulb
at the base of the brain which receives messages
from the skin and sets up appropriate reflex action
in the chest muscles. "A" denotes the vagus nerve.

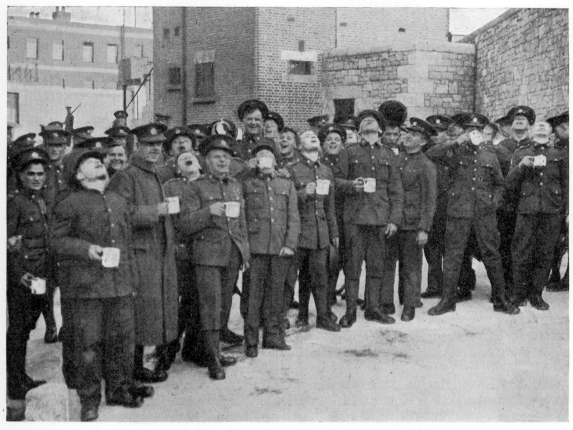

[Topical

THE " GARGLE PARADE "
Soldiers at Devonport gargling during an epidemic of sore throats and influenza.

We are to be congratulated on the fact that, in these latter days, great progress has been made in hygiene and in therapeutics (use of remedies). Fortiani's pneumothorax, already mentioned, is a method which consists in the introduction of air or of nitrogen gas into the pleural cavity. This ensures the compression and so the placing in a favourable condition for cure of unilateral focuses of tuberculosis of the lung, even in the acute stage ; also focuses of pulmonary gangrene. By this means, profuse hæmorrhage from the lung may be controlled.

Vaccination and vaccinotherapy which, thanks to Sir Almroth Wright, are extending more and more, prevent or contribute to the cure of broncho-pneumonia of various types such as those complicating measles, influenza, and those following serious operations, now rendered less dangerous by the application of local or regional anæsthesia.

The employment of what are called colloidal metals by Crede, Netter, Robin, is a valuable weapon against infection.

In another direction, in intratracheal infections (infections into the windpipe) my operation of tracheo-fistulisation with small tubes left permanently in the trachea without troubling the breathing, renders easier direct antiseptic applications to the respiratory tract.

Progress is taking giant strides. The American school, by demonstrating the general dangers ensuing from dental decay, has rendered a great service to our patients. Finally, young people have more and more taken a liking for health exercises and sports.

Curing a patient of a disease of the respiratory tract (we have often emphasised this point and we do so once again in conclusion) is not limited to merely paving the way to the cure and to the suppression of the symptoms of infection. Curing a patient means restoring to him the normal working of the lung, by means of breathing gymnastics, by physical culture methodically applied, by resort to sports, which, with sobriety and a due amount of sleep, constitute the most effective guarantee against deteriorations of the general health and the febrile complaints affecting the lungs.

THE URINARY SYSTEM

By GEORGE SOMERVILLE, M.D., D.P.M., Deputy Medical Superintendent to the West Ham Mental Hospital.

EXCRETION

THE working or functioning of the human machine is dependent upon the maintenance of the energy supply and this requires the intake of a sufficiency of suitable fuel—in other words, food. It is the purpose of the digestive system to modify the raw fuel and so to render it a convenient and available source of energy. Waste products are separated, and, as their continued presence in the body would be extremely harmful to it, they are got rid of, or excreted through the medium of the bowel.

The body cells receive their supplies of energy from the pure fuel prepared by the processes of digestion. All these cells have work to perform : they must maintain their own life and they must carry out their special organic function. Constant activity means constant change. Building-up and breaking down go on side by side. As with the machine, there is wear and tear and consequently waste products result. These are passed into the circulating blood, and, in health, are effectively got rid of by the action of the various excretory organs, namely, the kidneys, skin, bowel, and lungs. If, however, the excretory apparatus is not in working order, the waste materials accumulate in the blood. They act as poisons, and grievous harm may be wrought to the body machine ; its functions are impeded and distorted.

Excretion is a vital function of the body. By means of the sweat, urine, fæces, and expired air the tissue waste is removed. Efficient excretion is as essential to the human body as good ventilation and sanitation is to the dwelling-house. Hosts of minor and many major maladies are caused by impairment of this function. Its maintenance in health is almost entirely a matter of personal hygiene.

THE URINARY SYSTEM AND ITS WORK

The kidneys are two bean-shaped organs situated in the upper abdomen close to the vertebral column. They lie opposite the bodies of the last thoracic and the first three lumbar vertebræ. Their dimensions are roughly thus : length $4\frac{1}{2}$ in. ; breadth, $2\frac{1}{2}$ in. ; and thickness, $1\frac{1}{2}$ in. The kidneys are retained in position by a mass of fatty and fibrous tissue ; the large vessels which convey their blood supply and the intra-abdominal pressure are additional supports.

The Kidneys.

Splitting the kidney reveals two distinct layers of tissue. On the outside is the cortex which contains a mass of convoluted tubules and tiny blood capillaries. Internally is the medulla which consists of a number of " pyramids " with bases abutting against the cortex and apices projecting into the outlet of the kidney (commencement of ureter). The pyramids are formed by the parallel terminations of the convoluted tubes. The kidneys are supplied with relatively large arteries which are direct branches of the abdominal aorta. The corresponding veins open into the vena cava.

The ureters are the tubes that convey the urine to the bladder from the kidney. They are from ten to twelve inches long, and lie behind the peritoneum. Each tube, which is composed of fibrous, muscular, and mucous coats, begins in a funnel-like dilatation in the kidney called the renal pelvis, and then becoming narrower it reaches the under surface of the bladder which it enters by an oblique channel.

The Ureters.

This oblique tunnel through the bladder wall acts like a valve, and prevents urine being forced back from the bladder to the kidney.

The bladder when empty lies within the pelvis in the form of a " flattened tetrahedron." When distended it rises up behind the abdominal walls about five inches, but may extend much farther in cases of extreme distention. It is composed of a strong muscular coat, the fibres of which run in the length and round the organ in three layers. Outside it has a partial covering of peritoneum. Under the muscular coat are the sub-mucous and mucous coats. The latter is thin, smooth, and pink in colour, and it has no glands, while the sub-mucous coat is loosely attached to the muscular coat.

The Urinary Bladder.

When the organ is empty the lining is thrown into folds which disappear as it becomes distended. In children it is placed much higher up than in adults.

In front of the bladder are the pubic bone and the abdominal wall ; behind, the rectum in the male, and the uterus and part of the vagina in the female. The small intestine and colon rest on it above, and below in the male are the prostate gland, the seminal vesicles, and the ducts from the testes. On the floor of the bladder are three openings which mark the limits of a triangular space called the trigone. The foremost and lowest is at the apex of the trigone. This is the orifice of the water passage (urethra). The other two are the orifices of the ducts (ureters) through which the urine reaches the bladder from the kidneys.

The male urethra extends from the orifice in the bladder to the end of the penis. It is from seven to eight inches long, and is divided into a prostatic, a membranous, and a cavernous portion. It is composed of a mucous and sub-mucous coat, and, except during the passage of fluid, is closed in its entire length, being merely a small slit. The passage has numerous glands and pit-like recesses distributed all over it. When gonorrheal infection extends into these glands it is extremely difficult to get rid of it, as no applications to the lining membrane of the urethra are able to penetrate into the glands where the microbes of the disease have established themselves. In the female the urethra is about one and a half inches long. It opens immediately in front of the vagina, and behind the eminence of the clitoris. It has a muscular, vascular, and mucous coat.

The function of the kidneys is to extract certain waste substances, produced by body activities, from the circulating blood and to excrete them in the form of urine. Fine capillaries embrace the tubules and the selective power of the tubule cells permits the waste to filter through. Only the effete products are got rid of in health : the vital constituents of the blood are kept back. As the solid impurities can only be excreted in solution, this necessitates the filtration from the blood of considerable quantities of fluid.

From the kidneys the urine is propelled along the two muscular tubes—ureters—to the bladder. There it accumulates until a certain tension sets a reflex in action. The bladder muscle then contracts ; the sphincter of the urethra relaxes, and the urine is voided to the exterior. In the very young child this sequence of events is a pure reflex, *i.e.*, involuntary, but it very early passes under the control of the will.

The kidney function varies in activity in relation to the degree of skin functioning.* The excretion of urine is at its minimum during the night. This permits a vital organ a period of rest.

THE URINE

In health, the urine is a clear yellowish fluid, faintly acid and slightly denser than water. It contains in solution chlorides, sulphates, phosphates, and nitrogenous waste products, urea, uric acid, creatinine, and ammonia. Pigments, indirectly derived from the blood, determine its colour.

The average amount of urine passed per day by a healthy adult is about 50 ounces. ($2\frac{1}{2}$ pints). It varies in health according to

* See Skin and Kidney Interaction, section on Skin.

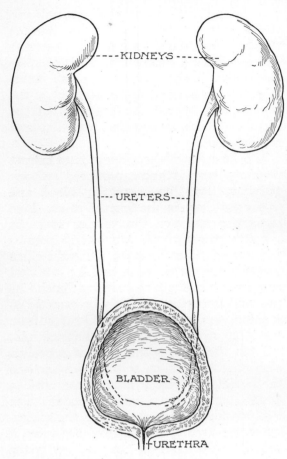

KIDNEYS

URETERS

BLADDER

URETHRA

THE URINARY SYSTEM
The excretion of the kidneys is conveyed by the
ureters to the bladder, and thence leaves the body
via the urethra.

the amount of fluid taken, exertion, and
the climatic conditions (temperature). Increase of urine is characteristic of certain
diseases, notably diabetes, chronic nephritis,
and hysteria. It is diminished in most fevers,
acute nephritis, and in heart disease.

Complete failure of the excretion of urine
is known as " suppression." It is a very
serious condition, rapidly fatal if not relieved,
and is usually caused by a very acute inflammation of the kidneys. Hot baths
to stimulate the skin and free purgation are
the methods of treatment adopted.

When there is a stoppage of urine from a
mechanical defect of the urinary apparatus
(stone, stricture, urethral spasm, prostatic
enlargement, weakness of the bladder),
" retention " of urine results. The urine

accumulates in the bladder and causes painful distention. Where spasm is the chief
factor, hot hip baths or hot fomentations
applied to the abdomen may give relief.
Mechanical obstruction will usually necessitate surgical intervention (catheterisation:
bladder puncture).

Incontinence of urine occurs when, owing
to paralysis of the sphincter muscle of the
bladder, generally from disease of the spinal
cord, the urine dribbles away as fast as it
is formed. Increased frequency of micturition is very common. The patient cannot
hold his water : the calls to urinate are too
frequent. The most common cause is local
irritation from inflammation of kidney,
bladder, or urethra as a result of tumour,
stone, tuberculosis, enlarged prostate, or too
acid urine. In children, worms or too long
a prepuce may cause frequency, especially
at night.

Nocturnal incontinence in children is a
troublesome disorder. It may be caused by
organic disease such as diabetes, but more
often it is related to general debility or local
irritation from stone or worms. If persistent
it may be associated with incipient mental
disorder or with adenoids where there is
deficient aeration of the blood and consequently very heavy sleep.

Certain abnormal substances may be
found in the urine and are indicative of
special diseased conditions. Albumen in the
urine is often a sign of serious heart or kidney
disease. It is also found in blood diseases,
febrile states, and sometimes in pregnancy.
A functional form, not associated with any
discoverable kidney defect, occurs occasionally in adolescents. Albuminuria is important not only because it is a sign of disease
but also because it is a serious drain on the
resources of the body.

Sugar in the urine (glycosuria) is constantly found in diabetes where it is associated with a great increase of the actual
excretion of urine. (It may amount to 400
ounces (20 pints) daily.) Thirst, voracious
appetite and progressive loss of weight are
accompanying symptoms. If a very large
quantity of sugar is taken in the diet

glycosuria may result. This, however, is transient and is soon rectified by alteration of the diet.

Blood may be passed in the urine. If it is intimately mixed with the urine, causing it to appear smoky, it is probably of kidney origin and frequently results from acute nephritis. If it is bright red and comes chiefly at the commencement of micturition it is of urethral origin (injury : urethritis) ; if at the end of micturition, and especially if in clots, it originates from the bladder (cystitis or stone).

The presence of pus in the urine is indicative of suppurative inflammation or ulceration of some portion of the urinary tract (urethritis ; cystitis ; pyelitis). Bile may make its appearance in the urine in the state of jaundice when, owing to some obstruction of the bile-duct, bile is absorbed into the blood stream.

The examination of the urine is of vital importance in medical diagnosis.

DISORDERS OF THE URINARY SYSTEM

The effects of kidney disease are reflected in alterations in the urine and in certain constitutional symptoms. Invariably when there is destruction of kidney tissue a state of general ill-health ensues. The patients experience malaise ; they waste and exhibit a typical waxy pallor. As a result of the retention of toxic nitrogenous waste products degenerative changes occur in the heart and blood vessels. The heart muscle, after an attempt to meet its increased liabilities, loses vitality and relaxes ; the arteries thicken and lose their elasticity. Bleeding from the nose, stomach and intestines may result. Rupture of a blood vessel in the brain may cause death (apoplexy). Breathlessness, sleeplessness, headache, defects of vision, and loss of mental vigour are commonly associated. The function of the gastro-intestinal apparatus is upset. There is lowered resistance to infections and consequently inflammations of the skin, mucous and serous membranes are common complications.

General Symptoms.

DROPSY (ŒDEMA) is a fairly constant feature of kidney disease. It is a condition where the serum from the blood exudes into the body tissues and cavities owing to the defective formation of the urine. Dropsy is also seen in heart disease and in anæmia, but, in contrast to these states, in renal disease it is of general distribution and is most noticeable in the early morning. Dropsy is absent in the variety of kidney disease where the supporting fibrous tissue is mainly involved (chronic interstitial nephritis).

Local pain is not a prominent symptom in kidney disorders. Sometimes, however, a dull aching in the loins may herald the onset of acute nephritis. Tumours and abscesses may produce lumbar pain and tenderness, and a floating kidney is often associated with a dragging sensation. Stone in the kidney or ureter may cause intense pain of a paroxysmal type. Backaches are of frequent occurrence, and are apt to be misinterpreted as evidence of kidney trouble. In women, congestion of the pelvic organs is a more common causal factor.

Uræmia is the condition which results from retention in the body of substances which in normal circumstances are elaborated into urea and excreted by the kidneys. It may occur in

Uræmia.

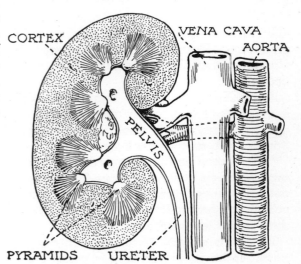

THE KIDNEY IN SECTION
Externally the kidney consists of a mass of tubules and tiny blood capillaries—the cortex. Internally is the medulla, formed by the pelvis, consisting of the terminations of the pyramids.

almost any disease of the kidneys—acute or chronic nephritis, tumour, abscess, or tuberculosis. The symptoms may develop within a few hours or may insidiously reveal themselves over a period of weeks or months. Persistent headache and dimness of vision, attacks of drowsiness during the day and sleeplessness at night are fairly early symptoms. Restlessness and muscular tremors, diarrhœa and vomiting supervene later. Paroxysmal attacks of breathlessness during the night are very characteristic. The acute symptoms may supervene at any stage when the patient passes into a muttering delirium and then into coma or convulsions. If he survives, blindness, deafness, and paralysis may ensue. It is in this way that many chronic kidney cases terminate.

To be of any value treatment must be prompt and energetic. It consists in stimulating the skin and bowels to take on the functions which the kidneys are unable for the time to perform. Hot-air baths, hot packs and diaphoretic drinks promote profuse sweating and purgatives produce watery evacuation of the bowels. Bleeding may be resorted to in combating the convulsions.

Sufferers from chronic kidney disease should avoid chill and should wear suitable attire. Diet should be under the supervision of a doctor ; vegetable proteins are preferable to flesh food ; alcohol is absolutely prohibited. Regular purgation is essential. Undue exertion, mental and physical, must be avoided.

Acute Nephritis (Acute Bright's Disease) is an acute inflammation mainly involving the cellular tissues of the kidney. **Acute Bright's Disease.** It may depend on chill, but a considerable proportion of cases supervenes on acute infectious fevers, most notably scarlet fever. Vomiting and headache may usher in the attack and sometimes there is febrile disturbance.

Dropsy is general from the commencement, varies in degree, and is usually first visible as a puffiness under the eyes. Fluid may accumulate in the body cavities. In the pleura it may seriously embarrass respiration. Digestion is disordered. The skin is waxy pale. Large quantities of albumen are present in the urine which may be turbid or smoky from the presence of blood. It is greatly diminished in quantity and in very severe cases may be entirely suppressed. This is a very grave sign and indicates the onset of uræmia.

The condition usually lasts from five to six weeks, and, when treatment is effective and the patient is nursed in hygienic surroundings, complete recovery is usual. Children as a rule make rapid recoveries. If the disease lasts longer than three months permanent damage to the kidneys is inevitable and a state of chronic nephritis develops. At any phase of the acute process death may occur from uræmia, heart failure, or any complicating acute inflammation.

Owing to the tendency of acute nephritis to become chronic, treatment must be carried out with the greatest care. The patient must be kept in bed in a room where an equable temperature can be maintained. Woollen garments and blankets are necessary to prevent chill. In brief, the outline of treatment is to relieve the kidney by giving non-irritating food ; to increase the action of the skin and bowels ; and to lessen local congestion. Diet must be the simplest and should consist solely of milk for the first week. Alkaline drinks appear to have a soothing effect on the kidney. Hot-air baths and hot packs produce free perspiration and are necessary if the onset of uræmia threatens. During convalescence diet still requires careful supervision and chill must be guarded against.

When an acute attack of nephritis passes off very slowly it is evidence that permanent kidney damage has resulted and **Chronic Nephritis.** that complete recovery is impossible. In this stage the patient becomes greatly debilitated, is very anæmic and dropsical, and large quantities of albumen appear in the urine. This disease cannot be cured ; treatment is similar to that of acute nephritis and at the best can only alleviate. At any time there is apt to be an acute exacerbation, or uræmia may manifest itself and prove fatal.

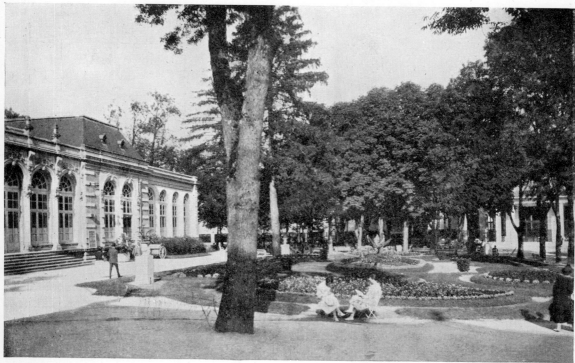

A SPA FOR KIDNEY TROUBLE
A view of Contrexéville, France, a spa with a great reputation for the treatment of stone in the kidney and other urinary complaints.

In this form it is mainly the cellular tissue of the kidney which has been destroyed by the inflammatory processes. When there is an overgrowth of the supporting fibrous tissue, another type of chronic nephritis results. It may be the final stage of the last mentioned type, or it may develop insidiously as a result of chronic intoxications—lead, alcohol, syphilis, gout, bowel stagnation. It is accompanied by widespread degenerative changes in all the blood vessels and with increase in size of the heart. The symptoms exhibited are mainly those of incipient uræmia. There is gradual impairment of mental and bodily vigour, headache, tremors and twitching of the muscles. The blood pressure is very high and hæmorrhages occur. The disease is progressive, and though treatment may diminish the strain on the kidneys and allow of a restricted life for some years, death eventually results from uræmia, cerebral hæmorrhage, or heart failure.

Pyelitis is a suppurative inflammation of the pelvis of the kidney. It may be caused by the presence of a stone or it may result from the extension upward of an inflammation of the bladder. Pain and tenderness in the loins, frequency of micturition, feverishness and general malaise are the most striking symptoms. Pus is present in the urine, and if the pyelitis is due to stone, blood may also be detected. Radical treatment depends upon the cause, but the symptoms may be relieved by rest, warmth, hot fomentations, and the administration of alkaline soothing drinks.

Pyelitis.

Pyelitis is important because extension to the kidney tissue may cause a SUPPURATIVE NEPHRITIS, a very serious condition which frequently terminates fatally. There is a hectic temperature, series of shivering fits and evidence of acute uræmia. Treatment is surgical.

Cystitis, or inflammation of the bladder may be caused by extension of a gonococcal urethritis, stone, decomposition of urine as a result of retention from stricture, or prostatic enlargement, and chill

Cystitis.

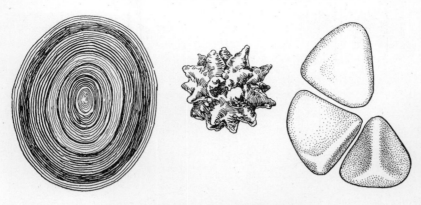

TYPICAL BLADDER STONES
Stones in the urinary system are deposits, in a variety of forms,
of solid matter from the waste products excreted.

in constitutional disorders such as gout or diabetes. In cystitis, micturition is frequent and painful (" scalding "). Fever and constitutional disorder occur. Pus is always present in the urine. The symptoms may be relieved by hot baths, and fomentations applied to the lower abdomen, along with a simple diet and a plentiful supply of bland drinks. Cure can only be made permanent by eradicating the fundamental cause ; otherwise the inflammation tends to recur or become chronic.

Inflammation of the mucous membrane of the urethra is most commonly caused by gonococcal infection. It is revealed **Urethritis.** by the constant oozing of pus from the uthera and by painful and scalding micturition. It is very important because it is apt to set up inflammation in the neighbouring organs and also to produce stricture owing to the healing of the ulceration by the formation of scar tissue. Gonococcal urethritis is an exceedingly infectious disease. Owing to its dangerous complications advice should be sought immediately and efficient treatment under medical direction should be carried out.

From the depositing of certain of the solids of the urinary excretion in the pelvis of the kidney, notably uric acid, **Kidney Stone.** urates, oxalates and phosphates, crystalline stones are formed. Various events may occur. The stone may remain in the kidney and cause a pyelitis ; it may produce attacks of renal colic ; it

may obstruct the ureter and render functionless the corresponding kidney ; if small it may be passed into the bladder (where it may cause cystitis) and eventually be voided to the exterior. Renal colic is characterised by paroxysms of lancinating pain which shoot down from the loin. It is often attended by vomiting, shivering, and collapse. Treatment is directed to the solution or removal of the stone. The bowels and liver should be regulated ; highly protein food diminished, and the urine kept diluted by drinking plenty of fluid—preferably alkaline water. Removal of the stone by surgical means frequently becomes necessary.

Invasion of the urinary organs by the tubercle bacillus is most commonly secondary to disease of the testicle. The **Tuberculosis.** disease advances insidiously. Both kidneys are usually involved. The symptoms resemble those of pyelitis, but there is often evidence of tuberculosis in other parts of the body. It is treated by the general methods adopted in all cases of tuberculosis, viz., rest, fresh air, and plentiful nourishment.

Floating kidney is of common occurrence, but it does not give rise to symptoms unless the degree of mobility is consider- **Floating Kidney.** able. It is responsible for many vague abdominal discomforts, and inveterate dyspepsias. Mental depression and neurasthenia are often associated with it. As it is sometimes related to the rapid loss of abdominal fat, attempts to fatten the patient may relieve the symptoms. Tonics and abdominal massage are also of great benefit, but it is usually advisable to wear a suitable belt.

Distention of the pelvis of the kidney (the funnel-shaped commencement of the ureter) is termed Hydronephosis, and this condition is a consequence of obstruction in some portion of the urinary passages. The commonest causes include impacted stone in the ureter, growths within the abdomen leading to pressure, enlarged prostate, and stricture of the urethra.

Distension of Kidney.

Following the obstruction, which is gradual, the pelvis of the kidney enlarges at the expense of the excretory tissue owing to the inability of the urine completely to escape, and ultimately there may be very little kidney substance left. The accumulated fluid naturally consists of urine—sometimes mixed with pus if any inflammation is present.

In mild cases there may be no symptoms, but, as a rule, a swelling makes its appearance in one loin which not infrequently disappears on the passage of urine. Should both kidneys be involved, with the destruction of kidney tissue, symptoms of uræmic poisoning will arise. In such cases the outlook is very unfavourable.

In treatment, it is clear that the first object must be to remove the fundamental cause, be it stone or tumour, and the sooner this is done the less likelihood is there of damage to the vital kidney tissue.

Abscess Around Kidney.

Suppuration or abscess formation may take place around the kidney (Perinephric Abscess) either as a result of spread of infection from that organ or from other organs in the vicinity —as from an appendix abscess, perforation of the intestine, pleural suppuration, or tuberculosis of the spine.

Dull, aching pain is experienced in the kidney region of the back, which is tender on pressure. The sufferer is generally feverish, but the constitutional symptoms vary in degree according to the cause. The treatment is surgical, the abscess requiring to be opened and drained.

Though simple tumours or growths occur in the kidney they are not very common.

Kidney Tumours.

The most important growths are of the malignant type, sarcomata, carcinomata or cancers, and hypernephromata, the last being an example of the embryonic " rest " tumour—which means that a portion of another organ (in this case the suprarenal gland) has, owing to some developmental error, become enclosed in the kidney and has commenced to grow erratically.

The chief symptoms of kidney growths are three, viz., localised pain, the passing of blood in the urine, and the presence of a palpable swelling in the kidney region. The outlook in such cases is invariably grave, and depends upon the successful operative removal of the affected kidney and upon the possibility of the other kidney carrying on the urinary function alone.

Cystic disease of the kidneys is a comparatively uncommon condition which, in most cases, is present from birth, though symptoms of the affection do not show as

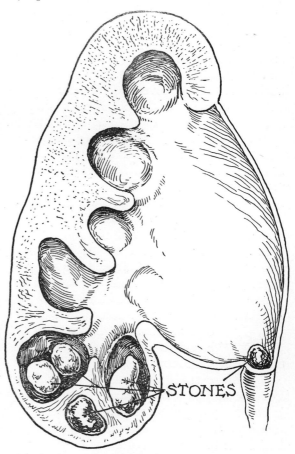

KIDNEY STONES

Kidney stones are formed in the pelvis of the kidney, where they may set up colic, or be passed via the ureter into the bladder.

a rule until about the age of forty or fifty years. In a few cases no evidence of the disease is present during life, and it is only detected accidentally on post-mortem examination.

Cystic Disease.

Both kidneys contain cysts or cavities of varying size and number. As a consequence, there is a considerable diminution of the kidney tissue available for secretory purposes. The cysts are filled with a clear or turbid fluid which contains albumen and phosphates. In some cases cystic kidneys may be accompanied by congenital deformities in other parts of the body, and may also be associated with cysts in the liver and spleen.

The symptoms of this affection—arising in middle age—include the occurrence of a swelling in both lumbar regions, the passing of blood in the urine, and evidence of chronic nephritis, viz., abundant secretion of pale urine containing a trace of albumen, thickened arteries with high blood-pressure, and enlargement of the heart. The patient's health may not be severely affected for some years, but, owing to deficiency of the kidney function, symptoms of uræmia are liable to ensue, the warning signs being headache, sleeplessness, tremors and twitchings of the muscles, and a gradual impairment of the mental and physical vigour. Death may result from the uræmia or from any other of the complications of chronic nephritis such as heart failure or apoplexy.

The treatment can only be palliative, and is similar to that adopted for chronic nephritis. Surgical operation is valueless.

In chronic nephritis numerous small cysts may arise as a result of obstruction of the fine tubules. In this variety the kidney is never so large as in the congenital condition.

Other Cysts.

Hydatic cysts may occur in the kidney, but are comparatively rare. The parasite is the " tænia echinococcus," a variety of tape-worm, which is only found in man in larval form. The disease is usually contracted from an infected dog. The detection of such a cyst is by no means easy unless it opens into the pelvis of the kidney, when the characteristic hooklets are found in the urine on microscopical examination. In some cases the hydatid cyst exists without symptoms for years, but in others it may rupture into the abdominal cavity or into the stomach or bowel—a relatively serious complication. The treatment is by surgical operation.

HYGIENE OF THE URINARY SYSTEM

The maintenance of healthy excretory organs is closely bound up with a sound personal hygiene. Regular exercise is a great aid to excretion. By speeding up the circulation, it causes the waste products to be washed out of the tissues. The interactions of the kidneys, skin, and bowels must always be borne in mind. Unhealthy skins and sluggish bowels throw additional work on the kidneys. Their effects, though slight at any one time, are cumulative. The vitality of the kidney cells is insidiously attacked and their functional activity is diminished. Chill, especially in the debilitated, must be avoided. Emergence from a hot to a cold atmosphere causes a constriction of the previously dilated skin blood vessels. Consequently large quantities of chilled blood flood into the internal organs and the delicate kidney cells are thus liable to be devitalised or damaged.

By careful supervision of the convalescence of patients suffering from infectious fevers, especially scarlatina and diphtheria, acute inflammation of the kidneys may be prevented. Such patients should be kept in bed, protected from chill and strictly dieted for at least three weeks. The periodic examination of the urine for the occurrence of albumen is essential, for early detection, and prompt treatment reduces the likelihood of permanent injury to the kidneys.

Certain poisons are known to have detrimental effect on the kidney tissue. Alcohol, lead, and the toxins of syphilis and gout not only cause degeneration of the heart and blood vessels but also lead insidiously to chronic kidney disease. Such causal factors are eminently preventable.

In order that the health of the body may be maintained the excretory organs must always function at their maximum efficiency.

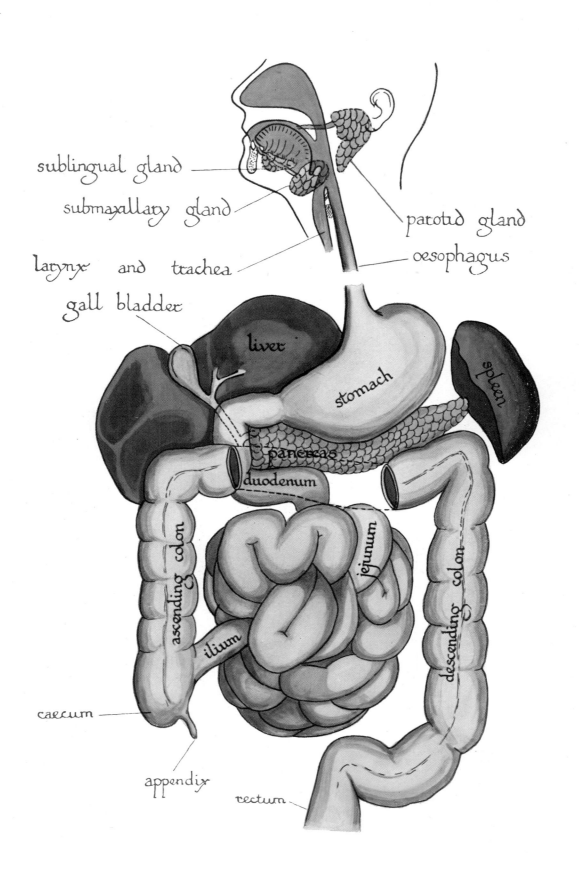

sublingual gland

submaxillary gland

parotid gland

larynx and trachea

oesophagus

gall bladder

liver

stomach

spleen

pancreas

duodenum

ascending colon

jejunum

ilium

descending colon

caecum

appendix

rectum

THE DIGESTIVE SYSTEM

THE DIGESTIVE SYSTEM

*By GEORGE SOMERVILLE, M.D., D.P.M., Deputy Medical Superintendent at the
West Ham Mental Hospital.*

THE NATURE OF DIGESTION

IT is the function of the organs which constitute the digestive system to modify and prepare food in order that it may be incorporated in the human body. By the processes of digestion the food is rendered soluble and diffusible, and so is capable of being absorbed by the circulating blood. The altered food is eventually assimilated by the living tissues and provides for their growth and repair. The mechanism of digestion is occasioned by certain chemical activities of the secretions of the digestive tract and its associated glands, and by certain physical activities whereby the food is pulped and propelled through the digestive canal.

THE DIGESTIVE TRACT

The digestive apparatus consists of a musculo-membranous canal, stretching from the mouth to the anus, and certain glands which pour their secretions into it. The digestive or alimentary canal comprises the mouth, pharynx, œsophagus (gullet), stomach, and small and large intestines.

The MOUTH is a cavity lined by a mucous membrane covered with epithelial cells. It contains the tongue, teeth, mucous and salivary glands. The cavity is bounded above by the hard and soft palates ; beneath the tongue it is bounded by a layer of muscles and soft tissue which forms the floor of the mouth.

The TONGUE is composed of muscle fibres running in various directions and covered by a mucous membrane which is studded with numerous papillæ or localised epithelial elevations. Three kinds of papillæ are described : " conical," " fungiform," and " circumvallate." The conical papillæ are found on the upper surface of the tongue and give it the characteristic roughness. They are minute sense organs and convey tactile impressions. The circumvallate papillæ are relatively large and number from seven to twelve. They are situated at the back of the tongue in a V-shaped line, with the apex directed backwards. The fungiform papillæ are numerous and are scattered over the upper surface and edges of the tongue near its tip. The circumvallate and fungiform papillæ are special sense organs. They possess " taste buds "—modified epithelial cells surrounded by nerve fibrils—which, on stimulation, originate impulses to be interpreted in the brain as tastes.

The TEETH are implanted in the jawbones and serve for grinding and pulping the food ; they also aid in speech. Each tooth consists of a " crown " which projects from the gums, and a root, consisting of one

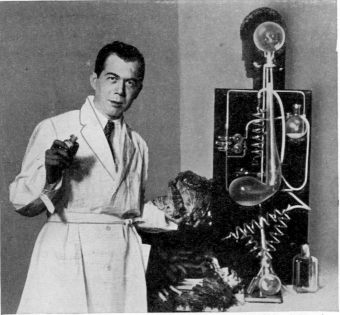

[*Pacific and Atlantic.*

THE DIGESTIVE SYSTEM—A WORKING MODEL
Dr. B. G. Hauser with his model of the internal organs of the body designed to demonstrate the process of digestion.

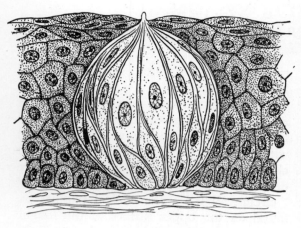

A " TASTE BUD "
One of the numerous tiny elevations on the tongue
which send impulses to the brain to be interpreted
there as tastes.

or more fangs, which is embedded in the bone. The main bulk of the tooth is formed by the ivory or " dentine " which is covered in the crown by " enamel " and in the root by a layer of bone. The centre of the tooth is hollowed out to lodge the " pulp "—a connective tissue containing bloodvessels and nerves.

Human beings have two sets—the temporary or milk teeth in childhood and the permanent or adult teeth which develop later. In the child the milk teeth consist of two incisors, one canine, and two premolars in each half-jaw (twenty teeth in all). The adult set consists of two incisors, one canine, two premolars, and three molars in each half-jaw (thirty-two in all).*

The SALIVARY GLANDS include the " Parotid Glands," situated in the deep spaces between the ears and the angles of the jaws ; the " Submaxillary Glands," placed under cover of the wings of the mandible ; and the " Sublingual Glands," which lie under the tongue.

Each gland is formed by branching tubes supported by connective tissue and lined by large cells which secrete the saliva. Small ducts lead from these tubes to unite ultimately as main ducts which open into the cavity of the mouth. The parotid gland secretes a clear watery fluid containing the

* See Section on The Teeth.

ferment " ptyalin " ; the sublingual gland produces a mucous secretion ; the submaxillary gland is a mixed gland and provides both types of secretion.

The salivary glands are supplied with nerves from the autonomic and sympathetic nervous systems. The flow of saliva during a meal is due partly to the mere presence of any kind of food in the mouth, and partly to mental factors which include appetite, with the varying effects of different foods, and the emotional state. (Extreme fear will completely inhibit the secretion of saliva.)

The mouth opens through the " fauces," the passage between the tonsils, into the pharynx or throat, where the œsophagus commences.

The PHARYNX is that part of the digestive apparatus which extends from the back of the mouth and nose to the top of the gullet. It is somewhat conical in shape and is composed of muscular and fibro-membranous walls. During the swallowing act it may be likened to the extended part of a funnel that ends in the gullet which spreads downwards from it. It has opening into it, above, the nasal cavities, in front, the back of the mouth, and below, the larynx and the gullet. Behind the fold which divides the front part from the back of the mouth on each side lies the tonsil. This is a mass of lymphoid tissue of sponge-like character owing to the presence of numerous pits or follicles. After puberty the tonsil becomes much smaller as a rule.

From the commencement of the œsophagus to the lower end of the rectum, the digestive canal is constructed on a similar anatomical plan. The interior of the tube is lined by a mucous membrane ; externally is a muscular coat which consists throughout of an inner circular and an outer longitudinal layer of muscle fibres. The mucous and muscular coats are united to each other by a layer of loose connective tissue, the submucous coat.

The ŒSOPHAGUS or gullet is the conduit for food which passes from the throat down to the stomach. It is a strong muscular tube about nine inches in length and consists of four coats : an outer or fibrous, a muscular, a submucous, and an internal or mucous. The œsophagus lies behind the trachea, aorta, heart, and roots of the lungs, in close relation to the vertebral column, and pierces the diaphragm just before its entry into the stomach.

The ABDOMEN is the largest cavity in the body. It is bounded above by the diaphragm which is spread like a dome over

The Abdomen. it and divides it from the cavity of the chest or thorax. A line drawn through the nipples roughly indicates its upper limit. Below it is bounded by the structure which completes the floor of the pelvis : that is to say, the levator ani and coccygeus muscles on either side.

It is divided into two parts. The upper or abdomen proper, and the lower or smaller part, the pelvis. It is bounded in front and at the sides by the abdominal muscles ; at the back, by the spine and the psoas muscles ; below by an imaginary plane at the level of the upper aperture to the pelvis, and above by the diaphragm. It contains the intestines, stomach, liver, pancreas, spleen, kidneys, and the suprarenal glands. It is lined throughout with a smooth membrane, the peritoneum, which covers the surface of the contained organs also, in such a manner that when it leaves the wall of the abdomen to cover an organ it passes to it on its upper side, spreads around and underneath it until it reaches the upper part which came from the wall. It then passes back on the underneath surface of this, being united to it. In other words, the peritoneum makes a suspending band, or ligament, which holds up the organ, and contains the blood vessels and nerves which pass to and from it.

The PELVIS is that part of the abdominal cavity below the abdomen proper which is contained within the bony ring known as the pelvic girdle. It is bounded behind by the sacrum and tail bone. In front and at the sides it is bounded by parts of the haunch or innominate bone (ilium, ischium, pubis). It contains the bladder, the rectum, and a small part of the colon above it called the sigmoid flexure, and a small part of the small intestine as well as some of the generative organs.

The abdomen proper is divided into nine regions by six lines drawn across it at equal distances on its front aspect. The middle zone is called the umbilical, the one on each side the right and left lumbar, the three above the right and left hypochondriac, with the epigastric in the middle, and below in the middle is the pubic or hypogastric, with the right and left inguinal, or iliac regions on either side.

The STOMACH is the most dilated part of the alimentary canal ; it is the receptacle for the food after it has been

The Stomach. masticated and swallowed. The gullet opens into the stomach above and to the left ; below and to the right the stomach becomes continuous with the duodenum or first part of the small

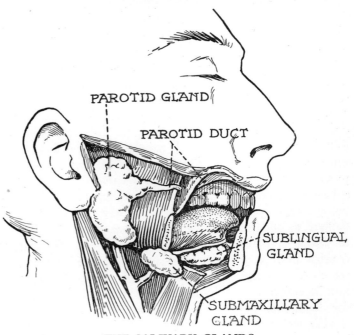

PAROTID GLAND

PAROTID DUCT

SUBLINGUAL GLAND

SUBMAXILLARY GLAND

THE SALIVARY GLANDS
A dissection of the mouth showing the important glands whose secretion begins the process of digestion.

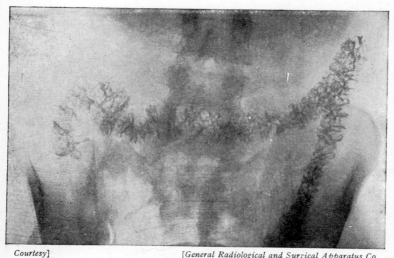

Courtesy] [*General Radiological and Surgical Apparatus Co.*

X-RAY PHOTOGRAPH OF THE COLON
Showing the transverse and descending colon containing a special preparation to render it opaque to the X-rays.

intestine. The stomach is pear-shaped, with a blunt left extremity called the " fundus " and a narrow right extremity or "ˌpylorus." The fundus is situated immediately below the heart and base of the left lung ; it is separated from them by the diaphragm. The pylorus is in relation to the lower surface of the liver. The form and position of the stomach are greatly influenced by the amount of food it contains and by the empty or distended state of the other hollow organs in its vicinity. The stomach lies between two folds of peritoneum (the lining membrane of the abdominal cavity) which allow of its free suspension.

The wall of the stomach consists of four coats—from without inwards—peritoneal, muscular, submucous, and mucous. The muscular coat is peculiarly thickened at the pyloric end to form a thick ring, a valve or sphincter. The mucous membrane has a honeycomb appearance and is loosely attached to the intervening submucous coat to allow of considerable displacement. It consists mainly of small tube-shaped glands which secrete the gastric juice. This secretion is composed of hydrochloric acid and the ferments, pepsin and rennin. Mucus is also secreted by the surface epithelium. The secretion of the gastric glands is regulated by the vagus nerve which is reflexly

stimulated by impulses received from other nerves.

Sight or smell of food, the anticipation of a meal, and the actual mastication of food produce, through the vagus, an abundant secretion. As with the salivary secretion, mental factors play a large part.

The gastric juice is antiseptic owing to the presence of hydrochloric acid. It "inverts," by the medium of the acid sucrose into glucose. It contains rennin which curdles milk, and a protein-splitting ferment, " pepsin."

The INTESTINE comprises that part of the alimentary canal which is situated below the stomach. It is a continuous tube—twenty-eight to thirty feet in length—suspended in loops by the peritoneum in the abdominal cavity.

The intestine is divided into the " small intestine " and the " large intestine." The former extends from the stomach to its junction with the latter at the cæcum. It is twenty-two feet in length and about one and a half inches in width. The small intestine is conveniently divided into three parts viz., the " duodenum," consisting of the first ten or twelve inches, into which the ducts of the pancreas and liver open ; the " jejunum " forms the next eight or nine feet, and is continued as the " ileum," which opens into the commencement of the large intestine.

The DUODENUM, so called because it is about equal in length to the breadth of twelve fingers, is the shortest, widest, and most fixed part of the small gut. It is curved on itself so that it nearly forms a circle. Beginning at the pyloric valve, it passes to the right under part of the liver, and then drops down for a short distance, embracing the head of the pancreas, from which it turns upwards and forwards towards the left side to end in the jejunum. The common duct of the gall bladder and pancreas enters the duodenum about three and a half inches below the pylorus. The jejunum, so called because it is always found empty after death, forms about two-fifths and the ileum three-fifths of the remainder of the small intestine. This terminates at the back of the large intestine in the middle line, where the cæcum and colon join, and from which it is shut off by the colic valve.

The intestine, like the stomach, is composed of four coats, serous, muscular, sub-mucous, and mucous. The serous coat is part of the peritoneum. This leaves the wall of the abdomen, passes forward and reaches on to the gut, with which it becomes intimately adherent, and then passes back to the abdominal wall. From this it will be seen that the gut is suspended in the abdominal cavity by a flat, fanlike membrane (mesentery), which owing to the extreme length of the gut and the short area of attachment to the wall, must be gathered. This arrangement also has the advantage that it leaves the intestine freely movable, while preventing it from tying itself into knots. The muscular coat is arranged in two layers, the outer longitudinal and the inner circular. The sub-mucous layer is composed of loose tissue containing blood vessels, lymphatics and nerves. The mucuous membrane is thick and richly supplied with blood vessels in its upper part, but it becomes thinner and paler lower down. The thick mucous membrane of the upper part of the small intestine is arranged in folds across the tube,

giving it somewhat the appearance of a pipe tapped for deeply-cut screw. These circular folds (valvulæ conniventes), serve to retard the flow and thus afford time for the completion of the complicated chemical and physical processes of digestion in the intestine.

The whole membrane is covered with little projections (villi) which give it a velvety appearance. They are composed of blood vessels, muscle fibres, gland cells and tissues, and have a central tube, or tubes, called lacteals, which play a very important part in digestion. Small tubular glands are also found there and these secrete a digestive fluid—the intestinal juice. Small areas of lymphoid tissue are scattered throughout the small intestine—"Peyer's Patches"—which are of special interest because they

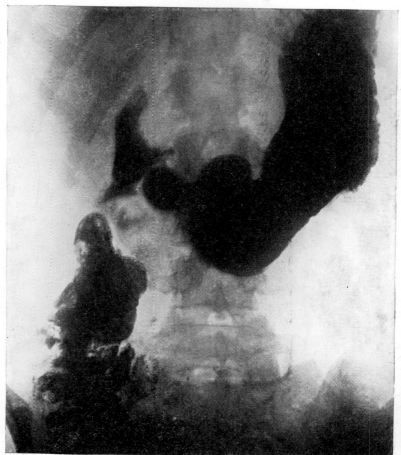

Courtesy]   *[Medical Supply Association.*

THE POSITION OF THE STOMACH
The stomach photographed after a bismuth meal. The lower ribs, backbone, and part of the intestine can also be distinguished.

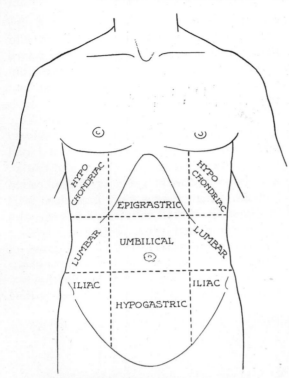

THE REGIONS OF THE ABDOMEN
The abdomen proper, bounded by the thorax above and the pelvis below, is divided in classification into nine zones.

become inflamed and ulcerated in typhoid fever.

Because of its mobility and elasticity the small intestine often escapes injury when the body is subjected to violence. The first part (duodenum) owing to its greater fixity and its position in front of the spine is that most frequently implicated. A violent blow such as a kick from a horse may rupture the gut, and peritonitis may be set up by the escape of its contents. Small wounds, even bullet wounds, are frequently not fatal. Removal of part of the gut for diseased conditions is often undertaken by the surgeon, and operations upon it are uneventful episodes in surgical practice.

The LARGE INTESTINE begins at the ileum and ends at the anus. It is about six feet in length, and of unequal calibre, being largest at the cæcum and gradually diminishing until it reaches a dilated part just above the anus, where it terminates. It is composed of four coats, serous, muscular, sub-mucous, and mucous, but the arrangement of the

muscular coat is peculiar. The longitudinal muscular fibres are collected into three bands, about half an inch wide, and so arranged that they gather the gut into a pouched or sacculated bag. The outer coat has numerous little fatty decorations (appendices epiploicæ) scattered over its surface. The cells of the mucous membrane are mainly directed to the production of mucus; this is essential for the lubrication of the food remains as they are propelled along the bowel.

The large intestine is divided into the cæcum, colon, and rectum. The cæcum is a pouch about two and a half inches by three inches. It hangs free in the right inguinal region, and has the ileum opening into it behind at the point where the ascending colon begins. The opening is guarded by the colic valve. This consists of two crescentic folds of mucous membrane which open to allow the contents of the small intestine to enter the colon, and under normal conditions prevent a return flow taking place. Below the valve is situated a minute orifice leading into the " appendix vermiformis." This is a worm-shaped tube about three inches long, and from one-quarter to three-eighths of an inch thick, closed at the end. It springs from the lower end of the cæcum, and has a fold of peritoneum attached to it for a considerable portion of its length. It has a very small canal extending throughout.

The colon is divided descriptively into five parts, namely, the ascending, transverse, descending, iliac, and sigmoid colons. The ascending extends from the cæcum to the under surface of the liver, where it bends to the left forming the right colic flexure. It is held to the abdominal wall by the peritoneum, which does not cover it at the back. The transverse colon passes across to the left side, sagging downwards as it does so owing to its mode of attachment and to the presence of the duodenum, pancreas, jejunum and ileum behind it. It has above and immediately resting upon it, the liver and gall bladder, part of the stomach and spleen. Under the spleen, which lies in the left hypochondriac region, it turns downwards (splenix flexure), and becomes the descending colon, which merges into the iliac at the level of the crest of the haunch bone. This short segment of the colon reaches as far as the plane of the pelvic brim, where it becomes the sigmoid, or pelvic colon, which is very freely movable, and sometimes becomes twisted upon itself, causing obstruction. At its lower end it becomes the rectum.

This is about five inches long, and curved to follow the sacral bone from which it is separated by blood vessels, nerves and muscle. In front it has coils of the small intestine resting upon it above, and below it is in close contact with the bladder and prostate gland in the male, and with the vagina in the female. The anal canal in which the rectum ends is about one and a half inches long. It is the narrow muscular passage closing the intestinal tract by its tightly contracted orifice, the anus. Its mucous membrane is thrown into longitudinal folds, and has a very rich supply of blood vessels.

Dilatation or varicosity of the veins in this area produces the condition known as piles, or hæmorrhoids.

The ANUS is the muscular outlet of the bowel. It is always tightly contracted except during the passage of fæces. It may be looked upon as a slit in the muscular floor of the pelvis. It is commonly the seat of external hæmorrhoids.

The LIVER is the largest gland in the body : it weighs about fifty ounces. It occupies the upper right-hand region of the abdomen. The upper rounded surface occupies the dome of the diaphragm : its lower surface rests on various abdominal organs, viz., the right kidney and suprarenal gland, the colon, the duodenum, and the stomach. The liver is maintained in position by ligamentous folds—thickened portions of the peritoneal membrane. On its under surface at the level of the right costal margin is a small sac, the " gall-bladder."

The liver consists of an enormous number of lobules. Each is formed by columns of cells radially arranged and is penetrated by capillary-like blood vessels which converge from the periphery to the centre. The blood vessels of the liver are peculiar. There are two sets of veins, the hepatic and the portal, and one set of arteries. The arteries supply blood for the nourishment of the organ itself. All the blood coming from the intestines charged with the products of digestion reaches the liver through the portal vein ; this immediately breaks up into smaller and smaller vessels until it ends in minute spaces around the tiny lobules. The blood from the portal vein here meets and mixes with some fresh arterial blood brought to it by the hepatic arteries. All this mixed blood filters between the cells of the lobule which extract and add materials to it in its passage to a central tube—the beginning of the hepatic vein which will ultimately convey the blood to the general blood stream by pouring it into the great inferior vena cava. Between the cells are little canals which form a network and eventually unite to form the bile ducts. Each lobule acts as a secretory unit. The liver cells absorb substances from the circulating blood, elaborate them into bile, and secrete this fluid by the bile capillaries. These small ducts unite to form the main liver duct which, on its course to the duodenum, gives off a branch to the gall-bladder—the temporary reservoir for bile.

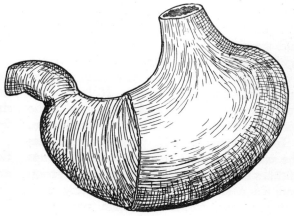

THE FOOD RECEPTACLE
The stomach dissected to show its inner muscular coat.

The functions of the liver are related to the general metabolism of the body. The liver serves as a store-house for glycogen (animal starch) which it builds up from the carbohydrate absorbed during digestion and which it changes into glucose and returns to the circulating blood in order to retain constant the percentage of blood-sugar. It transforms the waste substances derived from the used-up tissues of the body into urea and uric acid which, absorbed into the blood-stream, are excreted in the urine. It elaborates bile which continuously trickles into the intestine but is secreted in large quantities on the arrival of food in the duodenum. The amount of bile secreted daily varies from 500 to 1000 c.cs. (1 to 2 pints). It is a viscid fluid, golden brown in colour and possessing a bitter taste. The colour depends on the presence of the bile-pigments, bilirubin and biliverdin (derived from blood pigments). The bitter taste is due to the bile salts, the taurocholate and glycocholate of sodium. Bile also contains mucin, urea, and mineral salts. It is mainly an excretion, *i.e.* it is a medium by which the body gets rid of tissue waste. At the same time bile is an important factor in digestion : it aids the pancreatic juice in the splitting-up of fats. Bile salts have an important antiseptic function : they check the putrefactive processes in the intestine.

The PANCREAS (sweetbread) is a secretory gland situated in the back of the abdomen behind the stomach. The expanded end or "head" occupies the curve of the duodenum. It is continued to the left as the "body," and terminates as the "tail" which abuts against the spleen. The gland is traversed by a duct from left to right and gathers many tributaries en route. It leaves the pancreas at the head and, joining with the common bile duct, opens into the duodenum.

In fine structure the pancreas resembles the salivary glands. It is composed of groups of tubes lined by columnar cells. Each group ends in a small duct which, uniting with similar ducts, forms the main pancreatic duct.

The obvious function of this gland is the production of the pancreatic juice—one of the most important of the digestive secretions. The pancreatic juice is an alkaline fluid which contains four ferments, viz., "trypsin," which digests proteins ; "amylopsin," which converts carbohydrates into sugar ; "lipase," which splits up fats, and a milk-curdling ferment.

Scattered throughout the pancreas are collections of special cells known as the "Islands of Langerhans." These cells produce an internal secretion which is absorbed directly into the blood-stream. Disease of these "islands" results in the condition known as "diabetes."

FOOD AND THE BODY

The functioning of the digestive system is best understood by a preliminary consideration of the varieties of foodstuffs. To maintain the bodily activities expenditure of energy is necessary. Food, after digestion and absorption, is the normal source of this energy.

Foods may be classified in five groups, viz., "proteins," "fats," "carbohydrates," "salts," and "water."

The proteins are complex nitrogenous substances widely found in the animal and vegetable kingdoms. They are vital constituents of cellular tissues. Chemically they are compounded of numerous different amino-acids. Proteins are exemplified in lean meat, white of egg, fish, the casein of milk and cheese, the gluten of flour and oatmeal, and in the legumin of vegetables such as beans and peas. They are absolutely necessary for the growth and nutrition of the body tissues, and they are also a source of heat and energy. In the processes of digestion the complex proteins are split up into simple amino-acids by the action of certain ferments or enzymes (proteases).

The fats are salts formed by the combination of certain fatty acids (palmitic, stearic, and oleic) with glycerine. Fats are exemplified in butter, cream, lard, and olive oil. They are important energy producing foods, but require a certain proportion of carbohydrate and protein before they can be consumed in the body. Fats can only be absorbed after they have been completely digested into fatty acids and glycerine.

The carbohydrates include the sugars, starches, celluloses and gums. They are compounds of hydrogen, oxygen, and carbon. Before carbohydrate can be absorbed it must be digested into the simple form of sugar (glucose). Carbohydrate is the main source of muscular energy.

The salts comprise the chlorides, phosphates, and carbonates of sodium potassium and calcium, and also certain iron salts. They are essential to the health of the tissues.

Water is a general solvent and is necessary to hold in solution the various food substances and the waste products. Moisture is absolutely essential for the health of animal tissue.

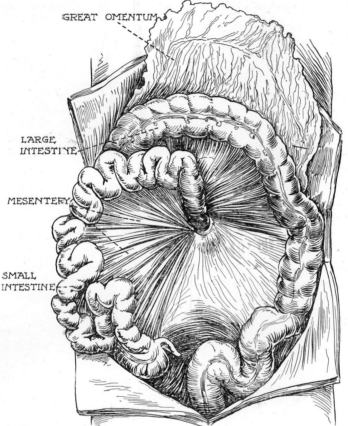

LARGE INTESTINE

GREAT OMENTUM

MESENTERY

SMALL INTESTINE

HOW THE INTESTINE IS SUSPENDED
The mesentery so anchors the intestine to the abdominal wall that it is freely movable, yet cannot tie itself into knots.

suitable—high temperatures destroy them, cold delays their activity.

The process of digestion commences when food is taken into the mouth. Saliva is immediately secreted and is poured into the mouth in considerable quantities. It is intimately mixed with the food which is ground up or chewed into a pulpy mass by the teeth, aided by the muscular movements of the cheeks, lips, and tongue. The saliva contains the ferment "ptyalin" which converts insoluble starches into soluble sugars. After mastication, the food, lubricated by saliva, is collected into a bolus by the tongue and pressed backwards against the roof of the mouth, through the fauces, to be grasped by the pharyngeal muscles and passed into the œsophagus. The transit of the bolus through the gullet is caused by rhythmic waves of muscular contraction (peristalsis) of reflex origin, and the food reaches the stomach through the relaxation of the circular muscle at its cardiac orifice. This series of events is known as the act of "deglutition" or swallowing.

When the food enters the stomach some time elapses before sufficient gastric juice is secreted to deal with it, and during this period the swallowed saliva continues its action of converting starches into sugar.

Salivary Digestion.

THE PROCESS OF DIGESTION

The chemical changes, whereby the various foods are digested and rendered suitable for absorption, are carried out by specific ferments or enzymes. These are products of living cells : their chemical composition is unknown. Certain conditions are necessary for the proper action of the body ferments. They can only act in the presence of water ; some act in an acid medium—others in an alkaline one ; the temperature must be

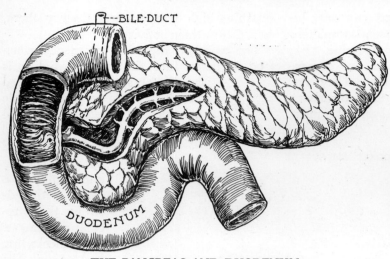

--BILE-DUCT

DUODENUM

THE PANCREAS AND DUODENUM

The first section of the small intestine—the duodenum—curves round the head of the pancreas, which pours a digestive secretion into it.

Within half an hour enough gastric juice is secreted ; ptyalin digestion ceases and gastric digestion commences.

The important ferment of the gastric juice is " pepsin." This only acts in an acid medium : it digests the relatively insoluble proteins into the more soluble " peptones." The free hydrochloric acid aids in protein digestion ; prevents putrefaction of the food by killing pathogenic bacteria ; inverts cane sugar into glucose ; and, by dissolving the envelopes of the fat-cells in adipose tissue, sets free the fat in preparation for the subsequent digestive action of the pancreatic juice. The protein of milk, caseinogen, is acted upon by the rennin ferment ; it is converted into insoluble casein which is precipitated and is eventually digested by the pancreatic secretion. The " lipase," or fat-splitting ferment, which is sometimes found in the stomach, is believed to originate from regurgitated pancreatic juice.

Gastric Digestion.

In the stomach the food is churned up and thoroughly mixed with the gastric juice by the rhythmic contractions of the muscular walls. It is reduced to a semi-fluid mass called " chyme." This is gradually pushed towards the pyloric end of the stomach where its passage into the duodenum is regulated by the contractions and relaxations of the pyloric sphincter. The control of the sphincter depends upon the reactions of the contents of the pyloric part of the stomach and of the duodenum respectively. When the acid chyme comes in contact with the duodenum the sphincter contracts and the flow of stomach contents stops until they are neutralised by the alkaline pancreatic juice and bile when the sphincter relaxes and permits the further passage of the chyme.

With an average meal, the stomach should be emptied within three or four hours ; with a heavy meal, six to seven hours may elapse before the stomach is emptied. Alcohol is the only substance absorbed to any extent from the stomach.

In the intestine the altered food, or chyme, comes under the influences of secretions derived from the liver, the pancreas, and the intestine.

Intestinal Digestion.

The pancreatic juice is poured along with the bile into the duodenum. It is an alkaline fluid and contains ferments which act on the proteins, fats, and carbohydrates. The protein ferment, " trypsin," only acts in an alkaline fluid and is a more powerful ferment than pepsin. It splits the proteins into their most absorbable form, *i.e.*, amino-acids. The starch ferment, " amylopsin," has the power of converting starch into sugar after the manner of ptyalin.

The lipolytic or fat-splitting ferment breaks up the fat into fatty acids and glycerine ; the fatty acids combine with the alkali to form soaps which are soluble and easily absorbed. The digestion of fats is augmented by the biliary secretion. Bile, by reducing the surface tension between fat and water, promotes the fine emulsification of fat and facilitates the action of the ferment ; it also helps to dissolve the soaps. On absorption by the epithelial cells of the intestine, the fatty acid and glycerine are re-synthetised. The fat is taken up by the lymphatics of the intestinal mesentery : it gives them a milky appearance, and they are known as lacteals. These fine channels eventually join the main lymphatic vessel —the thoracic duct—which opens into the large vein leading into the right side of the heart. Thus the absorbed fat reaches the blood-stream indirectly via the thoracic duct.

The secretory activities of the pancreatic and liver glands are occasioned by the chemical stimulus of a substance produced by the action of acid on the duodenal mucous membrane. This product is known as " secretin," and it belongs to the group of " chemical messengers " or " hormones " which are absorbed directly into the blood-stream and produce their effects on remote organs of the body.

The completion of the chemical digestive processes is effected by the intestinal juice. This secretion is produced by tubular glands occurring in the mucous membrane of the small intestine. " Secretin " is the stimulus for its production.

The intestinal juice is an alkaline fluid containing a number of ferments. " Maltose " completes the digestion of starch into sugar ; " invertase " and " lactase " convert complex sugars into simple ones ; " erepsin " acts on partially digested proteins and reduces them to amino-acids.

It will be noted that the terminal result of the action of the digestive juices on food-stuffs is their conversion into amino-acids, s i m p l e sugars (glucose), fatty acids, soap, and glycerine. Each stage of the

process is correlated with and is dependent on the preceding stage.

The small intestine, with its ridged mucous membrane and " villi," plays the most important part in the process of absorption. Each villus is covered with an epithelium which has a special selective function and is able to transmit products of digestion to the central lacteals or capillary blood vessels which form the core of the villus.

While digestion is proceeding the intestinal contents are slowly propelled along the gut towards the colon. At the same time these contents are subjected to a continuous mixing process. The onward movement is caused by progressive waves of muscular contraction and constitutes " peristalsis " ; the mixing action is produced by separate segmental or ring-like contractions. These movements can be observed in human beings by means of the X-rays after the administration of a bismuth meal.

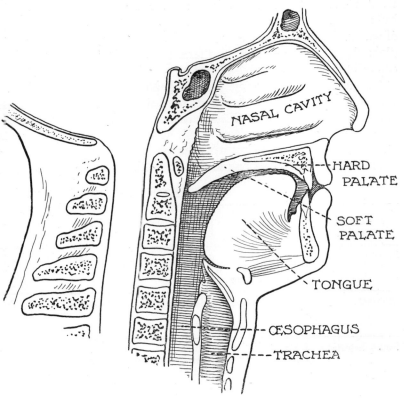

THE ACT OF SWALLOWING
A section of the head and throat during swallowing. Food is collected into a bolus by the tongue and pressed backward against the roof of the mouth, when the pharyngeal muscles force it into the œsophagus.

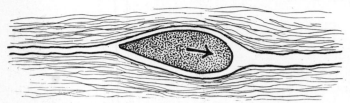

THE FOOD ON ITS JOURNEY
The food is collected into a " bolus " and forced on its journey through the gullet by waves of muscular contraction.

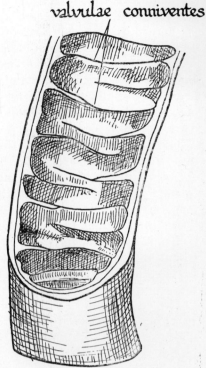

valvulæ conniventes

THE SMALL INTESTINE IN SECTION
The folds of the mucous membrane (valvulæ conniventes) control the passage of food and mix it thoroughly.

The muscle of the small intestine is controlled by fibres from the vagus and the sympathetic nervous system ; hence the influence of mental states on the bowels. Pain and anger may inhibit their activity ; anxiety and fear cause exaggeration.

About five hours after a meal the contents of the small intestine commence to pass into the large intestine. These contents are devoid of nutritive material and consist mainly of indigestible residue with waste substances excreted from the liver and intestinal walls. The large intestine is relatively short and its function is to reduce the bulk of the food residue by the absorption of water. Bacterial decomposition also takes place there ; putrefaction and fermentation occur with the formation of gases.

The residues are slowly propelled along the colon ; gradually become semi-solid and constitute the fæces. These are retained for some time in the colon until, usually after a meal, a certain quantity passes into the rectum. This gives rise to the desire for defæcation, and, by relaxation of the sphincter of the anus accompanied by contraction of the walls of the rectum aided by voluntary contraction of abdominal muscles, the contents of the rectum are evacuated. In the child defæcation is a pure reflex ; in the adult it is under voluntary control. The principal facts relating to digestion and absorption are summarised in the following table.

DIGESTION AND ABSORPTION

ALIMENTARY TRACT.	SECRETORY GLANDS.	SECRETION.	TYPE OF FOOD ACTED UPON.	CONVERTED TO.	ABSORPTION BY
Mouth	Parotid Sublingual Submaxillary	Saliva	Starches	Sugar	Capillaries of Intestinal Villi
Stomach	Gastric Glands	Gastric juice	Proteins	Peptones	Capillaries of Intestinal Villi
Small Intestine	Liver Pancreas Intestinal Glands	Bile Pancreatic Juice Intestinal Juice	Fats Starches Proteins	Fatty Acids Glycerine Soaps Amino-Acids	Lacteals of Villi Capillaries of Intestinal Villi
Large Intestine	Active digestion ceases with the small intestine. With the exception of water there is little absorption in the large intestine.				

DISEASES OF THE DIGESTIVE SYSTEM

By GEORGE SOMERVILLE, M.D., D.P.M., Deputy Medical Superintendent at the West Ham Mental Hospital.

LARGELY owing to faulty habits of eating, drinking, and personal hygiene, disorders of the organs related to the digestive system are very prevalent.

DISEASES OF THE MOUTH

The state of the mouth gives valuable indications of the general health of the body. The mucous membrane is pale in anæmia ; bronzed in Addison's disease, and yellow in jaundice. The tongue to some extent reflects the state of the alimentary tract. In dyspepsia it becomes flabby, thickly coated with fur and is indented by the teeth. In exhausting diseases, such as pneumonia or typhoid fever, the tongue may become brownish-red, dry, and cracked. Tremulousness of the tongue is very marked in cases of alcoholism and general paralysis. Offensive breath may be associated with dyspepsia, but is more frequently caused by pyorrhœa —a purulent infection of the gums.

Stomatitis, an inflammation of the mucous membrane of the mouth, may be due to **Inflamed Mouth.** microbic infection or to irritants such as tobacco, raw spirits, or over-spiced food ; in children it is commonly associated with dentition. Small painful ulcers are frequent in gouty dyspeptics.

Severe ulceration may occur in badly nourished children suffering from scurvy. The gums are swollen and bleed readily. Greyish-white ulcers form, which cause loosening of the teeth, and sometimes destruction of the margin of the jaw-bone.

Thrush is a parasitic infection of the mouth caused by a yeast type of fungus **Thrush.** which occurs in infants brought up under unhygienic conditions. Small white patches form on the tongue and cause local heat and pain. Loss of appetite and diarrhœa frequently result. Local treatment with borax and glycerine

rapidly alleviate. The strictest cleanliness must be observed when feeding the child.

Occasionally in young children, subsequent to an attack of measles, a very acute inflam-**Gangrene of the Mouth.** mation of the mouth which terminates in destruction of the tissue or gangrene may occur. The disease, which is known as " Cancrum Oris," runs a rapid course and is generally fatal.

The tongue may become inflamed as a result of an irritant, a septic wound, or the **Inflamed Tongue.** sting of a wasp or bee. Swelling occurs which may be so severe as to prevent swallowing and to necessitate incision in order to reduce the inflammatory œdema. This condition is known as " Glossitis."

Whitish pearly patches develop on the upper surface of the tongue in the condition

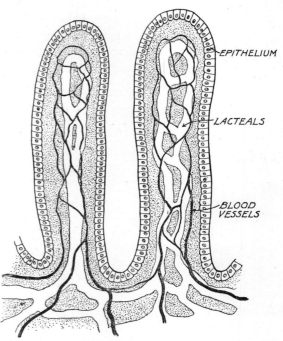

HOW NOURISHMENT IS ABSORBED
" Villi " of the small intestine, which absorb the nourishing factors from digested food through the epithelium, whence they are conveyed via the lacteals and blood vessels to all parts of the body.

known as "Leucoplakia." It is always associated with excessive tobacco smoking, and most frequently occurs in syphilitic subjects. It is important because, if untreated, it may develop into a cancer. In treatment it is essential to stop all irritants ; constitutional disease must be remedied ; locally the patches should be painted with silver nitrate solution from time to time.

Any ulceration of the tongue which is chronic and does not yield to any local treatment should be viewed with the gravest suspicion. It may be due to cancer, syphilis, or, more rarely, tuberculosis. The earlier the discovery is made, the better are the chances of effective treatment and cure.

DISEASES OF THE SALIVARY GLANDS

Excessive secretion of saliva follows the use of drugs such as mercury or tobacco. It is a common symptom in mental disease (dementia præcox), and often occurs in encephalitis lethargica (sleepy sickness). Diminished secretion may be produced by belladonna or atropin.

Inflammation of the parotid salivary glands is known as " Mumps " or " Infective Parotitis."* It occurs in epidemic form. A number of important complications are apt to follow, and chief among these is orchitis or inflammation of the testicles.

DISEASES OF THE PHARYNX

Inflammation of the throat (Acute Pharyngitis) is commonly associated with exposure
Simple Sore Throat. to cold in rheumatic, gouty, or debilitated persons. Infective organisms play a part, and the disease may assume epidemic form.

It reveals itself by heat and dryness in the throat with soreness on swallowing. There is slight fever, and aching of the back and limbs is commonly present. The neighbouring glands in the neck are often enlarged and painful. The tonsils may participate in the inflammation.

As a rule the condition subsides in a few days. Severe pharyngitis may be prevented by promptly taking a Dover's powder,

* See Section on Infectious Fevers.

followed by a hot bath and rest in bed. Gargling the throat with dilute Condy's fluid and inhalation of steam impregnated with pine oil afford considerable relief.

Septic Pharyngitis (Hospital Throat) is a very severe variety of throat inflammation
Hospital Throat. which is attended by ulceration and suppuration. It is due to organismal infection and occurs in individuals whose general health is poor. There is considerable fever and constitutional disturbance. The immediate application of carbol-glycerine relieves the local inflammation. The general health should be improved by suitable dietary, rest, and fresh air.

Chronic Pharyngitis (Relaxed Throat) is due to chronic congestion of the pharynx as
Relaxed Throat. a result of excessive voice-strain (CLERGYMAN'S THROAT) or the immoderate use of irritants such as tobacco or alcohol. There are no constitutional symptoms, but there is a chronic tickling cough with hoarseness and a constant feeling of dryness and irritation in the throat.

Avoidance of irritants and rest for the voice are the first principles of treatment. Locally, a solution of silver nitrate or Mandl's paint should be applied.

Acute Tonsillitis (Quinsy) is an acute inflammation of one or both tonsils which
Acute Tonsillitis. is sometimes associated with suppuration, and is of infective origin. Inflammatory involvement of the tonsils also occurs in scarlet fever, diphtheria, and other infectious fevers.

The onset is sudden : there is pain, swelling, and redness of the tonsils with fever and constitutional disorder. The glands in the neck are painful and swollen. Abscess formation may take place, but early incision will prevent it giving rise to serious trouble.

This disease usually subsides in the course of a week, but with a tendency in certain persons to recurrence during cold damp weather.

The tonsils should be painted with carbol-glycerine ; inhalation of steam and the application of poultices help to relieve the pain and discomfort. A brisk purge is advisable at the commencement of the illness. When suppuration occurs the tonsil will require immediate incision.

In Chronic Tonsillitis the tonsils are permanently enlarged. It is frequently associated with a similar enlargement of the adenoid tissue in the naso-pharynx. The disease is common in unhealthy children ; it may follow acute attack or arise subsequent to measles, scarlet fever, or diphtheria.

Chronic Tonsillitis.

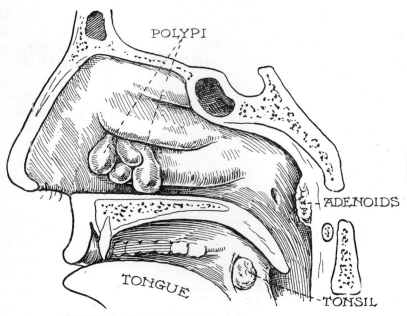

DISEASE SITES IN THE NOSE AND THROAT
Enlarged tonsils and adenoid growths obstruct the respiratory and digestive processes and are a serious menace to health.

Enlargement of the tonsils and of the other adenoid masses in this region gives rise to a characteristic group of symptoms. The mouth is open, the lips thickened with perhaps the lower one protruding. The nose is small, inclined to retroussé, with small nostrils which do not dilate during inspiration, while the bridge is broad and flattened. The upper jaw is narrowed, causing the incisor teeth to become prominent and the bony palate acutely arched : as a secondary consequence to this the permanent teeth are crowded owing to the deficient development of the jaw bones. Some deafness may be present owing to blocking of the Eustachian tube with adenoid masses. Foetor of the breath is nearly always present ; cough, especially noticeable at night, is frequent. This would appear to be due to the decomposing matter in the crypts of the tonsil which may be seen as yellowish patches. The voice becomes nasal in tone and the letters " m " and " n " cannot be pronounced. Facial spasm is at times apparently caused by enlarged tonsils.

Children of the adenoid type are prone to diphtheria, while they offer a poor resistance to other infectious diseases. There is a vacant expression. The child as a rule is listless or slow, perhaps irritable and inattentive. The breathing is snuffling and the sleep snoring or snorting, while sudden startings and cryings break its sequence. Wetting the bed is not unusual. Often attacks of an asthmatic character may occur. Owing to the obstructed breathing the chest becomes deformed ; either flat-chested and hollow or pigeon-chested. The spine becomes rounded, and the shoulder blades protrude (winged). The general mentality of the child, as well as its physical growth, suffers.

Chronically enlarged tonsils in childhood are a source of many dangers. Their removal by operation is essential. Improvement in the physical health and mental development rapidly ensue.

DISEASES OF THE ŒSOPHAGUS

Inflammatory diseases of the gullet are of relatively infrequent occurrence. Local injury may be produced by the swallowing of corrosive or scalding fluids. Ulceration is caused and is followed by the formation of a scar which is apt to narrow the passage

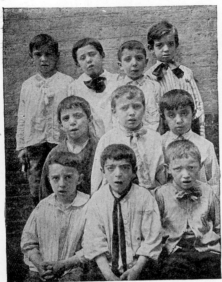

" Elementary Biology," Gruenberg (Ginn & Co.)
TYPICAL " ADENOID FACES "
The vacant expressions and listless bearing characteristic of children with enlarged adenoids.

and produce a stricture. This gives rise to pain and difficulty in swallowing, with regurgitation of food.

A more serious form of stricture is that which is caused by a cancerous growth at the lower end of the gullet. There is progressive difficulty in swallowing with a steady decline in strength. Owing to the inaccessible position of the cancer, treatment can only be palliative and is directed to nourishing the patient through an artificial opening in the stomach.

Stricture of the œsophagus may also be caused by the pressure of tumours or aneurisms within the cavity of the chest, and a spasmodic variety may occur in hysteria.

DISEASES OF THE STOMACH

The majority of stomach diseases, though of varied origin, exhibit a more or less common group of symptoms which are classed under the term " dyspepsia." Hence the diagnosis of individual disease entities is by no means easy.

A blow over the region of the stomach may cause death without any observable lesion.

Wounds. This is due to the shock from injury to the sympathetic nervous plexus. All wounds and injuries of the stomach are accompanied by intense shock, but although serious are not necessarily fatal. The fullness or emptiness of the organ, the character and position of the wound, the presence or absence of germs, the subsequent treatment and the general condition of the patient, all help to decide the issue. If food be present in the wounded stomach it may escape and set up general peritonitis. Many cases are on record where the stomach has been wounded by bullets and the victims have completely recovered. Injury to a large blood vessel may prove rapidly fatal. The stomach is frequently subjected to surgical operations for the relief of ulcer and cancer, and occasionally for the removal of foreign bodies.

Acute inflammation of the stomach (Acute Gastritis, Acute Catarrh) is most commonly

Acute Gastritis. caused by the ingestion of irritant, poisonous, or indigestible foods, *e.g.* flesh of crabs or lobsters, tinned food containing ptomaines. A surfeit of food and excessive indulgence in alcohol are also prominent as causal factors. Gout, rheumatism and other constitutional conditions such as liver heart, and lung disease are important predisposing causes.

Following the imprudent meal or drinking bout there is severe abdominal discomfort usually associated with nausea and vomiting. The tongue is thickly furred ; appetite is lost ; a degree of fever may be present. Headache, depression, and considerable prostration may result. Diarrhœa ensues in a few days as a rule. Recovery takes place in about three to six days, but repeated attacks result in a condition of chronic gastric catarrh.

In treatment it is first essential to remove the irritant from the stomach ; calomel followed by a seidlitz powder is very useful. Rest for the stomach is imperative ; complete abstinence from food for twenty-four hours, followed by a milk diet is the best remedy. Any constitutional factor must be appropriately treated.

Chronic Gastritis (Chronic Catarrh) may follow repeated attacks of acute gastritis or it may be related to the chronic engorgement associated with lung, heart, liver or kidney disease. The mucous membrane of the stomach becomes congested and thickened, and small hæmorrhages are apt to occur. Later an atrophy of the secretory structures of the stomach results and leads to further impairment of the digestive function.

Chronic Gastritis.

The symptoms include gastric pain or discomfort, flatulence, a constant feeling of nausea, occasional vomiting—especially in the morning, poor or capricious appetite, constipation, abdominal tenderness and gradual impairment of general nutrition.

The success of treatment depends upon the possibility of removing the cause. Diet must be carefully regulated. Milk, soups, white fish and a moderate amount of carbohydrate are advisable. Meals should be small but frequent.

Gastric and duodenal ulcers are of frequent occurrence. They are common between the ages of twenty-five to thirty. Gastric ulcers are more

Ulcers.

common in women ; duodenal ulcers in men. The actual causes are obscure and not fully understood.

In gastric ulcer as a rule, though not invariably, there is a history of long-standing dyspepsia. Aching pain occurs in the upper abdomen and is increased by pressure. Occasionally it may be referred to the right shoulder blade. The taking of food accentuates the pain and to relieve it the sufferer may induce vomiting. In duodenal ulcer the pain comes on two to three hours after taking food, and is often relieved by eating. The erosion of a blood vessel may cause vomiting of blood (hæmatemesis). The wall of the stomach or duodenum may be so corroded that perforation results, and this may lead to peritonitis.

The course of gastric and duodenal ulcers is extremely variable. The ulcer may heal completely or incomplete healing may take place and relapses are then apt to occur. The risk of serious hæmorrhage or of perforation

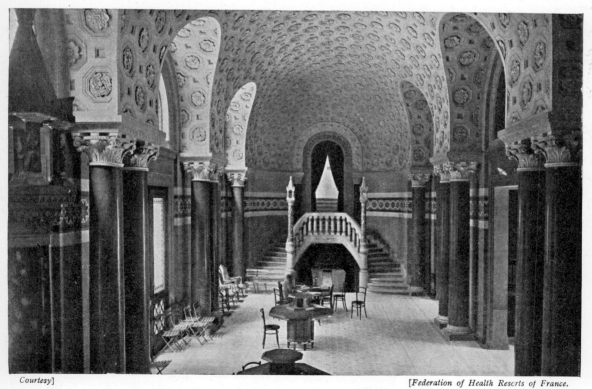

[Federation of Health Resorts of France.

IN THE BATHING ESTABLISHMENT, CHATEL GUYON
Dyspepsia and other diseases of the stomach and intestines are treated at this Spa in the Auvergne Mountains, France.

with peritonitis render these conditions dangerous to life. Cancer of the stomach frequently originates at the site of a chronic ulcer.

The most important feature of treatment is the careful adjustment of diet. This must be rigorously carried out under the direction of a doctor. For at least a week milk and cream must form the staple part of the diet. Later boiled egg, cereal foods, custards, creams of fish and chicken are permitted. Hæmorrhage or perforation demand *urgent* treatment.

Chronic Dyspepsia (Chronic Indigestion) is a condition of disordered digestive func-
Dyspepsia. tion not related to any gross change in the mucous membrane of the stomach. There are two main types : atonic dyspepsia and acid dyspepsia.

ATONIC DYSPEPSIA is the commoner of the two, and is due partly to a deficiency of the acid of the gastric juice and partly to defective motor power of the stomach.

The symptoms include a feeling of weight or distension coming on immediately after food associated with pain either in the upper abdomen or shooting up to the right shoulder ; eructations of wind ; diminished appetite ; languor ; depression ; palpitation.

This ailment is related to long-standing errors of dieting, imperfect mastication, anæmia, overwork, and mental anxiety. It is not a serious menace to life, but renders the sufferer miserable and wretched.

In treatment the main indication is to remedy the dietetic errors. Food should be simple, nutritious, and of little bulk. Bitter tonics should be taken to stimulate the gastric secretion. Rest before and after meals is important. The general health must be improved. Abdominal massage, electricity, exercises, and baths are useful curative measures.

In Acid Dyspepsia, which occurs in young nervous persons, there is an excess of
Acid Dyspepsia. hydrochloric acid in the gastric juice. Burning pain comes on one to two hours after taking food, and it is usually relieved by eating. It is associated with acid eructations and waterbrash. The appetite remains good.

Treatment is mainly dietetic : stimulating foods such as meat essences must be avoided ; cream and olive oil tend to lessen the secretion of acid and should be taken with each meal. Bicarbonate of soda quickly relieves the pain and discomfort.

Dilatation of the stomach may be a sequel to chronic gastric catarrh or it may be due
Dilatation. to an obstruction (cancer or contracted ulcer) at the pyloric end of the stomach. General debility, anæmia, and neurasthenia are predisposing factors.

Locally there is pain and discomfort, and, if the dilatation is considerable, there is vomiting at intervals of two or three days of large quantities of acid frothy material. The breath is very fetid and eructations of ill-smelling gas occur. Appetite is poor, thirst marked, the bowels constipated, and nutrition suffers greatly.

In treatment the endeavour is to keep the stomach as empty as possible. This may be attained by dieting—giving concentrated and predigested food, and by periodic

" CORSET STOMACH "
A deformity not uncommon in the days of tight-lacing. The stomach is displaced in the body and greatly constricted.

washing out of the stomach. Massage, baths, exercise, and tonics are necessary to brace up the general health.

Hæmorrhage from the stomach may be caused by ulcer or cancer, as already noted. **Hæmor-rhage.** It may result from disease of the blood vessels, and has followed operations for removal of the appendix, when it is of the gravest import. It is seen in chronic heart disease and in the liver disease (cirrhosis) of chronic alcoholics ; in some acute blood diseases, in certain poisonings, and infective fevers. Injuries from without or within may be the direct cause. The blood may be poured into the stomach from a ruptured aneurism, in which case death would probably be almost instantaneous, or it may come from an enlarged spleen. Here, too, the result is usually fatal. Blood from the stomach is vomited, not coughed up, is usually clotted dark coloured, and perhaps has food mixed with it. The patient will pass tarry-looking stools afterwards. Blood from the nose or throat may be swallowed and subsequently vomited.

CANCER OF THE STOMACH

By VICTOR PAUCHET, M.D. (Paris),
Surgeon to the Hôpital Saint-Michel, Paris.

CANCER of the stomach is the most common of all cancers. Most cancers of the stomach are preceded by ulcers. Consequently, if we discover the means to avoid ulcers of the stomach, or, when they are present, if we can cure them with tolerable certainty, we accomplish a beneficent work. Now, we can cure the ulcer by removing it, and we can often prevent the formation of the ulcer either by the observance of a few hygienic rules easily followed, by disinfecting the intestinal canal or by removing a chronically infected appendix.

The majority of cancers of the stomach follow old ulcers. Sir Arbuthnot Lane, **Causes of Cancer.** writing on the causation of cancer, stated that there were three necessary and affiliated causes ; if one of the causes were absent, no cancer resulted.

(*a*) A parasite, unknown at present, but very likely existing.

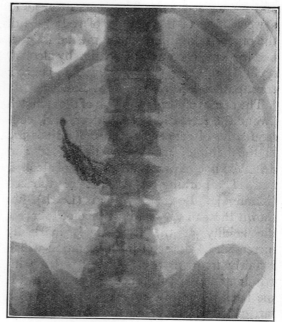

A CURIOUS OBSTRUCTION
A case for surgical operation—safety pins in the stomach revealed by the X-ray.

(*b*) Some constitutional trouble which lowers the vitality of the organism and prevents it from resisting the onset of the disease.

(*c*) A local irritation.

To make this clearer, it may be stated that a woman suffering from cancer of the womb has generally suffered from inflammation of that organ (metritis). In a man, cancer of the rectum is generally preceded by inflammation of that part of the large intestine (proctitis), or by piles. A woman suffering from cancer of the breast has had, previously, mammitis, that is to say, chronic inflammation of the mammary gland, caused generally by constipation. Similarly, cancer of the large intestine (above the rectum) has had, as a necessary forerunner, general inflammation of the colon or a local inflammation of the same. Cancer of the stomach is necessarily preceded by an ulcer or by gastritis (inflammation of the stomach). Finally, for the tongue to be affected with cancer, it is necessary that a period of irritation from carious or jagged teeth or tobacco should have preceded its development.

" Cancer is, therefore, a debit incurred,

and not an accident. The general causes of a weakening of the powers of resistance of the organism are physical or mental fatigue, bad hygiene, chronic intoxication by alcohol, syphilis, tobacco, and especially chronic constipation " (Sir Arbuthnot Lane).*

The causes of local irritation of the stomach favour the formation of an ulcer, and, consequently, of cancer. Some individuals are in the habit of swallowing their food and drink too hot, of partaking unduly of alcohol, and of absorbing the fumes of tobacco (inhaling). Lord Moynihan (Leeds) has shown that, under the influence of tobacco, the acidity of the stomach is markedly increased. A cause of local irritation which is fairly frequent and which has been incriminated is a substance allied to tar. If the back of a white mouse be rubbed with tar, cancer develops on the part rubbed.

For this reason, some surgeons have banned the eating of smoked articles of diet, such as smoked herrings, smoked meats, etc., seeing that certain parts of these contain tar which may favour the development of cancer. We have not verified this statement : we mention it for what it is worth. One cause of local irritation of the stomach which is but too frequent is a bad state of the teeth.

How can one diagnose ulcer of the stomach which precedes by some years cancer of that organ? Either by pain, vomiting, or hæmorrhage. But, in order to think of ulcer, we must not pin our faith on such obvious symptoms. There are three signs which are commonly present and which are sufficient for the diagnosis :—

(a) Stomach pains. They appear at a fixed time after meals, from one to four hours, according to the situation of the ulcer ; if it be seated in the duodenum, eating calms the pain ; if, on the contrary, it is in the stomach, eating would increase the pain. The regular and invariable time at which the pain appears is a very important symptom.

* Read *Le Chemin du Bonheur ; L'art de rester jeune*, published by Oliven, Paris ; *La Constipation*, by Dr. Victor Pauchet, published by Doin, Paris.

(b) This pain occurs in attacks during a few weeks or months ; they then completely disappear so that the patient believes himself cured. The intermittence of these attacks of pain is, thus, a very important sign.

(c) X-ray examination. Most ulcers are visible by the X-rays, but the radiologist must be a specialist in diseases of the stomach.

To sum up, in every patient who has occasional stomach pains, if these pains appear in connection with meals, at a regular time, and if there are intervals of apparent recovery, we must diagnose an ulcer of the stomach ; X-ray examination will generally confirm this conclusion.

Is the ulcer spontaneously curable (without operation) ? Treated from its first appearance with a severe dietary, for some months, the ulcer may heal, but in the majority of cases, it does not heal, and the attacks of pain recur without intermissions.

What are the possible consequences of an ulcer ? If it be situated in the duodenum it might give rise to serious hæmorrhage or a perforation may occur which might be fatal. If located in the stomach the same complications may arise, but another complication may arise some years later, namely, the development of cancer. The duodenal ulcer never becomes cancerous, but gastric ulcer frequently does so. A cured ulcer of the stomach may become cancerous ten, fifteen, or twenty years later. In the subject affected with ulcer of the stomach, one must consider the ultimate result of an operation ; removal of the ulcer is the only useful measure ; gastro-enterostomy (short circuiting the stomach to the intestine) is bad practice. For duodenal ulcer this latter measure may be useful ; for stomach ulcer it only relieves. Ulcer of the stomach must always be removed.

How can cancer of the stomach be diagnosed ? Formerly, cancer of the stomach Diagnosis was recognised by means of the of following signs :— Cancer.

(a) Gastric Stasis ; the pylorus (the entrance into the duodenum) being narrowed by the cancerous growth (the pylorus being the common seat of it), the stomach empties itself more slowly.

(b) Hæmorrhage. The vomiting of blood is fairly common, but more often it is absent.

(c) Examination of the Stools. This may show blood as a tarry liquid, but more often the blood is not visible. To recognise any blood that may be present the stools must be examined for several consecutive days.

(d) Examination of the Gastric Juice. This reveals a diminution of the normal acidity.

(e) Progressive Loss of the Appetite, more especially a repugnance to meat.

(f) Loss of Strength. The patient is unable to perform his usual duties; he has not the same physical and moral resistance; he has lost his former activity.

(g) Loss of Weight. The patient loses weight because he eats less; but even if he eats as much as formerly, he loses flesh from the general poisoning caused by the cancerous growth.

(h) X-ray Examination. Every person complaining of a diminution of digestive powers should be examined by a

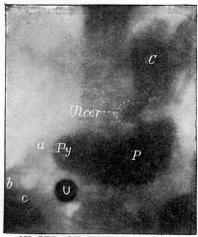

ULCER OF THE STOMACH

A typical case revealed by the X-rays, showing the ulcer and the resulting tight, hour-glass constriction. C.P.—cardiac and pyloric portions of the stomach; Py.—pylorus; a, b, c—parts of the duodenum; U—umbilicus.

specialist for this disease. At an early period the departures from the normal are very little marked. As a matter of fact, it hardly interests the surgeon to see an advanced case; the presence of cancer must be recognised at its beginning. X-rays show the growth at its early stage in insignificant signs, but these are sufficient.

The evolution of the symptoms is of paramount importance. In the case of an ulcer, these symptoms are transitory; treatment relieves them at once. In cancer medical treatment and dieting do no good. Every month or every three months the symptoms are aggravated; the doctor who recommends delay of surgical measures may be making a serious mistake.

Chronic appendicitis is often the origin of gastric and duodenal ulcers; in removing an infected appendix the surgeon prevents the development of the ulcer of the stomach, and, hence, of cancer. The infection of the appendix follows infection of the intestine; intestinal infection is itself caused by chronic constipation which must be corrected by pure mineral oil taken during meals and by re-education of the bowel. The action of the bowels must be solicited after each meal.

Grasp well the following facts :—

"Whenever I have operated for an ulcer

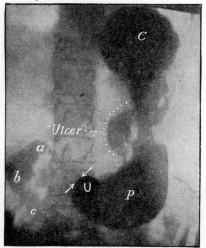

["Chronic Intestinal Stasis," A. C. Jordan (O.U.P.)

THE BEGINNINGS OF CANCER

The X-ray photograph in this case reveals lighter areas near the chronic ulcer, subsequently found to be due to nodules of cancer.

or for cholecystitis (inflammation of the gall-bladder), I have invariably found appendicitis which compelled me to remove the appendix. Consequently, patients who have ulcers of the stomach or of the duodenum, or who have cholecystitis, have an old appendicitis dating to a long-anterior epoch. It is probable that if the appendix had been removed ten, fifteen, or twenty years earlier, these patients would have had neither cholecystitis nor ulcer." (Lord Moynihan).

Therefore, when a patient tells you that he believes he had chronic appendicitis, but that he had consulted a doctor who told him not to have his appendix removed, and that he would recover without that, this patient risks the appearance one fine day of a stomach ulcer or of cholecystitis. The doctor who had advised against the removal of the appendix had done a very bad service to his patient. The removal of the appendix is a trivial operation ; it is an operation that lasts five minutes and recovery ensues in a week ; under local anæsthesia the patient runs no risks. Even if there be some doubt about the existence of appendicitis, the appendix must be removed.

To recapitulate : cancer of the stomach can be cured by the surgeon on the condition that the operation be performed very early, that the stomach walls be removed from a distance far away from the actual growth, and that by a very experienced operator.

Cure and Prevention.

The cure of cancer of the stomach demands its very early recognition. To do this, the appearance of obvious signs must not be awaited. It is sufficient that, in order to bring about the operation, *presumptive evidence* of its presence shows itself. The mere suspicion of cancer of the stomach should suffice for the performance of the operation. It is better to find no cancer but to cure a mild condition when the stomach is opened than to wait until one is sure of the presence of cancer, for, by that time, the case is too advanced, and, even if the operation be performed, relapse is to be looked for.

To avoid cancer of the stomach, ulcer of that organ must either be avoided or it must be removed. And, finally, if you would avoid gastric ulcers, keep the teeth in good order ; smoke and drink alcohol sparingly ; do not eat highly-spiced food, do not burn your stomach by eating very hot food or drinking very hot beverages ; see that your nose is healthy internally, and keep the same watch over your tonsils and your throat, for suppuration in those parts irritates the stomach and may favour the development of ulcers or cancer. If your doctor thinks you have chronic appendicitis, do not consult two others to confirm the diagnosis ; get a surgeon to remove the diseased appendix, for it is the cause of later developing stomach ulcers, cholecystitis, and various other chronic disorders. In having a doubtful appendix removed you run no risk and you have—eight chances out of ten—obtained great benefit from the operation.

DISEASES OF THE INTESTINES
By GEORGE SOMERVILLE, M.D., D.P.M.,
Deputy Medical Superintendent at the West Ham
Mental Hospital.

CONSTIPATION is the state wherein the intestine discharges its contents incompletely or too seldom. It signifies an insufficient action of the bowels with retention of fæcal matter.

Constipation.

The causes of constipation are multitudinous : they may be summarised thus :—

1. Dietetic.—Omission of food which leaves a residue (roughage) to stimulate peristalsis, *e.g.* oatmeal, wholemeal bread, fruit, and vegetables ; poor food or food insufficient in quantity ; deficient intake of fluid : change in quality of drinking water.

2. Deficient Peristalsis.—Sedentary habits; inattention to the calls of nature ; laxness of abdominal wall in neurasthenics, melancholics, the senile, the anæmic, the debilitated, women after pregnancies and convalescents after fevers or other diseases ; drugs—such as lead, opium, iron ; reflexly from uterine or ovarian disease.

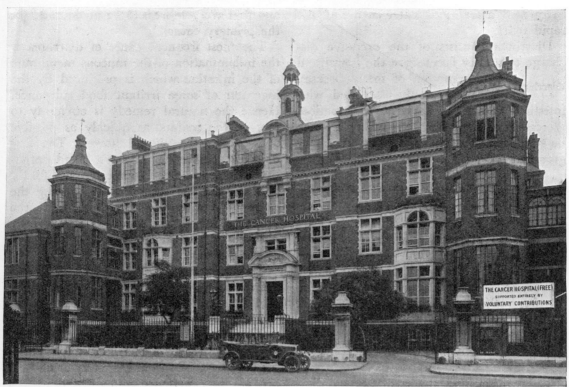

THE CANCER HOSPITAL
The hospital in Fulham Road, London, devoted to the prevention and treatment of cancer.

3. **Diminished Secretions.**—Excessive loss of fluid by skin or kidneys (diabetes) ; profuse vomiting ; deficiency of bile ; sluggish liver ; astringents—chalk, opium.

The symptoms which result from constipation are caused by auto-intoxication from fæcal stagnation. These include languor, depression, dyspepsia, headache, and skin eruptions.

The atonic overloaded bowel along with the lax abdominal muscles causes a drooping of loops of the intestine and results in bending or " kinking." This leads to further delay in the passage of the bowel contents (stasis) ; microbic life flourishes, and a profound toxæmia follows.

Treatment is entirely dependent upon the causal factors. The general methods include inculcation of good habits, exercise, massage, electricity, baths, and special dieting.*

*See Section on " Nutrition."

Intestinal Colic. Irregular and spasmodic contraction of the intestines gives rise to abdominal pain referred to as " colic." It is generally due to some irritant or indigestible material in the bowel (food or drugs) ; it may also be caused by fæcal masses in constipation or by gaseous distension from decomposition of the intestinal contents. Colic is an important symptom in certain bowel diseases, notably enteritis, dysentery, appendicitis, intussusception and cancerous stricture. In lead poisoning, colic is a common symptom : it is probably caused by the poisoned nerves.

The pain varies from slight spasms to severe and almost unbearable paroxysms which cause collapse. Treatment naturally depends on the causal factors. Colic is a symptom—not a disease. In ordinary cases of colic due to irritants, an efficacious purge —a full dose of castor oil—is necessary to clear out the bowel. Hot fomentations or a linseed poultice help to relieve the pain.

Frequently a soap and water enema affords rapid relief.

Diarrhœa consists of the excessive discharge of watery fæces from the bowel and is a symptom of many diseases. It is commonly associated with intestinal catarrh. As with constipation, the causes of diarrhœa are many : they may be summarised into primary and secondary groups.

Diarrhœa.

PRIMARY DIARRHŒA.—*Dietetic*—Ingestion of Irritants. *Poisons*—Mercury, arsenic, ptomaines. *Climatic*—Chill, sudden heat. *Nervous*—Hysteria. *Bacterial*—Infections.

SECONDARY DIARRHŒA.—*Infective Diseases* —Typhoid, dysentery, cholera, pyæmia, septicæmia, tuberculosis. *Chronic Circulatory Disorders*—Heart, lung, and liver disease. *Terminal conditions*—in nephritis, pernicious anæmia, and cancer.

(*For Diarrhœa in Children—see special section*).

Before discussing the treatment of diarrhœa, it is necessary to emphasise that this condition is merely a symptom common to a number of diseases and is in no sense to be regarded as a disease *per se*. Although diarrhœa frequently is evidence of some trivial indisposition, yet the possibility of its association with a grave complaint renders it a symptom which must never be regarded lightly. It is to be remembered that it is a principle of curative medicine never to treat a symptom without first endeavouring to investigate and treat the underlying cause. If this principle is lost sight of, much harm may be done, for a relieved symptom creates a false feeling of security and, the disease progressing under cover, valuable time and opportunity may be lost. For example, to stop the diarrhœa of a tuberculous enteritis by means of opium and bismuth and, ignorant of the fundamental disease, to imagine the sufferer is cured, is to court disaster.

Treatment of Diarrhœa.

Nevertheless, diarrhœa, as an inconvenient and distressing symptom, requires to be dealt with—always provided it is realised that it is the outward sign of inward disorder and that every effort is to be made to detect the primary cause.

The most frequent cause of diarrhœa is the inflammation of the mucous membrane of the intestine which is produced by the ingestion of some irritant food substance. Hence the natural remedy is obviously to remove the irritant as quickly as possible and to rest the injured bowel. The first object is achieved by giving a bland purgative such as castor oil (one tablespoonful for adults), and the second by restricting the sufferer to a purely fluid diet until the inflammation has subsided as revealed by absence of pain and diminished frequency of the motions.

Certain persons are peculiarly liable to diarrhœa from apparently trivial causes, and in such cases careful revision of the dietary becomes necessary. As a rule, the sufferer is aware of the offending foods and is able to limit his diet accordingly. Those who have suffered from dysentery or cholera are apt to experience attacks of diarrhœa on slight provocation such as exposure to cold or indulging in certain unwonted foods or varieties of alcoholic beverages. To avoid attacks such individuals should elaborate their own hygiene of food, drink, exercise, and clothing—a process of self-education.

When diarrhœa is fully realised to be a symptom, and the underlying cause is being dealt with, then it becomes necessary to check the condition, and this is generally accomplished by the administration of astringent drugs such as ipecacuanhæ, kino, chalk, or opium. An excellent pharmacopœcial preparation is pulvis cretæ aromaticus cum opio, which is given in doses ranging from 10-40 grains. Where ulceration is present, as in dysentery, rectal injections (enemata) of starch and laudanum or of silver nitrate solution are often given, but their effect depends upon the accessibility of the site of the lesion.

Diet is naturally of first importance in the control of diarrhœa—no matter the cause. In the acute stages barley water or milk with soda or lime water are indicated. Milk possesses mildly astringent qualities, and therefore is peculiarly suitable in the treatment of diarrhœa. As soon as the diarrhœa shows signs of abating—but not till then—eggs, arrowroot, or other milk puddings may be given and later white fish or chicken. The usual or average diet must be reached by careful and gradual additions, otherwise relapses are liable to occur and delay the ultimate cure.

Diarrhœa in children requires careful investigation, and treatment varies with the nature of each case. Care should be taken to detect any error in diet and the possibility of milk contamination should always be kept in mind. Most cases benefit by a mild dose of castor oil.

Enteritis. Inflammation of the intestines is most commonly caused by the ingestion of irritants, *e.g.* unripe fruit, decomposing meat or arsenic. Chill may give rise to a mild attack. During the course of acute fevers, such as pneumonia or influenza, it is often present. Chronic forms occur in Bright's disease, cirrhosis of the liver and heart disease.

The prominent symptom is diarrhœa; this is associated with abdominal pain usually of a colicky nature. Nausea and vomiting may occur. Thirst is suffered from, and the degree of fever is indicative of the severity of the inflammation. In severe cases blood and mucus are present in the motions.

In treatment it is best to commence with the removal of any possible irritant by a dose of castor oil. Rest in bed is necessary and fomentations may be required to relieve

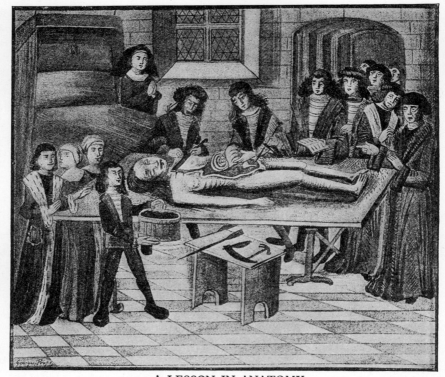

A LESSON IN ANATOMY
A quaint mediæval picture of a dissection of the abdomen in progress.

abdominal pain. Patients should be starved for a couple of days; this gives rest to the inflamed intestine. Later, diet should be restricted to milk, beef-tea, and chicken jelly.

Ulceration of the intestine may occur in tuberculosis, dysentery, typhoid, and cancer. Diarrhœa is common in all cases, and the motions contain blood, mucus, pus, and shreds of membrane; they are often very offensive. In ulcerative conditions there is always the danger of hæmorrhage or perforation and peritonitis.

Appendicitis. Inflammation of the vermiform appendix varies in degree and extent. Slight inflammation limited to the appendix gives rise to colicky pains—appendicular colic—and is often associated with a dyspepsia of reflex origin. It is frequently due to a small fæcal concretion blocking the lumen of the tube and is related to constipation. The appendix and the adjacent peritoneum become chronically inflamed, and at any time an acute attack may supervene. Severe inflammation may go on to suppuration or gangrene, and the appendix becomes the centre of an abscess ; local peritonitis may become general and constitute a serious menace to life.

An attack of appendicitis usually comes on suddenly. Acute pain is experienced in the abdomen ; it is first felt in the region of the umbilicus, but later it settles down in the right lower abdominal region. It causes the sufferer to lie on his back with his legs drawn up. It is associated with marked localised tenderness. Nausea is experienced, and

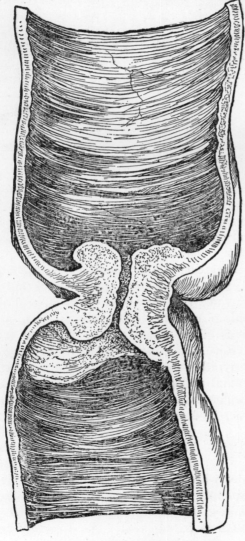

CANCER OF THE INTESTINE
A section of the colon showing the obstruction due to a cancerous stricture, with consequent distension of the bowel above.

vomiting often occurs. There is moderate fever and the pulse is rapid.

In a number of cases these symptoms prevail for a few days and then subside ; when the inflammation is severe and suppuration takes place, local and constitutional symptoms are intensified. Unless operation is immediately performed and the abscess evacuated, death may occur with startling suddenness.

Unnecessary risks should not be taken with cases of appendicitis ; operation at the earliest moment is desirable. Pending operation, the patient should be kept in bed with the pelvis lower than the rest of the body. No aperients or enemata should be administered. Only water is allowed by the mouth.

Intestinal obstruction or stoppage of the bowels may be " acute " when the canal is
Intestinal suddenly and completely blocked ;
Obstruc- or " chronic " when it is narrowed
tion. gradually.

Obstruction may be due to causes external to the bowel such as pressure from tumours of neighbouring organs ; or it may result from compression by bands of tissue produced by chronic peritonitis. A coil of intestine may twist round itself and kink, the condition being known as " volvulus." " Intussusception " or the invagination of one part of the bowel into another is a common cause in children. Within the bowel, a tumour or the contracting scar of an old ulcer may lead to constriction and eventual obstruction. Impacted fæces, gallstones, or foreign bodies may result in blockage. Strangulation of a knuckle of bowel in a hernial sac is a frequent cause in adults.

In acute obstruction there is severe abdominal pain associated with copious constant vomiting—firstly of stomach contents —then of bile, and lastly of fæces. There is a degree of collapse ; temperature is subnormal ; pulse rapid and feeble ; skin cold and clammy. Constipation is absolute after a few hours. Later, there is abdominal distension and tenderness.

In chronic obstruction, the symptoms are

similar but milder and extend over weeks or months. The abdomen becomes greatly distended. At any time an acute obstruction may supervene.

As there is a mechanical defect, operation without delay is the only possible method of treatment.

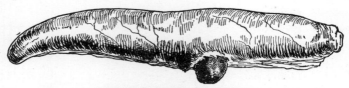

A PERFORATED APPENDIX
A highly dangerous development which may occur in the acute stage of appendicitis. Immediate operation is imperative.

THE PREVENTION OF CONSTIPATION

By ALFRED C. JORDAN, C.B.E., B.A., M.D., B.Ch., D.M.R.E., M.R.C.P., late Medical Radiographer to Guy's Hospital and the Royal Hospital for Diseases of the Chest.

CONSTIPATION is the cause of untold suffering and disease and the curse of civilisation. Man is the only constipated animal—if we except man's companions—the dog and the cat. If any one doubts the prevalence of constipation, let him reflect upon the fortunes that have been made by the sale of purgatives. Not all mankind is constipated. Some of the Indian hill tribes are not ; moreover, these tribes are far healthier than civilised races, and they are free from the digestive troubles that are rife among all civilised peoples. Not only are their digestions good, but they are spared the serious diseases which follow upon digestive disorder, among them appendicitis, gastric ulcer, duodenal ulcer, gall-stones, and cancer.

The amenities of our civilisation have become essential to our happiness ; we cannot return to barbarism. Must we regard chronic disease as the inevitable penalty of civilisation, or can we change our habits in some particulars so as to keep our bodies healthy while we continue to develop our mental and communal activities ? Does our choice lie between healthy savagery and unhealthy culture ? Fortunately not. In the first place an unhealthy body means a poisoned brain, an impaired memory, and an inability to concentrate. "A sane mind needs a healthy body." This is proverbial, and medical science confirms its truth.

Price of Civilisation.

I shall endeavour to show that the body can be kept healthy without sacrificing any essential of civilised culture. Why has civilisation brought disease in its track ? Because it has led to the adoption of faulty habits. Study the way of living of the Indian hill tribes. Their life is spent in the fields, actively engaged in agricultural and other open-air pursuits which involve energetic exercise. Their food is produced by their own labour. No tinned, bottled, or preserved food reaches them ; no packets from factories. They live on fresh grains and pulses, fruits, nuts, eggs, greens, and milk. Meat is an occasional luxury, for it is not often that they can afford to kill a lamb or a kid.

Some tribes are debarred by religion from eating meat. Corn is coarsely ground and made into cakes with water ; these are rapidly browned on both sides over a fire. The children have no sweetmeats ; they get all the sugar they want or need from ripe fruits and from the sugar cane which they munch. They can chew it all day without getting more sugar than is contained in an ordinary lump, and with it they swallow a quantity of vegetable fibre (which makes valuable " roughage "), and a lot of saliva which helps to digest the sugar. These tribesmen furnish practical proof of the way the bowels ought to act, for their bowels act three or four times daily and the motions are soft.

There are wide areas of rural Britain where it would be quite easy to imitate the habits and diet of healthy tribes. People must be persuaded to give up factory-made foods and drinks and subsist on the natural foods provided by their own toil and skill. There is need for a large-scale exodus from the overcrowded towns to the land, where there is room for many

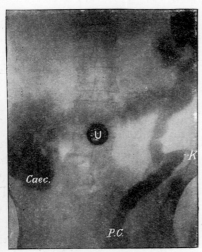

A KINKED INTESTINE

An X-ray of the whole of the large intestine showing obstruction due to a sharp kink (K). Cæc.—cæcum; P.C.—pelvic colon; U—umbilicus.

thousands of workers to produce the natural foods the nation needs.

Good housing and welfare work must accompany the trek to the land, while the millions who remain in the towns will benefit by an increased and cheapened supply of fresh natural foods. These millions of townsfolks must no longer be allowed to fill the hospitals with diseases that might be prevented. They must be kept healthy. So far as the Health Authorities are concerned, everything possible is done in a most efficient and successful way to keep down epidemic and acute diseases, but chronic diseases are more rife than ever, especially rheumatism, digestive troubles, and cancer.

People must be taught how to live so as to steer clear of digestive troubles and all their crippling consequences. How is it to be done? First and foremost, the digestive organs must be got into a healthy state and maintained in active function. What do we mean by active function? The usual reply is : " A visit to the closet once daily." The example of the healthy natives shows the insufficiency of this standard. If we eat three full meals daily, but eliminate waste matter only once, the result must be accumulation and stagnation of waste material, in a word, constipation.

Constipation is a deadly thing, for stag-

nation means putrefaction. Foul waste matters injure the bowel which contains them, and poison the entire system. Those who eat three meals daily should get rid of waste matters thrice daily. As Dr. Leonard Williams puts it, " we must make way for the increment by discharging the excrement." How is it to be done ? *Not* by taking purgative drugs. The habitual use of drugs is dangerous and should only be practised under medical supervision. This may seem an exaggeration, but I maintain it with conviction born of experience. The proper way to restore the bowel to healthy function is to restore its walls to a healthy state by ensuring that it contains no decomposing matters. The large intestine must then be re-educated to respond to the call of the full bowel. The time for the bowels to act is after meals ; this is proved by physiological experiment.

Reform in this matter must commence from the cradle. A healthy infant is a savage ! It gets rid of its waste at frequent intervals. Throughout the nursing period all would be well, but, unluckily for the little creature,

Infants First.

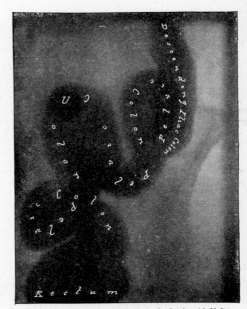

["*Chronic Intestinal Stasis*," *A. C. Jordan* (*O.U.P.*)]

THREATENED OBSTRUCTION

The pelvic colon, very greatly elongated, has formed three complete loops, any one of which may kink and cause acute obstruction.

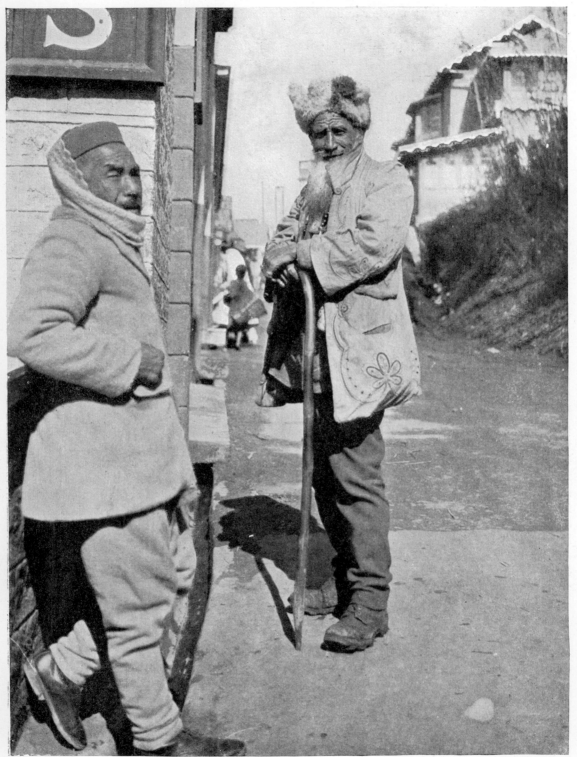

[W. F. Taylor.

A STALWART RACE
Tribesmen of the Indian hill country where, owing to the open-air life and fresh, simple diet, digestive troubles
are unknown.

509

it has to be " civilised " ; mother and nurse lavish loving devotion to the sacred task of rendering the darling constipated ! It is a dirty little darling if it soils its napkins ; it must be educated ! There is a right way to carry out this education, viz., to " hold out " the child after each feed ; but, too often, the misdirected ambition of the attendant ministers is to reduce the number of evacuations to the deadly civilised ideal of one daily.

Next comes the fateful day in a child's life when he is promoted to the water closet —an apparatus constructed with an hygienic ideal in view, but without the least consideration for physiological requirements— even for grown people. As for a small child, he is made to balance dangerously on the edge of a vast crater, poised high above the ground, with legs dangling so that they can give no support to the abdomen. While he was still allowed to use the pot-de-chambre, he was, at any rate, in a natural squatting posture, with thighs raised to help the abdominal muscles.

Then comes school, and " civilisation " reaches the decisive phase of rigid subjection to discipline and convention. Some of the biggest and most exclusive of the public schools are so meagrely equipped with sanitary conveniences that it is impossible for all boys to visit the closet even once daily, while a boy who often asks to " leave the room " is regarded with suspicion and displeasure. Recently I was told by a dyspeptic patient that he attributed his years of suffering to his school days. The lavatories were in a basement infested with huge sewer-rats which terrified him so that he would pass days in the greatest discomfort from a full bowel rather than face the horrors of the dark, dank basement.

After school comes, for most men, an office or a factory, and too often convenience or expediency is allowed to come before physiological righteousness.

To summarise this part of the subject of constipation :—(1) At all ages a visit to the lavatory is due after each meal.

(2) A natural " squatting " attitude should be assumed for the purpose ; a child can do so by using a " chamber " ; a grown up must improve upon the ordinary closet by placing a stool on either side so as to raise his feet, or by installing some form of adjustable foot-rest. This is a temporary expedient ; the proper course is to reform the construction of water-closets.

How should a man conduct his life so that his three daily visits to the lavatory shall not be paid in vain ? Firstly and chiefly by his diet ; secondly, by " exercise." The food which contains the vitamins and salts needed to keep the tissues healthy is also the food which remains " sweet " in the intestines, so that it does not injure the bowel-wall or produce poisons which injure the system. This food contains enough insoluble " roughage " to stimulate the bowel to healthy activity without producing the slightest irritant action.

Diet and Regime.

Man's digestive apparatus was meant, by Nature, to deal with natural foods. Cooking, is, after all, a new thing in the evolution of the human race—merely a matter of a few thousand years. Man's tastes have altered, but his stomach and intestines have remained as they were. Man must revert to natural, uncooked foods ; he must relegate cooked foods to the position of luxuries, to be indulged sparingly now and then.

As a concession it may be allowed that some foods (*e.g.*, eggs) do not suffer much change by careful cooking and may be classed with the natural foods. Quite briefly, the foods to take are dairy produce, including milk, butter, cream, cheese, eggs ; garden produce, such as potatoes and greens, especially raw greens and salads ; ripe fruits and nuts ; grains and pulses. Bread should be wholemeal, made of coarsely-ground wheat, with fresh yeast to make it rise. White flour and white bread should be abolished. Puddings should be given up in favour of fresh fruit or fresh fruit salad and cream. Potatoes should be cooked in their jackets ; green vegetables should be steamed, not boiled.

At every meal, fresh raw garden produce should be taken ; there is plenty of variety —lettuce, radishes, cucumber, tomatoes,

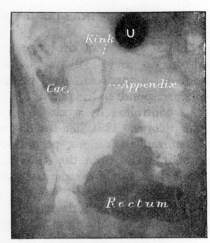

A KINKED APPENDIX
An X-ray photograph in which the appendix is revealed in its full length, with a pronounced kink.

celery, chicory, endives, batavian, mustard-and-cress, and many others. Fresh fish is permissible in moderate amount ; meat is not necessary for perfect health, and nobody is entitled to eat meat unless he is able to "work it off" promptly by vigorous open-air exercise. If meat or poultry is eaten it should be young and fresh and cooked no more than need be. Excess of sugar is to be avoided, especially in the popular form of sweetmeats and chocolates, too often indulged in freely between meals. Honey is an excellent natural sugar food—vastly to be preferred to jam and marmalade.

Meals should be moderate in amount, well-spaced through the day, and eaten slowly to allow of sufficient mastication. Between meals the stomach should be allowed complete rest from food.

The best drink is water ; it should be taken at bed-time and on rising ; also between meals. Little drink should be taken during meals ; food should be thoroughly masticated, never "washed down."

Most native races spend many hours a day in the practice of dances and exercises.

Exercise. Undoubtedly they improve their health and condition immensely by this means. Obviously, any one who tried to persuade civilised men and women, actively engaged all day in working for a living, to imitate the life of the natives

in respect of dances would meet with complete failure. There are, at the present time, thousands of young people who spend many hours of the night dancing, but, unfortunately, our dances have no hygienic value and are carried on in unhygienic rooms and in unsuitable attire.

While conceding that it is not possible for us to hold hygienic dances as the natives do, it is, nevertheless, perfectly feasible to spend a few minutes—night and morning—in exercises in the bedroom or the bathroom. The exercises should not be strenuous or fatiguing. They should start with a few ordinary limb and bending exercises to loosen the joints, but most of the time should be devoted to the muscles of the trunk and the abdomen. When possible (too seldom, alas ! in this country) the exercises should be carried out in the open air or at a wide open window in sunshine.

Week-ends and holidays should be spent in the open air and in the sun as far as possible. As regards attire, the most suitable holiday wear for men is the increasingly popular open-fronted flannel shirt, flannel "shorts," and shoes. Girls, also, are finding out the best attire, which is loose and allows free air-entry.

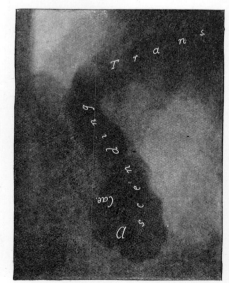

["*Chronic Intestinal Stasis,*" A. C. Jordan, (O.U.P.)]
A RESULT OF CONSTIPATION
An X-ray photograph taken after a bismuth meal to show the displaced cæcum doubled back behind the ascending colon.

HUMAN SANITATION

By Sir W. ARBUTHNOT LANE, Bart., C.B., M.S., F.R.C.S.

THE sanitary arrangements in dwelling-houses are more or less familiar to all. There is the pan of the water-closet whose effluent is controlled by a flap, the contents of which are discharged from the pan into a syphon trap, from which they are carried by a long pipe into the cesspool in the area. The cesspool discharges its surplus into a drain in the street. When the contents of the pan of the closet are evacuated by pulling up the plug, an amount of material corresponding in quantity is discharged automatically from the cesspool into the main drain.

Any block to the discharge of material from the cesspool to the drain in the street, if sufficient, is followed by a corresponding over-distension of the cesspool and an accumulation of material in the house drain and in the syphon trap. In consequence of this stagnation, material accumulates in the pan of the closet, and if it is allowed to remain for some time the fæcal matter ferments, decomposes and evolves offensive

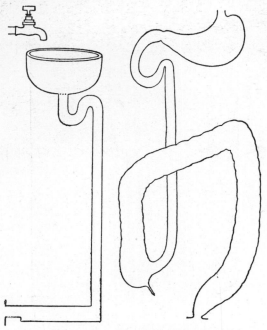

THE HUMAN DRAINAGE SYSTEM

A comparison between the drainage scheme of a house (left) and the gastro-intestinal tract.

gases, dangerous to the health of the people in the house.

The human system of drainage is constructed on an almost identical pattern. The stomach, a muscular bag, practically a pump, corresponds to the pan of the closet. Its exit is controlled by a circular muscle called the pylorus. This, like the flap in the closet in normal conditions, permits of the passage of material from the stomach into the syphon trap, but prevents its regurgitation. The commencement of the small intestine, which corresponds to the house drain, is arranged in the form of a syphon trap precisely similar to that in the house, so that the passage of material through it shall be delayed to allow of the secretions of the liver and pancreas being diffused through it. This human syphon trap is called the duodenum. As the contents of the syphon trap escape they enter a long coil of small intestine which corresponds to the house drain. This discharges into the large bowel or colon, the effluent of the small intestine being controlled by a muscle and valvular arrangement which, while permitting of the discharge of the matter in the small bowel at intervals, in normal conditions prevents any regurgitation of the contents of the colon or human cesspool.

The material as it enters the colon is of a fluid consistence, and it is carried through its length till it forms a puddle of porridge-like consistence above the circular muscle, called the sphincter, which controls the orifice. The presence of the fluid or pasty material in this situation sets up a reflex which results in its expulsion. If, however, this reflex has been controlled by habit and education, material is delayed for an excessive time in the colon, its fluid contents being absorbed into the circulation and leaving a firm mass or even a hard lump. In proportion as this mass becomes deprived of its fluid contents, so its capacity to stimulate the muscle coat of the bowel to propel it along its length diminishes, and the tendency to set up the reflex action of evacuation becomes less and less marked. Just as in the case of the drain in the house, the

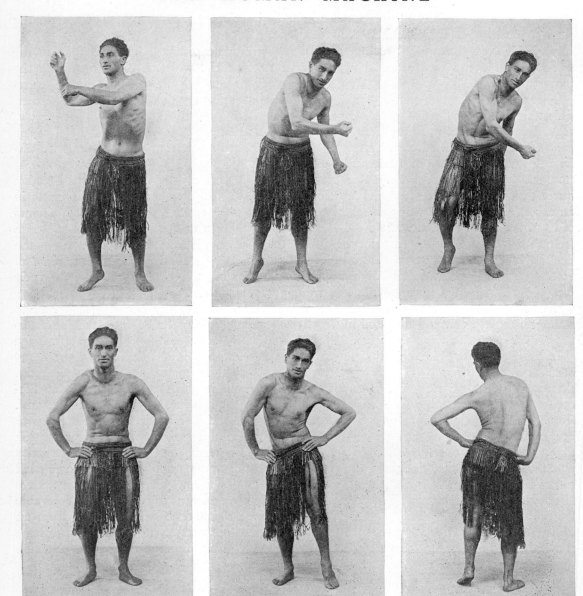

Courtesy]   ["*Native Exercise,*" *E. A. Rout (Mrs. E. A. Hornibrook) Heinemann.*

NATIVE DANCES—A FINE NATURAL EXERCISE

Two Maori dances which form excellent exercises for strengthening the abdominal and pelvic muscles and stimulating the organs of digestion and excretion. Movements of rotation, swinging, contraction and expansion are included. *Above:* The paddle dance in three positions. *Below:* The hura dance, front and side contractions and back view.

stagnation and accumulation of material in the cesspool or large bowel is followed by a damming back of the fluid contents of the small bowel, whose weight is increased in proportion to its bulk. The strain exerted upon the end of the human syphon trap or duodenum by the overburdened heavy small intestine results in the kinking of the bowel at this point, since, unlike the solid drain in the house, it is of a soft consistence and is readily kinked.

The effluent from the duodenum or syphon trap being controlled in this way, and material continuing to be pumped into it from the stomach, it becomes over-distended, and its mucous lining gorges with blood over the area of greatest strain. Later this surface bleeds, becomes abraded and then ulcerated. This ulcer may become so deep as to perforate the wall of the bowel and may cause death.

These ulcers do not persist for a long time, since the pylorus, which prevents regurgitation, after a time becomes spasmodically contracted and ceases to permit of the forcible expulsion of the contents of the stomach into the duodenum. The consequent over-distension of the stomach throws an excessive strain on the mucous membrane of its upper part and about the muscle controlling its effluent, so that it, as in the duodenum, bleeds, becomes abraded and ulcerates. If nothing is done by surgical or medical treatment to meet the mechanical condition which exists, the ulcer remains, and, after a time, it serves as an excellent soil in which the cancer germ can live and thrive.

In a normal state of health any deleterious organisms swallowed with the food are destroyed by the gastric juice, so that those contents of the stomach which are expelled from it into the duodenum or syphon trap are sterile. The food material is further digested by secretions formed by the liver, pancreas and mucous lining of the small intestine, and from this is absorbed into the circulation such constituents as are required for the nutrition of the body. Before being utilised for this purpose they are treated by the cells in the liver and modified so that they can be carried safely through the circulation.

Any waste products which remain in the fluid material which is discharged into the colon or cesspool are acted on by innumerable organisms which break up the residues, and, being deprived to a varying extent of their fluid components, are carried along the length of the large bowel and are discharged.

While this represents the normal action of the gastro-intestinal tract as it exists in robust native races, living in their normal surroundings, and eating the food to which they have always been accustomed, the process is greatly modified in the case of numbers of civilised communities, to their great detriment.

While a native mother suckles her child it evacuates from its bowel a motion automatically after each feed, the drainage scheme of the infant exhibiting the same mechanical sequence as the house drain. This habit is perpetuated through the lifetime of the individual by means of diet and exercise, and is regarded by the natives as of most vital importance to the preservation of their strength and vigour and capacity to lead the strenuous life their condition requires of them. Therefore, these natives never suffer from any of the innumerable diseases which result mechanically from an acquired obstruction of the drainage scheme in civilisation, the most terrible of which is cancer.

THE PREVENTION OF APPENDICITIS

By Sir W. ARBUTHNOT LANE, Bart., C.B., M.S., F.R.C.S.

THAT appendicitis is become more and more frequent is patent from the large number of operations that are being performed for this condition. To most of the public the affection is only realised when they complain of a more or less severe abdominal pain, with associated symptoms, as vomiting, etc., when they may be told that an operation is called for without delay, or, if the case

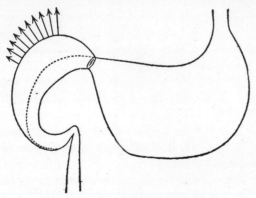

THE HUMAN SYPHON TRAP

The stomach and duodenum, showing how stress is exerted upon the latter when its end is kinked. The dotted line represents its normal outer margin.

is not so urgent, that one should be performed as soon as is conveniently possible.

The vast majority of people have no idea what the appendix is, what part it plays **Disease of Civilisation.** in the physiology and anatomy of the individual, what appendicitis really is, and what conditions cause it to develop. They recognise that it is quite a common disease in civilised life, and are surprised to learn that it never exists among nations living on the same simple food eaten by their ancestors for thousands of years and following the same habits common to them and all animals existing in a state of nature. A doctor who had lived for thirty-four years in South Africa among the natives, who up to that time had avoided the contamination and consequent physical and moral deterioration which follows so rapidly upon association with the white man, assured the writer that he never saw one case of appendicitis in a native race during the whole of that period. He said that as the native got into the employ of the white population he rapidly imitated their food and habits and developed their gastro-intestinal diseases, among which appendicitis is conspicuous, since it suddenly imperils the life of the sufferer and calls for prompt surgical measures for its eradication.

The appendix is a structure exactly like a worm in appearance and varies from **Structure.** two to three, four, or five inches in length. It is a tube which is lined by mucous membrane which secretes a glairy (viscous) fluid. This tube opens into the commencement of the large bowel near the aperture through which the contents of the small intestine are discharged into the big bowel. The contents of the small intestine which run into the large bowel consist of food from which almost all the nutrient materials have been extracted. These residues are broken up by organisms in the large bowel which plays the part of a destructor and cesspool.

If the contents of the large bowel are not discharged at sufficiently frequent intervals they collect in the whole length of this

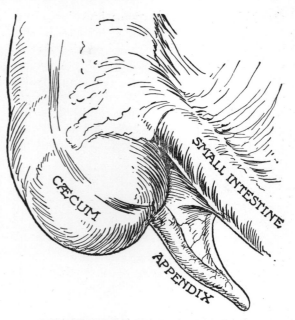

THE POSITION OF THE APPENDIX
The appendix, a useless relic of man's earlier structure, issues from the cæcum at its junction with the small intestine.

bowel and decompose and irritate its mucous lining membrane, producing an inflamed **Colitis.** condition which is called *colitis*. This infection or inflammation of the mucous lining of the large bowel readily extends to the lining of the appendix which opens directly into it, and may result in a blocking of its opening into the bowel, because of the swelling and engorgement of its mucous inner coat. Even solid masses may form concretions in it which are too large to escape from it. Either the pressing of the solid fæcal mass in its interior, or the tension resulting from the drawing back and accumulation of its secretions in it may cause tension and inflammation of the entire tube. This may vary in degree, from a state of engorgement or slight inflammation, to such a condition of acute inflammation as may bring about gangrene or perforation of the appendix. Both these calamities call for immediate operation, while the milder degrees of inflammation may pass unnoticed and be regarded merely as stomach ache.

Since the risks involved in every form of appendicitis may be serious, a medical man should be consulted at once when abdominal pain and tenderness are experienced, and no attempt should be made on the part of parents or friends to control the condition by purgative or other medicine before seeking expert advice. Too often a purgative is administered with the result that the poisonous contents which have escaped from the appendix are distributed broadcast

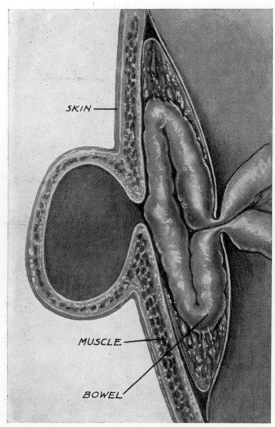

A STRANGULATED HERNIA

Showing one of the dangers of trying to reduce a strangulated hernia without operative treatment ; the protruding loop of bowel has been forced back through the abdominal muscles, but is still constricted by the peritoneum.

through the entire abdomen, when the risk of death is very great. In no condition is surgical treatment called for more urgently or is followed by greater benefit than it is in appendicitis, since the patient may be snatched from certain death.

The prevention of appendicitis is on all fours with that of all the other conditions which result directly or indirectly from constipation, such as adenoids and large tonsils, etc. *The bowel should be evacuated at a reasonable period after each meal,* and the usually accepted idea that it is necessary to accumulate the products of twenty-four hours' digestion and to allow it to putrefy in the big bowel, to irritate and inflame its mucous lining and to poison the body by the absorption from it, or from material dammed back by it in the small bowel, of filth, is obsolete.

Prevention.

There is nothing new in this, it is merely the fact that we have ceased to follow the diet and habits of our early ancestors. Hippocrates over two thousand years ago insisted—and he impressed this in very plain terms on the Greeks—upon the vital importance of eating correct foods and having an evacuation after every meal. With us a single daily motion is merely a habit, a very bad one and largely a matter of convenience to our fellow creatures as well as to ourselves. We are all so busy. One cannot insist too strongly on the utterly disgraceful disparity of water closets to boys in the large majority of schools, and on the totally insufficient time afforded for their use. This is a crying evil and must be met, not only by the children's parents, but by the community in general. We must alter our diet and habits in such a manner as to ensure health at all costs, unless we are prepared to pay the penalty of debility, disease, and premature death.

As far as appendicitis is concerned, let the public remember that the mode of its prevention rests entirely with them.

HERNIA

By GEORGE SOMERVILLE, M.D., D.P.M., Deputy Medical Superintendent to the West Ham Mental Hospital.

HERNIA is the term applied to the protrusion of any organ or part of an organ into or through the wall of the cavity in which it is naturally contained. Although hernias of the lung and of the brain do occur, they are relatively infrequent and the word is commonly used to signify an escape from the

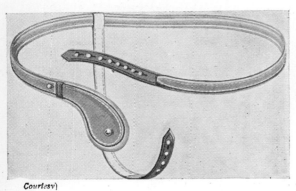

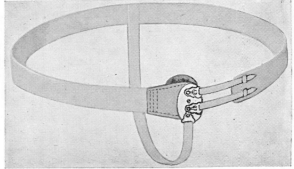

Courtesy)   *[John Bell & Croyden.*

FOR THE RELIEF OF HERNIA

The truss, a mechanical device used when operative measures are inadvisable, varies in form with the type of hernia to be treated. On the left is a truss for femoral hernia, and on the right an elastic band truss.

abdominal cavity of some part of the intestine or its appendages.

In certain parts of the abdominal wall, especially in the groin region, there are weak spots through which a knuckle of bowel is liable to be forced as a result of straining. These weak spots are natural openings, namely, the "inguinal canal" through which the testicle descends in fœtal life and which transmits the spermatic cord; the "femoral canal" which lies parallel with and on the inner side of the great femoral vessels as they pass out of the abdomen into the thigh. The region of the umbilicus and the vicinity of an operation scar are also structurally weak spots, and hernias are of common occurrence there.

Accordingly, abdominal hernias are described as "inguinal," "femoral," "umbilical," and "ventral."

Umbilical and inguinal hernias may exist at birth, and are then described as "congenital." In the case of an inguinal variety, the hernia descends along with the testicle towards the scrotum; it is commonly associated with mal-descent of the testicles.

A hernia may make its appearance suddenly following some very violent muscular effort, but more commonly it develops gradually. Occasional pain or a dragging sensation is experienced in the region of the hernia, and it is often accompanied by a peculiar feeling of weakness. A soft rounded swelling appears which, when the patient

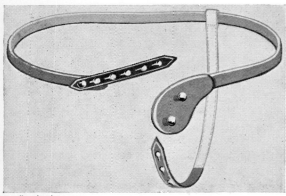

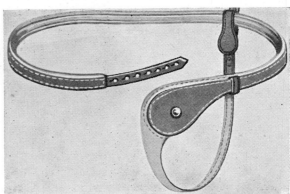

Courtesy]   *[John Bell & Croyden.*

TWO TYPICAL TRUSSES

A truss consists of a supporting belt or spring and a pad to cover the hernial opening. *Left :* A bath truss covered in celluloid ; *Right :* A truss for advanced inguinal hernia, with a stout spring in the belt, and a cork pad covered with chamois leather.

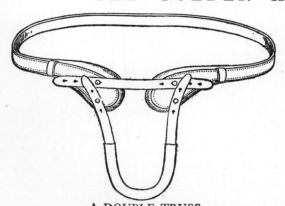

A DOUBLE TRUSS
Although there is a pad for both sides, this type of truss is often worn for a one-sided hernia, especially by stout people.

strains or coughs, presents an expansile impulse known as the " impulse on coughing."

In the early stages, as a rule, the swelling can be made to disappear by pressure over it and it is described as a " reducible hernia." At any time, either from a sudden increase in bulk of the hernia or as a result of the formation of adhesions, the hernia may be unable to be returned to the abdominal cavity and it is then known as an " irreducible hernia." Irreducibility is a constant source of danger. The portion of bowel may become compressed by the sides of the aperture through which it has escaped, and consequently the circulation of the blood is seriously impeded. The hernia is then said to be " strangulated " and it involves serious risks to life because of bowel obstruction or infective complications (peritonitis). Urgent symptoms supervene. Pain is acute and is attended by sweating, a feeling of coldness and prostration, followed by nausea and vomiting which may become fæcal. The symptoms are essentially those of intestinal obstruction. If the condition is not relieved by immediate surgical operation, it rapidly proves fatal.

Inguinal hernia is by far the commonest variety of hernia ; it occurs most frequently in men, and tends to descend along the spermatic cord into the scrotum. Femoral hernia is the next commonest form and it occurs most frequently in women. Umbilical hernia occurs in children, usually

appearing some weeks after birth, and in adults—chiefly corpulent women who have borne numerous children. Ventral hernias occur in any part of the abdominal wall that is the seat of a scar resulting from a wound or from suppuration. It is apt to follow too short a period of rest in the recumbent position after operation.

In the treatment of hernia the choice lies between the use of a mechanical support or " truss " which will control the hernia, and an operation designed to repair and strengthen the abdominal wall. In children and in adults who wish to live an active life recourse to operation is advisable in the majority of cases. In the elderly, the advisability of operation depends on whether the hernia can be adequately controlled by a truss and upon the general physical condition. A threatening or actual strangulation renders an operation absolutely necessary in order to preserve life.

Trusses vary in form according to the hernial opening they are destined to control, but essentially a truss consists of a supporting belt or spring and a pad to cover the opening.

Hernial Trusses.

In inguinal trusses, a stout spring contained in a belt encircles the pelvis, and the pad, made of cork covered with chamois leather, through which the force of the spring is transmitted, guards the inguinal ring and upper part of the inguinal canal, and thus restrains the intestine or omentum within the abdominal cavity. Such a truss should restrain the hernia under all circumstances and should be perfectly comfortable. To give satisfactory service a truss should be light and yet strong, should fit accurately, and the pad should remain in position in all movements. Too light a pressure on the part of the spring will mean that the truss will fail to retain the hernia ; too heavy a pressure causes discomfort and enlarges the hernial opening by leading to a wasting of the muscle of the abdominal wall.

Hence, in measuring for a truss it is of first importance that accurate figures are obtained and it is advisable that at first the truss should be applied and tested by the surgeon. The truss is usually placed in position when the patient is recumbent in bed (assuming that the hernia is reduced—within the abdominal cavity) and the pad should be made to exert pressure in an upward and backward direction. So long as the sufferer is in the erect posture the truss should be worn, though it may be discarded when he goes to bed at night, unless chronic coughing necessitates its constant application.

A double truss, having a pad for both sides, may be worn for a one-sided hernia for the reason that such a truss usually sits more comfortably and can be worn without understraps ; thus they are advisable in stout persons. Vulcanite, lacquered metal, or other waterproof material may be used in the construction of trusses for bathing ; those who perspire profusely may prefer them for general use—they are also convenient for children.

Femoral trusses are constructed similarly to the inguinal variety. The spring belt may encircle the pelvis on the same side as the hernia or on the other side (when it is known as an "opposite-sided" truss). Should difficulty arise in controlling the hernia the pressure of the pad may be rendered more efficient by attaching it to a thigh piece which can be laced on the outer aspect of the thigh. It is to be noted, however, that any form of femoral truss interferes with the freedom of movement of the limb and is an irksome handicap.

Ventral trusses for the control of umbilical and ventral hernias consist of an abdominal belt provided with a large, round, or oval, flattened vulcanite or aluminium shield which should widely overlap the hernial opening. Such trusses require to be specially constructed and adapted to each particular case.

Regarding trusses in the treatment of hernia, it must be emphasised that they are only palliative measures : they do *not* cure hernias—they control them and prevent their becoming worse. The use of an effective truss lessens the liability to a surgical emergency such as strangulation, though it does not entirely exclude such a happening. In otherwise healthy adults treatment of hernia by a radical operation (simple and without risk) is the sole and only satisfactory method of obtaining relief and cure.

DISEASES OF THE RECTUM AND ANUS

THE terminal segment of the bowel, the rectum, is subject to a variety of diseases, minor and grave, partly because it forms the place of lodgment of the fæces prior to evacuation and is therefore subject to considerable irritation, and partly because it is exposed to harmful external influences.

The commonest deformity of the anus is the absence of an opening due to its occlusion by a thin, fibrous membrane. It is found in newly-born infants, and, if unrelieved, symptoms of peritonitis ensue and death follows.

Malformations.

Occasionally, from an error in embryonic development, communications may exist between the rectum and the vagina, the bladder, or urethra. As a rule there is no urgency for treatment and operation may be delayed until the child is old enough to stand the strain.

From the nature of its contents, the rectum is especially exposed to bacterial infection, and this is accentuated by the irritation produced by hard masses of fæces, foreign bodies, intestinal parasites, or by the use of drastic purgatives or enemata.

Inflammation.

Ulceration is a common sequel to the various forms of inflammation of the rectum (proctitis), but is particularly liable to follow dysenteric and tubercular inflammations of the bowel and may sometimes arise during the course of gonorrhœa and syphilis.

All the varieties of ulceration occur in middle life and are more frequent in women than in men. The patient complains of a feeling of weight and heat in the bowel, of pains radiating to the loins and a constant painful desire to empty the bowel (tenesmus). The motions are thin, watery, contain much mucus, and may be tinged with blood. The skin around the anus becomes irritated by the discharge and is excoriated and

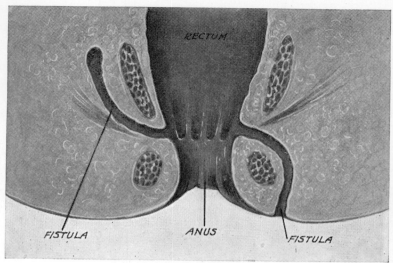

FISTULA OF THE ANUS

A section showing the interior of the rectum and anus with a fistula on each side. Occurring as the result of an abscess, a fistula is an abnormal channel which passes through the tissues in the vicinity of the rectum and anus.

to walk. A hot, red, and tender swelling develops on one side of the anus. Should the abscess burst, the symptoms abate rapidly. Poultices or other local applications are of little avail; free incision, as early as possible is the best method of treatment.

FISTULÆ, as already indicated, are a common sequel to suppuration in the vicinity of the rectum. They represent the irregular and tortuous tracks of abscesses making their way to the surface and which are prevented from healing owing to imperfect drainage or the reinfection of the raw surfaces by the passage of the fæces. Fistula is often associated with tubercular infection. Pain is continually suffered; the bowels are loose and thin fæces escape from the openings uncontrolled. A state of mental depression is apt to ensue. Treatment of fistula is surgical; the whole length of the track must be freely laid open and the wound allowed to heal slowly from its deepest part.

ANAL FISSURE is the term applied to a small irritable ulcer or abrasion at the lower end of the anal canal. It is a condition found in adult life and is more prevalent in women than in men. The characteristic symptom is an intense cutting or tearing pain accompanied by spasm during and after defecation. In severe cases the pain may be more or less continuous. The motions are often streaked with blood and there may be difficulty in passing water. Fissure is commonly associated with piles, fistula, polypus, or other rectal affections.

In the treatment of slight cases, the careful regulation of the bowels with special attention to personal cleanliness and the use of vaseline before an action of the bowels may result in cure. In more severe cases a minor

painful. If the ulcer be very chronic, it may lead to a narrowing and obstruction of the bowel (stricture) which necessitates operative measures. Treatment is directed to removing the cause if possible. Hot hip baths and enemata of starch and opium give relief. The bowels should be moved regularly by means of some bland aperient such as liquid paraffin. Ulcers may require surgical excision.

Suppurative processes are common in the region of the rectum and anus. In most cases, a localised abscess forms in
Abscesses. the cellular tissue at the side of the rectum and the pus usually finds its way to the nearest skin or mucous surface, producing irregular sinuses or fistulæ. Injury, mechanical irritation, exposure to cold or wet or other debilitating influences predispose to such suppurations. They often arise during the late stages of tuberculosis.

Superficial abscesses give rise to itching and throbbing pain aggravated by sitting or defecating. The parts are very tender to touch. Deep abscesses (ischio-rectal) are associated with more severe symptoms. There may be shivering fits with marked constitutional disorder. The pain is aching and throbbing, and the patient is unable

surgical operation is advisable; the ulcer is excised or scraped.

In pruritis ani there is intense and persistent itching in the vicinity of the anus associated with an excoriated, moistened, and thickened state of the skin. Itching is a symptom of many rectal affections including worms, piles, fistula, fissure, and eczema. It is fairly common in subjects of gout and diabetes. Occasionally it is of nervous origin. The irritation may be incessant, is worst at night, and prevents sleep. The discomfort may produce marked mental irritability and depression, and may render life unbearable. In treatment any local or general disease must be attacked. Scrupulous cleanliness must be adopted and the parts kept dry by an antiseptic dusting powder. All stimulants and dietetic condiments should be avoided. Exposure to X-rays may be beneficial when other remedies fail.

Pruritis Ani.

"Piles" or "hæmorrhoids" is the term applied to a varicose and often inflamed condition of the veins at the lower end of the rectum and anal canal. Two varieties are described: "internal piles," which originate in the lower part of the bowel and anal canal which is covered by mucous membrane; and "external piles," which occur in that part of the anal canal which is lined by skin. Frequently both varieties co-exist and are described as "mixed piles."

Hæmorrhoids (Piles).

Many factors contribute to the production of piles. They are apt to develop in middle-aged people who live a sedentary life—over-indulge their appetites, and who suffer from habitual constipation. Any cause of "straining" such as enlarged prostate, urethral stricture, or stone in the bladder is liable to induce congestion and overfilling of the hæmorrhoidal veins which, it should be noted, are not provided with valves. It must be realised also that, in a number of cases, piles may merely be evidence of any morbid condition which produces backward pressure in the venous circulation. Thus they commonly complicate heart and liver disease, and the pressure of abdominal

tumours, and of the pregnant uterus, acts in the same way. (Piles are of frequent occurrence during pregnancy, but generally pass off on its termination).

External piles may exist for years and cause little trouble other than an occasional burning sensation when a costive motion is passed. Examination of the part reveals a bluish cushion-like ring round the orifice of the anus and a turgescence of the veins is visible when the patient strains. In consequence of chill or injury they may become inflamed; they become enlarged, very tender, red, and give off a thin blood-stained discharge; they may even suppurate. Such an "attack of piles" subsides within a week, but is apt to recur.

Internal piles vary in degree. They may remain within the anal orifice and only occasion slight bleeding; they may form distinct fleshy masses which are protruded during defecation and give rise to a continuous oozing of blood with a discharge of mucus and to considerable pain; they may

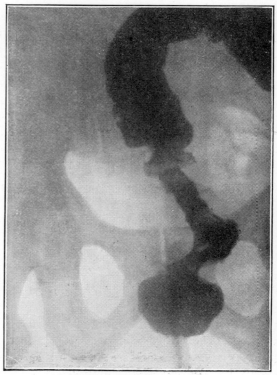

TUMOUR OF THE RECTUM
An X-ray photograph of the rectum revealing obstruction due to malignant tumour.

remain protruded—can only be returned with difficulty, if at all, and cause a profuse discharge of mucus which is associated with pruritis ani. As a result of the loss of blood, a serious anæmia may result ; such sufferers exhibit a clay-like pallor and are apt to become irritable, anxious, or depressed. Periodically internal piles may become the seat of an acute inflammation ; the extruded mass becomes swollen, red, and painful ; it may be so tightly grasped by the sphincter that " strangulation " occurs and the piles may suppurate and slough off. This occurrence is accompanied by severe pain and constitutional disorder.

In the treatment of piles, palliative measures should be adopted in the first instance. The bowels should be carefully regulated by the use of bland aperients such as liquid paraffin or castor oil. Drastic purges must be avoided. The diet should be simple and include plenty of fruit and vegetables ; alcohol is prohibited. Locally, scrupulous cleanliness is essential. Defecation may be rendered easier by lubricating the passage before the act with vaseline or by the injection of an ounce of olive oil. Sponging the perineum with cold water after defecation is useful in toning up the rectal muscles. If the piles come " down " and are inflamed, a hot hip bath followed by a morphine suppository will give relief. Should these measures fail and the patient continues to lose blood and becomes very anæmic, surgical interference is necessary. The piles are excised or cauterised.

In prolapse of the rectum a portion of the rectum is protruded beyond the anal margin. It is fairly common in weakly children after exhausting illnesses, and in elderly women who have suffered some injury to the pelvic floor as a result of childbirth. Prolapse of the bowel is liable to develop in any condition which induces straining, such as constipation, diarrhœa, worms, polypus, or phimosis. Violent coughing, as in whooping cough, may determine prolapse in a weakly child. A fold of bright red mucous membrane is protruded, usually after evacuation of the bowels, which at first can easily be returned but which later becomes more and more difficult to reduce.

Prolapse of the Rectum.

In treatment, any irritable condition of the bowel or other exciting cause of straining must be corrected. The child should be made to defecate while lying on the back, and should always rest after the act. Reduction is effected by raising the pelvis, smearing the prolapse with vaseline, and applying gentle pressure over it. A soft pad should be worn to restrain subsequent descent. Attention to the general health is necessary. In adults, as a rule, operative measures are necessary to effect a cure.

Innocent tumours, adenomata or polypi, may arise in the rectal mucous membrane ; they are sometimes traceable to the local irritation produced by worms. They are usually single, but in children may be multiple. Polypi give rise to pain, tenesmus, bleeding, and itching ; the constant straining frequently induces prolapse, especially in children. Their removal is a simple surgical operation.

Tumours.

Malignant disease of the rectum is fairly common. It is a disease of adult life and is of equally frequent occurrence in the two sexes. The tumour commences in the mucous membrane and gradually infiltrates the other coats of the rectum, invading neighbouring organs and setting up secondary growths. Ulceration associated with bacterial infection is apt to occur on the free surface and causes a characteristic offensive slimy blood-stained discharge which is usually the first symptom of the condition. Later there is a gradually increasing difficulty in obtaining a regular action of the bowels. Attacks of constipation may alternate with attacks of diarrhœa. Tenesmus or painful desire to go to stool is nearly always present, but actual pain does not occur till late in the disease. There is gradual failure of health revealed in emaciation and general weakness. As a rule the tumour can be palpated by digital examination.

Cancer of the Rectum.

In early cases, where the disease is confined to the bowel and there is no indication of secondary growths, a radical operation (assisted by exposure to radium) is the only measure to be adopted. When it is impossible to eradicate the disease surgically, relief may be afforded and life prolonged by " colostomy," an operation in which an artificial opening is made in the bowel above the tumour so that the fæces are discharged from that point and prevented from irritating and infecting the cancer.

DISEASES OF THE LIVER AND GALL BLADDER

JAUNDICE is a condition characterised by a yellow coloration of the skin and mucous membranes due to some hindrance to the normal outflow of bile.

Jaundice.

It originates most frequently from some obstruction of the bile-duct; the bile is unable to escape into the intestine in the usual way but is absorbed directly into the blood stream. A common cause is the extension of a catarrhal inflammation of the stomach and duodenum to the opening of the bile-duct. The flow of bile is obstructed and a transient attack of jaundice results. Foreign bodies, gall-stones, worms, or cancerous stricture may similarly block the duct, or pressure from tumours of neighbouring organs may cause a narrowing of the passage. Compression of the fine ducts within the liver by fibrous tissue—as in " cirrhosis "—is likewise a cause of chronic jaundice.

In the commonest type, *i.e.* " catarrhal jaundice," there is generally a history of some dietetic indiscretion. Dyspeptic symptoms are followed by the yellow pigmentation of the skin and mucous membranes. The colour varies from a pale yellow to a deep olive or bronze. It is associated with severe itching. The motions are clay-coloured and offensive in smell; constipation is usual. The urine is greenish-brown in colour. The pulse is slow; temperature sub-normal. Drowsiness, lassitude, depression, or irritability are common mental accompaniments.

Simple catarrhal jaundice clears up in a few days. Naturally, the causal gastritis must be relieved. Careful dieting and a dose of calomel, followed by a saline purge are helpful remedies; the skin irritation may be allayed by warm soda baths.

Intermittent attacks of jaundice are suggestive of gall-stone obstruction; a gradually progressive chronic jaundice is most often seen in relation to malignant disease (cancer). In these cases careful medical investigation is essential. It should be clearly understood that jaundice is a symptom and not a disease.

A degree of jaundice may also occur in various toxic states such as pernicious anæmia, malaria, typhoid, and yellow fevers, phosphorus and arsenical poisonings. It depends on the rapid destruction of the red cells of the blood associated with a disorganisation of liver function so that the bile is not excreted into the ducts but is absorbed directly into the blood stream.

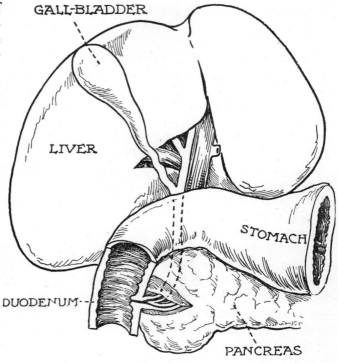

THE LIVER AND GALL BLADDER
The liver rests on the stomach and duodenum, and the gall bladder lies on its under surface.

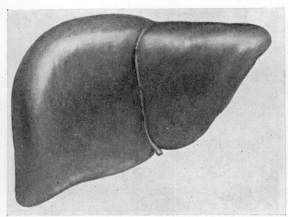 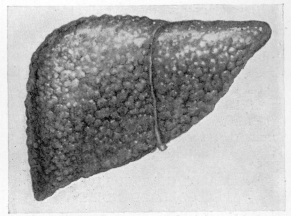

A WELL-KNOWN LIVER DISEASE

In cirrhosis, or " hobnail " liver, the organ shrinks and its surface becomes nodulated. *Left :* normal liver ;
Right : a liver in cirrhosis.

Inflammation of the gall-bladder is apt to occur in those who lead an indolent or sedentary life—in those who eat too much and exercise too little.

Gall-stones. Stagnation of the bile results : the pigments are deposited, producing " bile sand " and the subsequent irritation along with migrated organisms from the intestinal tract cause an inflammatory catarrh. The bile sand, rendered cohesive by the thick mucus, collects in small masses and eventually gall-stones are formed.

In acute catarrh of the gall-bladder, pain and tenderness are experienced under the ribs on the right side. A slight variable degree of jaundice is commonly associated. In chronic catarrh the general health is poor ; severe dyspepsia is suffered from, and " bilious attacks " are of frequent occurrence.

The presence of stones in the gall-bladder is not necessarily attended by symptoms or signs. As a rule, however, recurring attacks of pain with vomiting—" bilious attacks "— are apt to occur. The symptoms are those of chronic gall-bladder inflammation with periodic acute exacerbations.

Should a stone be forced through the narrow bile-duct towards the intestine, spasm of the muscle in the wall of the tube is set up (unless the stone is a very small one) and agonising pain—" biliary colic "— is experienced. This may be so severe as to cause collapse. Later, owing to the bile-duct obstruction, jaundice sets in and per-sists until the stone is forced into the intestine or is removed by operative measures.

Strict adherence to the hygienic laws of diet and exercise is the main principle of treatment and prevention. Meals should be simple, easily digested, and should contain a minimum of meat protein. Water in large quantities should be taken, and the bowels should be regulated with frequent saline purges and an occasional more powerful purgative such as calomel. Systematic exercise and massage are beneficial. Spa treatment is of value.

For an attack of colic a hot bath or hot fomentations may give relief : if very severe the doctor may be required to give an injection of morphia.

Gall-stones in the gall-bladder are insoluble. If they are quiescent, operation is not indicated ; if repeated attacks of biliary colic occur, or if there is complete obstruction of the bile duct with progressive jaundice, an operation, in which the gall-bladder is opened, cleaned out and drained, is of vital necessity.

Cirrhosis of the liver is a disease in which the vital secretory cells degenerate and are replaced by a passive fibrous tissue.

Cirrhosis. It is caused by a great variety of toxins or irritants, and chief among these is alcohol. Malaria and syphilis are also important causal factors.

The disease occurs in middle-life, and men are more frequently affected than women.

THE HUMAN MACHINE

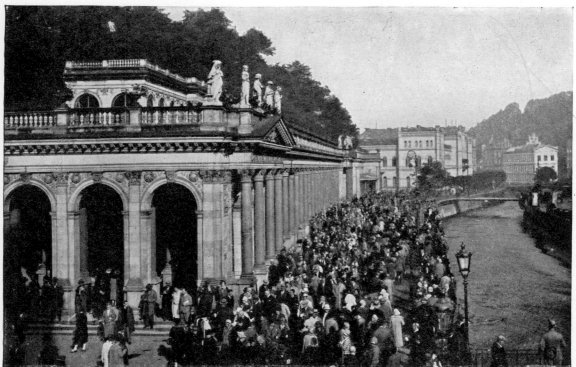

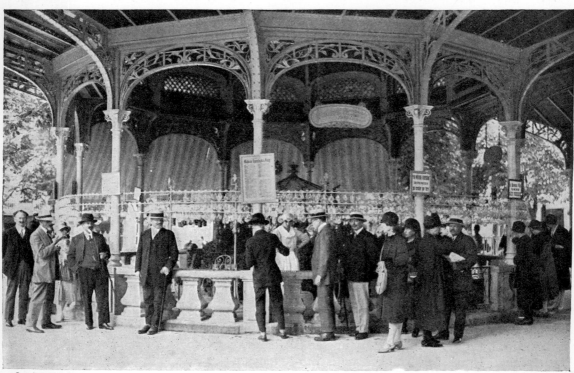

TAKING THE CURE

Drinking the waters at Karlsbad, Czechoslovakia (*above*) and at Vichy, France, two spas specially noted for the cure of liver complaints.

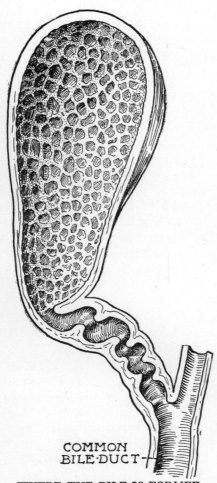

COMMON
BILE-DUCT

WHERE THE BILE IS FORMED
The interior of the gall-bladder and the bile-duct, the blocking of which gives rise to jaundice and "bilious attacks."

In the early stages of the disease the liver may be enlarged, but later it is markedly diminished. It becomes hard and small; the surface is nodulated—hence it is known as "hobnail" or "gin-drinker's" liver. The fibrous tissue compresses the blood vessels and dropsy results.

The onset of cirrhosis of the liver is insidious. The early symptoms are those of chronic gastritis; later, dropsy of the abdomen develops and bleeding from the stomach is apt to occur. The spleen is enlarged, and a slight degree of jaundice is nearly always present. The disease is progressive, and towards the terminal stages a restless delirium and coma supervene and death rapidly follows.

The outlook in cirrhosis of the liver is always unfavourable. Once the secretory cells have been destroyed they cannot be regenerated. In treatment the causal poison must be eliminated. The associated chronic gastritis must be relieved by dieting; regulation of the bowels by saline purges reduces the tendency to dropsy. Careful personal hygiene is essential.

DISEASES OF THE PANCREAS

Owing to the inaccessible position of the pancreas and the impossibility of examining its secretion, the detection of pancreatic disease presents considerable difficulty.

Acute inflammation, a rapidly fatal condition, is fortunately comparatively rare. Chronic inflammation may be associated with chronic disease of the gall-bladder. It leads to a failure of digestion and to deterioration of the general health. Vague pains and tenderness are experienced in the upper abdomen.

Degeneration of the "Islands of Langerhans," as already mentioned, leads to the occurrence of diabetes. Abscesses, tumours, and cysts occur in the pancreas as in any other organ.

DISEASES OF THE PERITONEUM

Peritonitis, or inflammation of the investing membrane of the abdominal and pelvic cavities and their contained organs, may be acute or chronic, localised or diffused. The extent and character of the peritonitis vary with the causal conditions.

Peritonitis.

ACUTE DIFFUSE PERITONITIS is usually caused by the lodgment within the abdominal cavity of micro-organisms. These include the colon bacillus, the streptococcus, the staphylococcus, the gonococcus, and the pneumococcus. Frequently there is a mixed infection.

Infection may originate in any of the organs covered by or adjacent to the peritoneum—or organisms may gain entrance through wounds. Among conditions of the gastro-intestinal tract which frequently result in peritonitis are appendicitis (first in frequency), perforating ulcer of the stomach, duodenum, and intestine, foreign bodies ulcerating through the bowel, and various forms of enteritis. Abscesses, or any form of suppuration, in the liver, gall-bladder, pancreas, uterus, and Fallopian tubes (in relation to childbirth) may spread to the peritoneum and produce a serious septic inflammation. In certain cases it is probable that the infection originates from the blood stream (septicæmia), as in the pneumococcal and staphylococcal forms.

The symptoms of acute peritonitis are usually superadded to those of the primary disease, but rapidly overshadow them. The patient complains of abdominal pain of a peculiarly severe and sickening character, accompanied by great tenderness. This pain is usually most severe over the organ from which the infection has originated. The face is pale, drawn, and has an anxious expression. The sufferer lies on his back with the knees drawn up in an endeavour to relax the abdominal muscles which are rigidly contracted. Respiration is rapid, shallow, and solely thoracic (the abdominal muscles take no part in it as in health). In the early stages the pulse is rapid, and though the temperature may be raised in the later stages, it becomes subnormal. Vomiting is seldom absent, and in severe inflammations it is continuous and persistent. The abdomen becomes distended by the formation of gases within the bowel and this further adds to the patient's distress.

As the inflammation spreads, the toxic symptoms become more and more marked. The pulse becomes small and running ; the face pinched and clammy ; the abdomen very distended. Collapse takes place, and death rapidly follows. The disease usually lasts four or five days, but, when the peritonitis is due to perforation, as in gastrric or duodenal ulcer, fatal collapse may set in within twenty-four hours. The puerperal form is very deadly ; it is generally accompanied by a septicæmia.

Should recovery take place the general toxic symptoms improve before the local. The physical signs gradually disappear or may become localised in the form of a circumscribed abscess. The outlook in cases of acute peritonitis is always very grave, and depends on the virulence of the infection, the strength of the patient, and the success of treatment.

Surgical operation is indicated in most cases of acute peritonitis with the object of attending to the condition from which the infection originated. The earlier this is carried out, the better are the chances of recovery. Pending operative measures the patient should lie recumbent on his back, with a pillow beneath the knees to bend the thighs and relax the abdominal muscles. An ice-bag may be applied to the abdomen

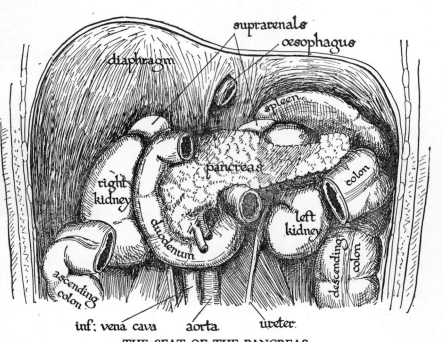

THE SEAT OF THE PANCREAS
A section of the abdomen, showing the inaccessible position of the pancreas.

to relieve the pain. Only fluid should be given by the mouth.

In localised forms of acute peritonitis adhesions form and limit the spread of the inflammation. Should the tissues overcome the organisms any inflammatory exudate is absorbed and recovery ensues ; but if the exudate becomes purulent, a circumscribed abscess is formed. The symptoms are similar to those of diffuse peritonitis but less severe. If abscess formation occurs, a defined swelling forms in the region of the organ affected. At any time the abscess may rupture into the general peritoneal cavity and give rise to an acute diffuse peritonitis. The only rational treatment is operative, with the object of allowing the pus to escape.

GONOCOCCAL PERITONITIS may occur as a sequel to gonorrhœa, and is met with chiefly in females. The infection spreads from the Fallopian tubes and the peritonitis may be limited to the pelvis. Although the symptoms are severe at first they soon abate and recovery is usual. Operation is not always indicated.

PNEUMOCOCCAL PERITONITIS occurs chiefly in female children between the ages of five and fifteen. It may be subsequent to pneumonia, pleurisy, or meningitis. The onset is very acute and is attended by rigors, persistent vomiting, severe pain, and sometimes convulsions. Natural recovery may occur, but it is usually necessary to open the abdomen and establish drainage.

CHRONIC PERITONITIS may arise in syphilitic and actino-mycotic infections, but is most commonly of tubercular origin, being secondary to tuberculosis of the bones, joints, glands, or bowels. Long-continued inflammations in certain abdominal organs may also give rise to a chronic peritonitis which, by the formations of adhesions and bands, may cause kinking, twisting, or strangulation of the intestine and so endanger life.

TUBERCULAR PERITONITIS is most common in children and young adults, and seldom exists as an independent disease. Infection spreads to the peritoneum either by way of the blood stream or the lymphatics. There may be considerable exudation of fluid (tubercular ascites), or it may exist as a dry form associated with adhesions and matting of the organs. The symptoms are abdominal pain and distension with the usual evidence of tubercular toxæmia, fever, emaciation, and loss of strength. Treatment is that which is generally applied to cases of tuberculosis. Inunction of a mercury ointment into the abdomen has been found to be beneficial. Improvement after operative treatment is often remarkable.

Cancer. Primary malignant disease (cancer) may occur in the peritoneum, but more commonly it is the seat of secondary growths derived from the stomach, intestine, or ovary.

THE HYGIENE OF THE DIGESTIVE SYSTEM

The hygiene of the digestive system includes the care of the mouth and teeth ; the science of dietetics ; the regulation of bowel function ; and the art of physical culture.*

It must be emphasised that of all the diseases to which human flesh is heir, those related to the digestive system are the most preventable, yet at the same time they are the most prevalent. It is a sad reflection that those diseases whose origins are understood and whose onset can be avoided should account for so large a proportion of human suffering.

Civilisation imposes on the majority of people artificial habits of diet, and the consequences are disastrous to health. The human engine will not run smoothly and efficiently on low grade fuel, but will become clogged ; and not only will the running be impeded, but the life of the machine will be materially shortened.

Colonel M'Carrison's pregnant words should ever be kept in mind : ". . . For myself, I work on more and more amazed, day by day, by the extraordinary effect of faulty food on the human organism. I begin to think that faulty nutrition is the bed-rock cause of the vast majority of tissue ailments."

* See section on Exercise.

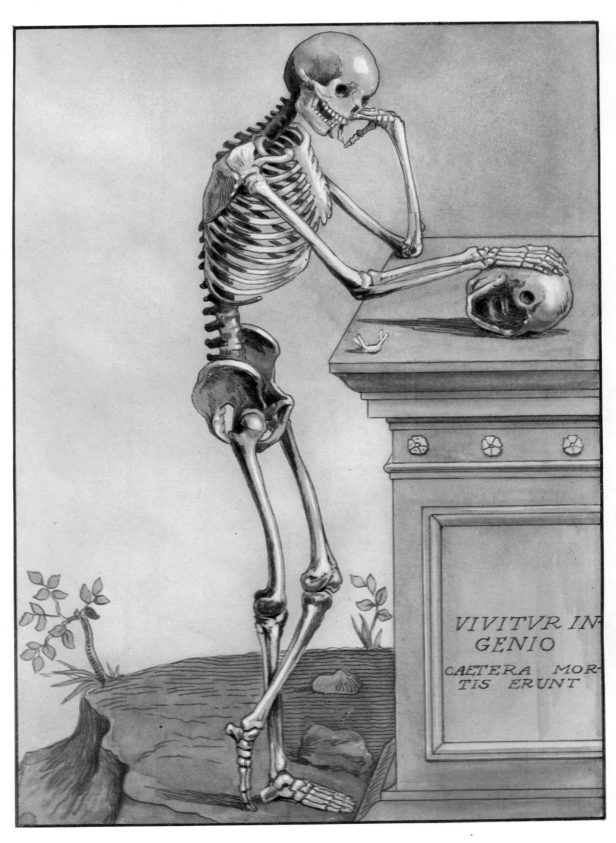

VIVITVR IN
GENIO
CAETERA MOR-
TIS ERUNT

THE HUMAN SKELETON.

From an engraving in a work by Vesalius (1543)—a beautifully and dramatically posed figure of remarkable
anatomical accuracy.

THE TEETH

THE STRUCTURE OF THE TEETH

By W. H. HORNIBROOK, F.R.C.S., L.R.C.P., D.P.H. (Irel.), Late Medical Officer of Health, Mackenzie County, New Zealand.

ADULT man should have thirty-two teeth in his mouth. The infant at birth is toothless, but the teeth are there waiting to erupt at their proper dates. In childhood the mouth is provided with twenty teeth, divided thus : on each side from the central line backwards are two incisor teeth, one canine, and two molars. The number is the same in both jaws.

The main structure of a tooth consists of dentine or ivory, which is a softer material than enamel but harder than bone ; hence arises the necessity for the skin or crusta on the outside of the root in order to afford a better attachment to the periosteum which lines the recess in the jaw occupied by the tooth. The exposed part above the gum is covered with a thin coating of enamel which is thickest on the grinding surface, but becomes thinner or worn off by use. The surface of the root of the tooth is clothed with a thin bony layer (crusta petrosa) in the same manner as the crown of the tooth is clothed with the enamel.

The interior of the tooth is hollow, and contains a mass of blood vessels and nerves which act as a sensory organ and provide the nutriment for the tooth itself. This is effected by filtration of fluid through minute canals existing in the dentine. The part above the gum is called the crown, the part within the jaw bone (alveolus) the root, the narrow area dividing the two the neck.

The teeth have special names ; thus, the eight central teeth are called incisors, they are chisel-edged and are designed for biting food. The four canines are longer than the incisors and pointed. In carnivorous animals they are well developed. The twelve molars have their surfaces divided into cusps, and are thus adapted to the grinding of food.

The temporary, or milk teeth, are smaller than the permanent ones and are twenty in number. That is to say, there are eight incisors, four canines, and eight molars. They appear in the lower jaw a little earlier than in the upper. The dates of their eruption are approximately as follows :—

Lower Central Incisors - -	8-10 months.
Lower Lateral Incisors and	
First Molars - - -	15-21 ,,
Canine - - - -	16-20 ,,
Second Molars - - -	20-24 ,,

The permanent teeth erupt at the following periods, the lower jaw again having the precedence :—

First Molars - - -	6th Year.
Two Central Incisors - -	7th ,,
Two Lateral Incisors - -	8th ,,
First pre-Molars - -	9th ,,
Second pre-Molars - -	10th ,,
Canines - - -	11th to 12th Year.
Second Molars - -	12th to 13th ,,
Third Molars - -	17th to 25th ,,

The temporary teeth begin to fall out at the sixth year, when the first of the permanent teeth erupts. During the eruption

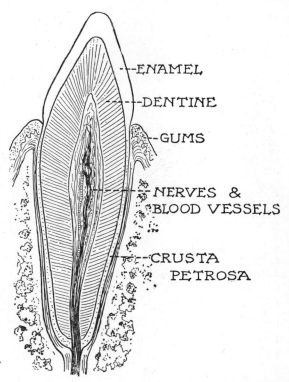

A HEALTHY TOOTH IN SECTION
The tooth draws its nutriment from the blood vessels through minute canals in the dentine.

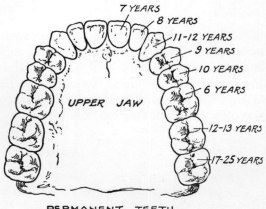

7 YEARS
8 YEARS
11-12 YEARS
9 YEARS
10 YEARS
6 YEARS

UPPER JAW

12-13 YEARS

17-25 YEARS

PERMANENT TEETH

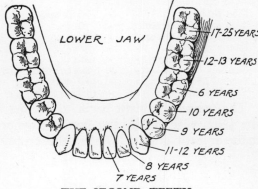

LOWER JAW

17-25 YEARS
12-13 YEARS
6 YEARS
10 YEARS
9 YEARS
11-12 YEARS
8 YEARS
7 YEARS

THE SECOND TEETH
Indicating the age periods at which second teeth
normally appear.

of the teeth, change is occurring not only in the jaw but in the whole constitution. Some of the disturbances of infancy are aggravated by the eruption of the teeth and the physiological processes in connection with it ; but to this common natural phenomenon has been attributed by the popular mind nearly every ailment of childhood.

DENTAL DISEASES AND THEIR PREVENTION

By C. BOWDLER HENRY, M.R.C.S., L.R.C.P., L.D.S., Surgeon-Dentist to the West-minster Hospital.

THE tenet that " prevention is better than cure " applies more forcibly to diseases of the teeth than to almost any other human ailment. To be effective, however, prevention in the first place must be instituted very early in life, as early indeed as the suckling infant. Secondly, it should be borne in mind that no cure, no technical device or operation, which the dental surgeon has yet devised, can approximate to the perfection of Nature. The ideal, which we should strive to develop and maintain in each individual of the community, is that of a normal set of teeth, each one healthy and unblemished, all placed in a normal relationship to one another and supported by healthy gum and bone.

"A clean tooth will not decay." Dental decay is never seen upon those smoother surfaces of a tooth which are exposed to the cleaning action of the lips and tongue and the tooth brush, and no doubt, were it possible to ensure that the many and complicated surfaces of the teeth were always as clean as the front surfaces of, say, the lower incisor teeth, dental decay would be a disease of the past, even with our present day tooth-destroying diet.

The Carious Cavity.

Dental decay is brought about through the agency of stagnation of the sugary and starchy foods in the various crannies around the teeth. Wherever these foods stagnate in the mouth, fermentation quickly sets in. The acid which is formed dissolves its way into the tooth in exactly the same way as acid dissolves chalk. A carious cavity may not be formed at once, but the surface of the hard protecting substance, which we call enamel, is damaged. Its surface, formerly smooth, is eroded and roughened, and the stagnation of food upon it is facilitated. Further fermentation and acid formation with resultant destruction take place, until a cavity is produced.

This is the beginning of the end. Decay proceeds rapidly under cover of the enamel, spreading out in all directions—the " nerve," technically and more correctly described as the " pulp "—the little vascular, exquisitely sensitive organ inside the tooth which is nourished by it, becomes infected and forthwith dies. Its decomposition is followed by putrefaction, and the poisons which are formed escape partly into the mouth, whence they are carried down with the saliva and food into the bowel ; but, more seriously still, the remainder penetrate through the fang into the bone around the tooth and thence directly into the blood stream, by which they are carried to all the vital tissues of the body.

In these circumstances the best that can happen is that an acute abscess should form, necessitating attention to or even **Germs in the Bone.** the removal of the offending tooth. Even then the hostile germs, which have gained entrance into the bone, are not eliminated. It depends upon the health of the individual at the time, and subsequently, whether these germs are removed from the bone. If the defensive mechanism of the body is good, the residual germs are destroyed once their source, the infected tooth, has been removed. If weak, then these germs may linger in the bone for years, still producing poisons, which now have no escape, save, from the patient's point of view, the worst possible—that is, directly into the blood stream.

If a cavity in the tooth be discovered early enough, the decay can be removed and the hole filled in with stopping material. The earlier the better. Every one, therefore, should visit his dental surgeon regularly, in order that the teeth may be examined. Small cavities in out-of-the-way places are perceptible only upon close scrutiny, even by the trained eye, and in the early stages cause no twinges of pain. And it is in these same out-of-the-way places that stagnation and cavity formation are most prone to occur.

The smaller the hole, and the more skilfully the operation of **Filling.** filling is performed, the more effectively is the tooth restored to its normal functional state ; but no one, least of all the dental surgeon,

would assert that a tooth, once it has been affected by decay, however beautifully it is filled, is so valuable to the individual as a healthy unblemished tooth.

Pyorrhœa creeps into a mouth so surreptitiously that it may have become deeply seated and have been in progress **Pyorrhœa.** for many years before the average individual detects anything abnormal. Pyorrhœa is a chronic disease, which manifests itself by a progressive destruction of the bone supporting the teeth. It is not a disease of the teeth themselves. If the jaw bone be likened to a piece of wood and the teeth to so many nails driven halfway into it, then pyorrhœa may be compared to a pest, which gets in by the side of the nail and gradually rots the wood around it until the nail becomes loose and falls out.

That teeth affected by pyorrhœa ultimately fall out is unimportant. The loss of a tooth or of a whole set of teeth is insignificant compared with the damage to the general health which is done during the process of loosening. The pity is that teeth

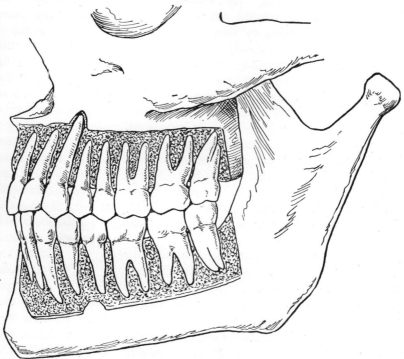

NORMAL TEETH IN THE JAW BONE
A dissection of the jaws showing the roots of the teeth in place.

so affected are not lost earlier. Unlike dental decay, which sooner or later gives rise to premonitory twinges of pain, pyorrhœa is entirely painless. In the last stages only, when an abscess may form under the affected tooth, is any real discomfort felt. To the uninstructed eye, the gums may appear normal in colour and outline, and there is even a subtle form of this disease, by no means rare, wherein even the skilled eye of the dental surgeon may detect nothing wrong. Yet an X-ray photograph of the bone may show considerable destruction around the roots of the teeth.

A small abscess forms on the end of a root of a dead tooth, or of a diseased tooth in which the nerve or pulp is dead, but it causes the patient no pain, soreness, or discomfort. There is no swelling, and neither the patient nor the dentist may know that there is an abscess there. Often the patient has beautiful bridgework, crowns, or fillings in his mouth and they cause him no distress or annoyance. Yet the abscess is constantly and insidiously supplying germs to the blood. They are sealed up in the bone. They cannot get out. They must go somewhere, so they find a way into the blood by slowly destroying the bone. At first there may be but a few of them. They may be members of a very weak family of germs. And the germ-destroying power of the blood kills them. But germs multiply very rapidly, and an ever-increasing army of them passes into the blood. This continues day after day and year after year, until the power of the blood to kill these germs becomes exhausted. Then the blood will sweep live, strong germs to a joint, in the fluid of which they multiply with exceeding rapidity.

The joint swells and becomes painful, the limbs are pulled into unnatural positions ; the joints become fixed. The patient has arthritis deformans, that strange disease which deforms the joints.

The physician may find no cause for the disease. He calls in the dentist and the X-ray, and they find these little abscesses on the ends of dead teeth. The same germs are found on the ends of the diseased teeth as are found in the joints, and to be safe, the abscesses must be destroyed.

These little abscesses are dangerous for another reason. They poison the nervous system. Small constant contributions of the germs found in these abscesses or the poisons the germs manufacture are distributed to the nervous system. Sometimes only a small group of nerves is affected, such as the nerves supplying the jaws, the ears, the eyes, the hands, or the arms. Sometimes it is the spinal cord, and sometimes the brain. One of the most frequent signs of this nerve poisoning is a prickly or numb feeling in the fingers, sometimes there is neuralgia, headache, fatigue and lassitude, or profound depression.

If this disease alone is to be checked it is essential that every member of society, from infancy upwards, should go at least once a year to his dental surgeon for examination and advice. The prevailing factors, which bring about the onset both of decay and of pyorrhœa, are much the same. Any factor which tends to lower the resistance of the teeth or the gums on the one hand, or on the other tends to promote the stagnation of food in the mouth, favours the onset of these diseases. Some of these factors are hereditary and are counteracted with great difficulty. One such is the proportionately diminishing size of our jaws, which is not accompanied by a proportionate reduction in the size or number of the teeth. The result of this is an inherent tendency in all of us to have crowded or irregular teeth, which are more difficult to keep clean than a perfectly regular set.

Mouth-breathing is a habit acquired usually as a result of nasal obstruction, the most common cause of which is **Mouth-breathing.** adenoids. If the adenoids become enlarged early in infancy and persist for more than a few weeks, the evil resulting from them in the dental health of the individual will remain throughout life. Normally, the upper jaw is slowly developed in size from birth until adult life is reached, in order to accommodate the increasing

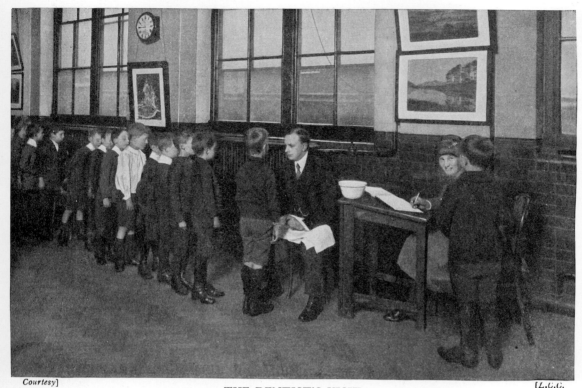

Courtesy]   [L.C.C.

THE DENTIST'S VISIT
Regular dental inspection—an essential measure for preserving healthy teeth—has been instituted in many schools.

number and size of the teeth which ultimately form the full complement of the adult set. The most active growth takes place between birth and the age of fifteen.

As the average person's jaw is racially too small for the teeth it has to support, it will readily be understood that any interference with its fullest development will lead to still further lack of accommodation for the teeth in their proper alignment. The teeth are cramped in the bone, where they are being developed, and erupt into faulty positions. The ultimate result is a set of crowded, tilted, and irregular teeth, difficult to keep clean artificially, and meeting their fellows of the opposite jaw so faultily as to derive little of the natural cleansing of mastication. The individual's ability to chew his food is also considerably impaired.

Unless artificial means of expansion are resorted to, the jaw once under-developed remains so and never picks up the growth which has been lost. The upper jaw is developed from the front backwards. The effects, therefore, of adenoids in early life can be seen in an under-development of the front portion of the mouth, with crowding and overlapping of the incisor teeth. The habit of mouth-breathing, if continued, leads to a pinching of the palate by the cheeks, and the side teeth are unable to come through in proper alignment. The growth of the upper jaw, therefore, controls the arrangement of the teeth.

It is folly to suppose that irregularities of the teeth will right themselves. Clinical experience shows that they do not, and further, that owing to the pressure of other teeth trying to erupt, slight irregularities in childhood become worse in adolescence, and even gross when maturity is reached. The importance of early treatment of irregular teeth cannot be over-estimated. The earlier it is performed the more easily and the more effectively can it be accomplished.

Adenoids may disappear spontaneously, or

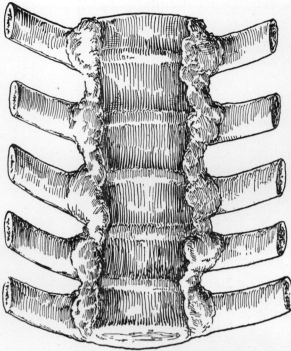

A DEFORMITY DUE TO DENTAL DISEASE
Arthritis deformans of the spine, in which outgrowths of bone bridge over the intervertebral spaces, is often due to poisons conveyed by the blood from septic teeth.

they may be removed by operation, but in either case the child, having lost the function of nasal respiration, may be left with a habit of breathing in and out through the mouth. In the daytime children should be drilled to keep their lips closed, when at rest, and at night it should be the duty of every mother or guardian to visit the sleeping child and, if necessary, gently close his mouth and prop the clothing under the chin.

The direct harm of mouth-breathing to the teeth is the hindrance of the normal flushing of the mouth by the constant flow of the saliva. Solutions of sugary foods, not washed away by the saliva, remain hanging between the teeth. Fermentation and acid formation take place, leading to an increase in the incidence of decay.

The gums are also affected by mouth-breathing. Around the front teeth, for example, the festooned margin of the gum upon close inspection is seen to be slightly pinker. It may even be red and congested, and the triangular portions between the

teeth may be swollen. If dried with a dab of the handkerchief this portion of the gum, instead of presenting the fine, velvety surface of health, will be seen to be shiny.

In a still later stage, pressure with the finger, or brushing with the tooth brush, causes a slight amount of blood, and perhaps a little yellow pus, to exude between the gum and the tooth. This condition of the gums represents a slight chronic inflammation, and its presence always denotes mouth-breathing. Also, it is a danger signal, for it constitutes the first stage of pyorrhœa, to which persistence in mouth-breathing invariably leads.

DIET AND DENTITION

The harmful effects of unsuitable feeding are both indirect and direct.

In the first place, the growth of the upper jaw, which is so important to the ultimate arrangement of the teeth, in its initial stages can only be attained fully by breast feeding. *In Infancy.* In recent years the advent of the boat-shaped bottle and improvement in design of the teat have done much to disperse the mechanical evils of artificial feeding. An infant at the breast does not suck. It munches the nipple and swallows the milk which has been thus expressed. In this early stage of its life a baby's bones are soft and easily moulded by muscular action. Any form of feeding which necessitates sucking causes the palate to be pinched by pressure of the cheeks, and leads to the formation of a contracted arch of teeth, with the attendant difficulties of cleansing.

The breast is the proper medium on which an infant's jaws should be exercised, and should invariably be preferred to any substitute. Furthermore, so far as diet is concerned, the assimilation of lime salts for the proper formation of the teeth must surely be easier from an infant's natural diet than from any substitute, many of which have been proved definitely to be harmful in this respect.

In parenthesis, attention is called to the " dummy " or " comforter," which, fortunately, is disappearing from the nursery. In France its manufacture and sale have now been forbidden by law. Dummy-sucking, thumb-, finger-, tongue-, lip-, or toe-sucking, if persisted in, will invariably pull a baby's jaw out of shape, and should be firmly prevented.

At the time when the teeth are beginning to be cut, and onwards, the child should be allowed to exercise its jaws upon such resistant substances as a crust of wholemeal bread or a chicken bone. Later on, a hard tough diet is to be preferred to a soft one. Children should be encouraged to masticate their food thoroughly. The tough diet and the exercise of their jaws both tend to develop a good arch of strong teeth. A diet which leads to stagnation of food around the teeth is a potential source of greater harm than one which is quickly and easily removed during mastication and does not linger in the crevices of the teeth.

The most harmful portions of our diet are the soft, sticky, starchy, and sugary foods. **Biscuits and Sugar.** White flour, especially in the form of sweetened cakes or biscuits, is pre-eminently harmful to the teeth. It is glutinous, when moistened by the saliva, and tends to stick to the teeth, where the sugar and starch contents of it are fermented into destructive acids. The pernicious practice of giving a child food in bed, especially bread and milk or biscuits and sweets, is culpable. During the night the salivary currents are stilled, the jaws are not active, and the fermenting food is enabled to remain undisturbed in the teeth.

Add to this the habit of mouth-breathing, which interferes still further with the salivary

lavage of the mouth, and it is small wonder that very few teeth escape destruction by decay. Biscuits produce a typical form of decay, which, as might be expected, involves mostly the crowns of the molar teeth. After eating a gingerbread biscuit, a large residue is left in the crowns of these teeth and the tongue wanders around from one to another endeavouring to dislodge it.

Sugar alone, on the other hand, be it in the form of boiled sweets, chocolate, or sweetened dishes such as stewed fruit, forms a solution in the saliva and tends to hang as a droplet between the individual teeth. Sweet-eating, accentuated by mouth-breathing, always presents a typical picture, namely, of decay occurring between the teeth, especially the front ones.

The next point of consideration in diet is the mechanical cleaning of the teeth by the friction of the food during mastication. Foods, therefore, which encourage prolonged mastication and which contain a tough and fibrous element, are beneficial. Wholemeal flour is better than white flour, because it is not so glutinous and is more easily washed away by the saliva, and also because of its

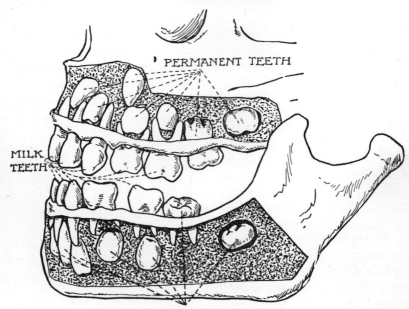

PERMANENT TEETH

THE FORMATION OF PERMANENT TEETH
Interference with the proper development of a child's jaw cramps and displaces the permanent teeth which are waiting to come through.

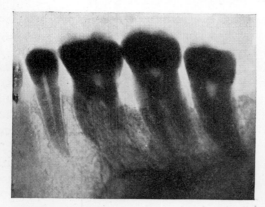

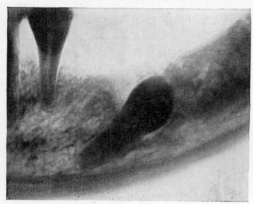

TEETH UNDER THE X-RAY (i)
Above : an X-ray of teeth affected by pyorrhœa.
Below : a tooth which has never emerged from the gums.

bran element, which, being tough, requires more thorough use of the jaws to masticate it and acts upon the teeth as a scouring agent. Other fibrous foods, such as salads, fruit, and celery, are similarly useful.

Fruits are useful in another way. The action of the acid fruit

Fruit.

juices in the mouth is to cause a reflex abundant flow of watery saliva, which is alkaline, in order to neutralise them. To finish off a meal by eating a hard, sharp-tasting apple is thrice beneficial. Firstly, the coarseness of the skin and pith have a definite cleansing action ; secondly, the sharpness, or acidity, promotes a profuse flow of saliva, which mechanically washes food debris and sugar solutions away from the teeth ; and thirdly, the

alkalinity of saliva counteracts not merely the acidity of the fruit juice, which may be regarded as harmless to the teeth, but it also neutralises the harmful acids produced by fermentation.

A bland diet, as typified by sand-cake, is everything that is harmful.

So much for the local and mechanical effects of diet. The general effects operating by assimilation of the food upon the structure of the teeth themselves are even more subtle and no less potent.

There is every reason to believe that the teeth, like the bones, are continuously nourished, and that by very slight changes in the diet they can be made harder or softer, more resistant to decay or less so.

So far as the growth and development of the teeth are concerned, it has been demon-

Growth and Lime Salts.

strated clearly that in certain articles of diet there are substances, vitamins, which influence very materially the growth and calcification of the developing teeth in a child. Their function is to assist the body in making the fullest use of the lime-salts in the foods. If these vitamins are absent, a greater amount of lime-salts must be ingested in the food ; but even then the structure of the teeth is not so good as when the helping vitamins are present.

Foremost among foods containing vitamins is cod liver oil. When it is added to the diet, poor in every tooth-forming respect,

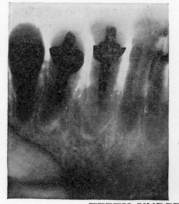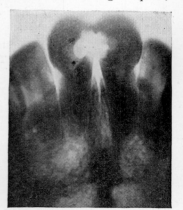

TEETH UNDER THE X-RAY (ii)
Left : teeth which are stopped but apparently healthy, really developing abscesses (shown by the lighter patches) at the roots.
Right : an advanced stage of caries with abscesses at the roots

of puppies, for example, the teeth which are formed are fine, strong, and hard, with white, glistening enamel. Puppies of the same litter fed upon the same diet without the cod liver oil have poorly formed teeth, soft, structurally badly made, with rougher, discoloured enamel. Other puppies of the same litter fed upon the same diet, but with the addition of a large amount of lime-salts, have teeth intermediate between these. The results of these experiments point therefore to the value of cod liver oil as a regular addition to the food from infancy upwards. When the child suffers from rapid decay of the teeth, the institution of a course of regular small doses of cod liver oil appears to harden the teeth, and the incidence of decay rapidly diminishes.

Lastly, so far as pre-natal influences are concerned, it is well known that the developing child in the womb absorbs for its growth a great deal of lime from the mother. In some cases her bones, by the loss of lime-salts, become soft, and even bend under the weight of her body. Her teeth also appear to share in this resorption of lime, for it is well known how prone to decay are the teeth of a pregnant woman. Every expectant mother, therefore, should take, if she can do so, cod liver oil, so that she may assimilate from her food as much lime as possible.

When a mother is expecting a child she should visit her dental surgeon at least three times during the pregnancy to take his advice upon the extra care of her own teeth and to receive helpful instruction on the care of the future baby's. When the child is three years old the first visit to the dentist should be made. Even though the teeth appear white and sound, a great deal of helpful advice may be obtained upon diet and mouth-hygiene. Even at this early age, signs may be detected of approaching undergrowth or deformity of jaws, which will assuredly ead to trouble later, and measures may be taken to avoid or circumvent them.

The Expectant Mother.

To bring up children with a full set of healthy teeth, set in perfect alignment in wide, fully functioning jaws, is not an unattainable ideal.

Provided that the teeth are perfectly normal in structure and alignment and that efficient nasal respiration is present, by simple attention to the diet it is possible for the teeth to keep clean of their own accord. Any factor, such as mouth-breathing, faulty

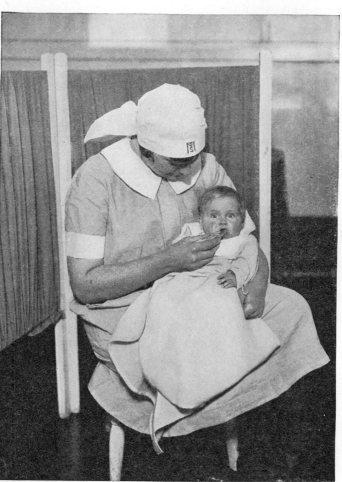

DEVELOPING BABY'S JAWS

As soon as the teeth begin to appear, baby should exercise his jaws upon some hard substance such as a crust of bread.

diet, or misplacement of the teeth, which interferes with the self-cleansing action of the mouth, renders artificial measures of hygiene necessary.

In this connection it should be mentioned that the teeth of each jaw are like bricks in an arch, and, if one be lost, movement takes place in those which are left. The disadvantages which accrue are that the teeth adjacent to the gap left by the missing tooth incline towards one another, and stagnation of food occurs under the tilt of their crowns. In the normal circumstances of a full set of teeth, each tooth closely abuts upon its neighbour, and the wedging of food between them is prevented.

When a tooth is lost, the teeth on each side of the gap become slightly spaced and food is apt to wedge between them and their further neighbours. If this food-stagnation continues, sooner or later decay, or pyorrhœa, or both, occur in these places. It may be a matter of years, but ultimately the trouble becomes evident. Thirdly, a tooth lost in one jaw leaves a part, or a whole, of a tooth in the opposing jaw functionless. It has nothing upon which to chew, whereby it loses the valuable cleansing of mastication,

and food stagnates upon it. In due course it, too, becomes unhealthy.

So evident has this become, that in children it is the recognised practice of a great many dental surgeons to remove the opposing tooth, even if sound, at the time that the decayed tooth is extracted.

In adults this treatment is considered too drastic. In childhood, under suitable conditions, where judicious extraction has been performed, the gaps will close up, or new teeth will come to fill them. In adult life the gaps remain, closing only partially by tilting of the teeth. This undesirable tilting and drifting of the units of the dental arch may be remedied by some artificial restoration, not because it is needed for mastication, but to keep all the other teeth in their proper position for functioning.

DENTAL HYGIENE

By Sir HARRY BALDWIN, C.V.O., M.R.C.S., L.D.S., Hon. Dental Surgeon to H.M. the King.

GUM-BRUSHING is the most important part of dental and oral hygiene. Brushing can make the gums healthy. If the gums are healthy the teeth will mostly take care of themselves. Very few gums are healthy—the reason being that they are not brushed.

Gum-brushing.

Gums *must* have friction. Every square inch of them, behind and before, should be vigorously brushed with a moderately hard tooth brush, using a fairly light hand, at least once a day and preferably oftener. Every square inch of gum, before and behind, should be brushed in this manner with at least fifteen double strokes, *i.e.* fifteen backwards and fifteen forwards.

In the main the strokes should be horizontal, as they are easier to do than vertical strokes, and thus more friction will be achieved. The brush should be frequently dipped and actively shaken, during the process, in saline water. A heaped-up egg-spoonful of common kitchen salt in half a tumbler of water will suffice.

After use the brush should be dried by hard friction on a towel. If any part of the

A CROWDED JAW
Poor development of the jaw—often due to defective breathing or mastication in childhood—commonly results in over-crowding of the teeth.

gum is sore that is a reason for brushing it until it loses its soreness.

Sometimes the gum is attached in such an irregular line to the necks of the teeth that some isolated points of the gum may get much more than their fair share of the friction and may become sore through actual abrasion. This is rare and must be met by using a softer brush for this part of the gum and a milder friction.

Friction is a most important part of the treatment of chronic congestion and inflammation of the gum. Friction is essential when a gum is healthy, to keep it so and to prevent pyorrhœa.

Gums should be pale pink, hard, tight, attached to the necks of the teeth with a very small amount of " free edge " and free from tenderness. Friction will induce all these signs and symptoms of health.

No inter-dental tartar should be present under the free edge of the gum. Friction on the gum will prevent its deposition. With proper friction on the gum from childhood up there should be no such thing as pyorrhœa.

The condition of the mouth, the character of the saliva, the kind and quantity of bacteria and other micro-organisms in the mouth, are all affected by the general health. In robust health the mouth is naturally cleaner than in lowered health. The oral condition will vary from day to day " pari-passu " with the general health. In lowered health the oral conditions are such as to conduce to dental caries. Dental caries then must be combated partly by maintenance of general health and vigour, by every available means, and specially by an ample supply of vitamins in the food. The worst and most unnecessary offender, as a devitaminised carbohydrate, in our food supply is the extremely white flour generally supplied, with its derivatives, white bread, pastries, etc. The other worst offender, as a devitaminised carbohydrate, is ordinary sugar and sweets.

One of the chief objects to aim at is to prevent the accumulation and retention of particles of carbohydrate (such as bread)

Vitamin Feeding.

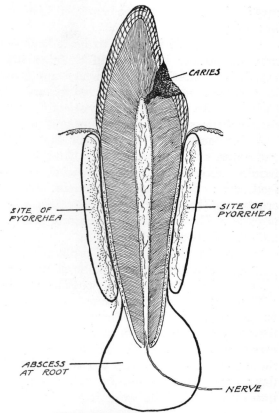

A DISEASED TOOTH IN SECTION
Abscesses at the root and early evidences of pyorrhœa are often only revealed by X-ray tests, which should supplement external examination in all doubtful cases.

upon and between the teeth, as fermentation of these particles produces the lactic acid which is the actual destroyer of the teeth. Therefore detergent foods, such as fruit, should be eaten. They should be eaten at every meal, and particularly at the end of the meal. They act beneficially both mechanically and physiologically. The mastication of raw vegetables and firm fruit removes the adherent particles of carbohydrate from the teeth, and mechanically cleans the teeth of sticky foodstuffs. The adherent particles of carbohydrate are the chief source of the acids which cause decay.

Fresh Fruit.

Physiologically, fruit increases the amount and the alkalinity of the saliva, and also increases the total alkalinity of the body. These are all to the good. Raw vegetables and firm fruit also supply certain very valuable vitamins, and, incidentally, their mastication affords a very beneficial friction to the gums.

A clean mouth is likely to be a healthy mouth, and the best way of cleaning the mouth is to masticate foods which are firm in texture and contain no sticky carbohydrate. Such foods are, pre-eminently, certain fruits, such as raw apples and pears.

Active mastication is good for the teeth and gums, and besides fruit any food which requires active chewing is beneficial. Such foods are : Swedish rye flat-bread, toasts, crusts, pull-bread or zweiback. Also raw vegetables like cucumber, watercress, celery, and all salads are valuable.

Dentifrices will always hold a place in the affections of the public, if only for brightening and polishing the teeth, but they are not to be relied on to prevent dental decay. Brushing the teeth and gums with saline water after every meal is the ideal. At the least, this should be done after the last meal of the day ; and that generally resolves itself into meaning just before going to bed.

Brushing the Teeth.

The teeth should be brushed all over, behind and before, and the masticating surfaces of the back teeth should be brushed as well. The idea in brushing is to clear out all interspaces and crannies, and to leave no particles of food adhering to the teeth. For this reason the teeth should be brushed horizontally and vertically, but especially vertically, using the brush, as has been aptly said, like brushing out the teeth of a comb ; or, as has been no less aptly said, using the brush like a series of toothpicks. Then comes the all-important *gum-brushing* already described.

SUMMARY OF PRINCIPLES OF ORAL HYGIENE

1. Vigorous and thorough gum-brushing.
2. Eating wholemeal bread, using wholemeal flour and stone-milled white flour for cooking ; eating fresh and natural foods to ensure a good supply of vitamins. Avoiding ordinary white bread and extremely white flour in all its forms, *i.e.* in bread, pastry, cakes, biscuits, puddings, etc.

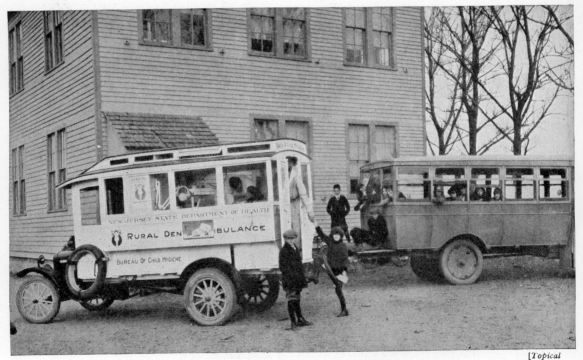

[*Topical*

A TRAVELLING DENTAL CLINIC
School children being treated in a dental ambulance in rural America.

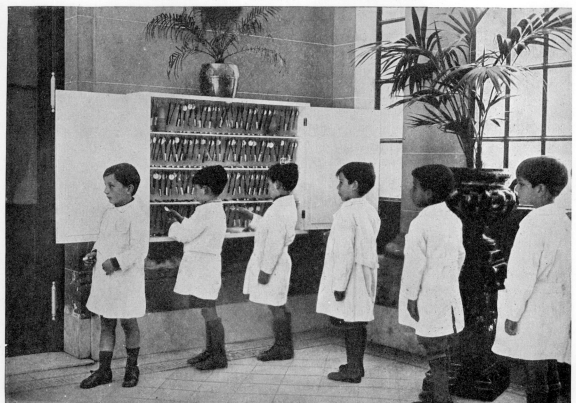

THE TOOTH-BRUSH PARADE *[British-Continental*
The children in this school must clean their teeth every morning before class.

3. Eating fresh firm fruits, like apples, pears, and nuts, or raw vegetables, like celery, at the end of meals.

4. Eating a fair proportion of other firm foodstuffs.

5. Tooth-brushing with saline water last thing before going to bed at night. Tooth-brushing and gum-brushing would be best practised after every meal, but the most important time is before going to bed at night.

6. Added to all these measures the teeth should be inspected, and, if necessary, treated, quite regularly by a dentist twice a year. If any damage is detected it should be repaired at the earliest possible moment. The repairing of damage prevents more damage, and so is a truly hygienic measure.

If the measures in dental hygiene here outlined were adopted and intelligently and steadfastly pursued from early years, very few teeth would ever be lost, and there would be little to fear from either of the two great dental evils ; dental caries and pyorrhœa.

THE CARE OF ARTIFICIAL TEETH

By JOHN CAMPBELL, Ph.D.

THE essentials in a plate are lightness and comfort, and no pains should be spared to secure the latter, although it may mean at first many visits to the dentist. A properly fitting dental plate does not after a time manifest itself either by the sense of touch or action, but even old plates require at times slight re-adjustments in order that they may retain a perfect fitting.

The most scrupulous cleanliness is necessary in the care of dental plates. Unless there are special reasons they should be removed at night, washed, brushed, and placed in a non-staining disinfectant ready for replacement in the morning after the usual cleansing of the existing teeth and mouth has been performed.

In cases where, under special instructions, it may be necessary during temporary periods for the plates to be retained during the sleeping hours, they should be removed for cleansing every night before retiring, and again in the morning.

When practicable, great comfort will be experienced if the plates are removed after a meal and washed in running water. It is a good plan to have plates in duplicate to be worn alternately. Continuity of comfort and appearance can thus be maintained when repairs are necessary. Replacements of single teeth and other repairs should be effected immediately.

As to the material of the plates, the wearer must be guided by the advice of the dentist, but practical experience has shown that vulcanite or one of its modifications fulfils quite well all ordinary requirements, and has many practical advantages in its favour.

When complete sets are fitted the colour of the teeth may be white and uniform, but in partial sets it is best to match as nearly as possible the colour of the natural teeth.

When plates are worn, foods like grapes, figs, raspberries, strawberries, nuts and preserves containing seeds should be avoided when dining out, and where there are no facilities for removal and cleansing of the plates. The hard seeds and particles are apt to intrude between the palate and the plates, producing great discomfort and even pain.

Antiseptic mouth washes are very refreshing for general rinsing purposes and for use before and after meals, and to keep the breath sweet and fresh. The following is a good prescription :—

Commercial alcohol	- -	6 ounces.
Thymol	- - -	¾ ,,
Tincture of myrrh	- -	¼ ,,
Oil of peppermint	- -	a few drops.

For use add a small teaspoonful to a tumbler of warm water.

Tenderness of the palate or gums, or the development of sore spots, indicates that the fitting of the plate may require readjustment, and skilled attention should immediately be sought before more serious developments arise.

Occasionally peroxide of hydrogen, one to seven of water, may be used as a mouth wash and to brush the teeth. This is especially useful where there is a tendency for the teeth to become yellow and dull, but it should not be used as a daily dentifrice.

The art and science of modern dentistry have been brought to a high state of efficiency, and have added considerably to the span of human life as well as the joy of living.

TOOTH POWDERS AND PASTES
By FRANCIS D. DONOVAN, L.D.S., R.C.S. (Eng.), Surgeon-Dentist to the Royal Household.
THE main purpose of dentifrices is to clean and polish teeth mechanically by removing food particles and other matter left on the tooth surface after each meal.

The tooth's most natural cleanser, and therefore the best, is the saliva. This has aptly been called " Nature's own mouth wash," and it is in itself an ideal dentifrice. The saliva is secreted from three glands situated in various parts of the mouth, and has certain properties to combat those forces which are responsible for decay. In its natural state it is very fluid, so that it may bathe the oral cavity constantly, washing away all adhering dangerous matter. Saliva is secreted into the mouth to the extent of several pints a day. It contains a very complex chemical compound known as ptyalin. This has the property of quickly digesting starch and sugar food particles, which would in time, through the activity of microorganisms found in the mouth, change into acids which attack and dissolve the main chemical substance of the tooth.

Saliva is also normally alkaline in character, and as such would neutralise and render ineffective any mouth acids already formed. Another substance in the saliva is mucin, which is gelatinous in character, and whose function is to mix thoroughly with the masticated food to lubricate its passage to the stomach to undergo digestion. An excess of this mucin would mean its deposition on the tooth surfaces and crevices, to accumulate and produce a condition which is to-day regarded as one of the most potential sources of dental decay. Excess of mucin would also make the saliva more sluggish in its washing and bathing action, thus robbing it of fulfilling one of its most important functions. It is these mucin deposits which absorb stain, giving the teeth a dingy, dirty appearance. The tooth substance itself does not stain. Mucin deposits are also the breeding places of decay-producing bacteria.

It must be realised, therefore, that in the study of dentifrices, their action on the salivary flow must be given very important and careful consideration. A dentifrice must not interfere with natural salivary secretion, but must stimulate it and maintain it in its normal natural condition. A dentifrice which retards or depresses this salivary flow, although apparently capable of giving the teeth a polish, defeats its own object, inasmuch as any beneficial action it may have would only be momentary, for the essential constant protecting power of the saliva would be very materially effected and reduced.

Artificial dentifrices are divided into two main classes—those which are acidic in character and those which are alkaline. The former are based on the theory that when mild acids, such as those of fruit, are introduced into the mouth, the mouth " waters " copiously, due to the excess of saliva which is stimulated. The alkaline dentifrices are based on the theory that the mouth acids, which attack the teeth and produce decay are neutralised by the large percentage of alkaline substances of which they are composed. Acid dentifrices are believed to stimulate and maintain a natural flow of saliva, whereas the action of alkaline dentifrices is only momentary, and is effective only on application. Alkaline dentifrices usually contain a large percentage of soap in their composition. The soap is believed to have a detergent action generally in the mouth, on account of its frothing and foaming properties, which allow for its penetration to all parts of the mouth and tooth structure.

There is another type which may be either acidic or alkaline, known as the antiseptic dentifrice. This type contains certain chemicals as ingredients which are used in the hope that they will kill the bacteria in the mouth which are responsible for decay.

The essential ingredient of any artificial dentifrice is its so-called polishing agent. This is in reality the substance which cleans and polishes the teeth. To be ideal it must not be harsh enough to injure any part of the tooth structure or the soft tissues of the mouth, but must be hard enough to remove adhering matter from the tooth surface. For this reason hard abrasives, such as powdered cuttle fish bone, pumice or carborundum must never be used, for their daily application would eventually wear away and destroy the all-important enamel of the tooth, which, if once removed, cannot be naturally replaced. Exposed portions of

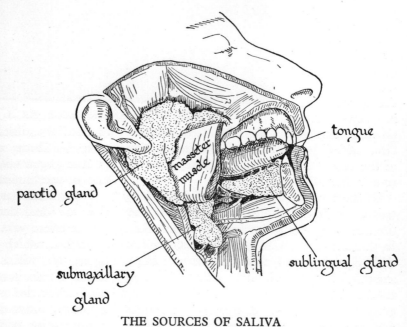

THE SOURCES OF SALIVA

Saliva, the digestive fluid secreted by the glands of the mouth, forms a most effective natural mouthwash.

the tooth under destroyed enamel are very quickly attacked by the bacteria of decay.

Many substances in the past have been used as polishing agents, the most common being powdered dry roots, burnt horn, charcoal and soot. The best known polishers of to-day are chalk (carbonate of lime) and phosphate of lime, which is chemically identical with the main tooth substance. Chalk is alkaline, whereas phosphate of lime is neutral and is the basis of some acid dentifrices. The effectiveness of any dentifrice is only complete when it is applied with the tooth brush in the correct way. The motion of application must be a rotary one, and always away from the gums to the biting surfaces of the teeth—that is, down in the upper jaw and up in the lower. The dentifrice must be forced by the tooth brush bristles well between the teeth, as it is here food particles and mucin deposits often accumulate, which would lead to the destruction of the tooth, and which, therefore, must be removed at all costs.

Of the three forms of artificial dentifrices, paste, powder, or liquid, the paste is to-day the most popular presented for application. In this form the main ingredients are mixed with glycerine and other liquids to form a smooth, bland product, which is very stable. The polishing agent is also very evenly and finely distributed throughout the dentifrice in paste form, which greatly enhances its effectiveness in carrying out its purpose in cleansing and polishing.

Pastes have only been popularised within recent years, the old-fashioned form being powder. The liquid form has never been generally popular in this country. Some powder dentifrices are to-day, however, put up in attractive upright tin containers, with a slot arrangement in the neck, which provides for only a sufficient quantity of the powder being used at each application. This is distinctly an advantage over the old-fashioned flat, round tin containers, when much of the powder was lost on each application.

Liquid dentifrices are usually only regarded in the light of mouth washes. They are incapable of giving a polish to the teeth, and the work of removing food and other debris is left to the bristles of the tooth brush, which are not always effective. Since all the substances in the composition of such dentifrices are soluble, they have no polishing agent with which to perform the function of mechanical cleansing and polishing.

From what has been said, it would seem that an ideal dentifrice is one which does not interfere with the natural secretions of the saliva, which possesses an ideal polishing agent, and which is manufactured in paste form. At the same time I would emphasise that, while the use of a good tooth paste is a pleasant aid to dental hygiene, the effective manipulation of the tooth brush is the way "par excellence" to a clean and healthy mouth.

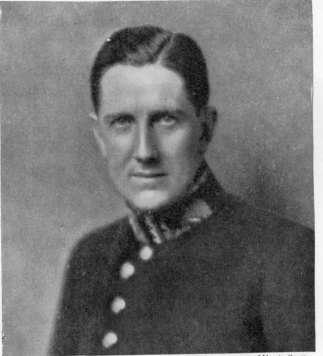

[Hugh Cecil

FRANCIS D. DONOVAN, L.D.S., R.C.S.

DIET AND DENTITION IN THE PUNJAB

By Lieut.-Col. H. HALLILAY, I.M.S., M.B., M.R.C.S., L.R.C.P., Civil Surgeon, Rawal Pindi.

ONE of the first things to strike the Medical Officer whose lot has fallen to practise in the Punjab, is the excellent condition of the people's teeth. This is especially true with regard to the country population who are engaged in, or dependent upon, agriculture for their livelihood. I must emphasise the fact that the statements made in this article refer to the people of the Punjab, the Land of Five Rivers, from which the bulk of the recruits for the Indian Army are drawn, and not to India as a whole.

To a stranger in the land it is a constant source of wonder to see those big, bearded men drinking milk with all the relish of a Devonshire carter for cider ; the country people regard it as a most strengthening and muscle-building food, while the professional wrestlers train on milk and almonds, which are considered invaluable for strength and endurance.

Because the Punjab is populated in the main by a sturdy race of small farmers, peasant proprietors, all of whom keep their own cows and buffaloes, milk is plentiful and within the reach of nearly every member of the village, although in the large towns it is extremely dear and bad.

One of the peculiarities of the diet of the Punjabi is its richness in mineral salts, owing to the large quantity of wholemeal bread which he consumes, with an abundance of milk and vegetables.

The abundance of mineral matter is reflected in the excellence of his teeth, an excellence which is ensured in the first instance by the admirable quality of his mother's milk, which in turn is the outcome of the highly vitalised, or vitaminised nature of the maternal diet, reinforced by a plentiful supply of mineral salts, essential in the business of building teeth and laying down bone. The diet of this people contains a quantity of hard food, and the excellence of their teeth has been attributed to this by some authorities.

The tooth brush is, of course, unknown amongst them, though many of them use a twig of the babool or nim trees for this purpose ; the datan, the chewed end of the stem, making a sort of bristle. I am confident that the use of a tooth brush never averted caries in any one ; indeed, it is possible to live one's whole life long without caries, though a tooth brush has never touched the teeth. Dental caries seems to be the special luxury of man and the domestic animals, in other words, of those persons and creatures who live on food for which their teeth were never intended.

I make this statement with the greater confidence because of the observations which I was able to make at first hand on so many of our poor relations in the Simla Hills, the brown hill monkey and the langur. These animals, though they do not use tooth brushes, do not suffer from dental caries. They have a dental chart which for all practical purposes is identical with that of man, both as regards number, shape, and arrangement. Their diet in their wild state is purely vegetarian, and their supply of the important " A " and " D " vitamins must be exclusively derived from green leaves, and from occasional egg-yolk, for I am afraid that they do not scruple to plunder the nests of any birds which they may discover.

Rickets is unknown amongst them ; I have never seen a deformed monkey. Of all animals, I should say that they are the most intrepid, the most insolent and active.

So we are faced by the fact that those animals whose physiology and whose structure most nearly resemble that of man are entirely vegetarian in their diet.

The Sikhs do not, as a general rule, get meat more than, say, once a fortnight in their homes, and then only in small quantities. In short, with them as with the rest of the inhabitants of the Punjab, bread is the staff of life, the wholemeal, unleavened flat cakes which every one in the Province eats, and of which the flour or " Ata " is in many instances ground in the house from the whole grain.

THE LOCOMOTORY SYSTEM

By GEORGE SOMERVILLE, M.D., D.P.M., Deputy Medical Superintendent at the West Ham Mental Hospital.

THE COMPOSITION OF BONE

BONE is composed of two layers of tissue. Externally is a dense ivory-like layer—the " compound bone " ; internally is a bony lace-work arrangement—the " cancellous or spongy bone." The rigid compact tissue forms an outer supporting case; it is tunnelled by tiny canals through which run the nourishing blood vessels, nerves, and lymphatics. The cancellous bone is rich in blood vessels; its meshwork supports the "red marrow "—a blood-forming tissue.

All bone is closely invested with a tough fibrous membrane called the " periosteum." It is richly supplied with blood vessels and nerves, and, by its property of forming new bone, it plays an important part in the repair of fractures.

Chemically, bone has a basis of animal matter (fibrous tissue) impregnated with certain earthy salts (the phosphates and carbonates of lime and magnesium). The relative proportions of the animal and earthy matters vary at the different phases of life. In childhood the animal tissue predominates ; in adults the earthy matter is increased. Hence the bones of children are tough and do not break readily : they bend when subjected to strain and a so-called " green-stick " fracture may result. With advancing years the bones become more brittle and consequently the liability to fracture is increased. The earthy matter gives hardness and solidity to bone ; the animal matter gives elasticity and toughness.

For descriptive purposes bones are described conveniently under the headings "long," "short," "flat," and "irregular."

The long variety is typified in the bones of the limbs. Each consists of a shaft and two expanded ends. The shaft is simply a tube of compact bone ; it encloses the medullary cavity—where reserves of the body fat are stored (yellow marrow). The expanded ends, consisting of cancellous tissue filled with red marrow enclosed in a thin shell of compact bone, are lined with a smooth layer of cartilage and go to form articulations or joints. The long bones mainly serve the purpose of locomotion.

The flat variety are typified in the skull bones. They are composed of inner and outer tables of compact bones with intervening layers of cancellous bone. Flat bones have a protective function.

Short bones are typified in the bones of the wrist and ankle ; they consist of cancellous bone thinly encased by compact bone. They contribute strength to joints of limited movement.

Irregular bones are so called because they do not fall into the other descriptive categories. The vertebræ are irregular bones.

Bones grow in thickness by the activity of the periosteal cells. Long bones grow in length by the constant activity, in the developing years, of a layer of bone-forming cartilage situated between the shaft of the bone and its expanded end. Injury to this cartilage in childhood may hinder the growth of the bone and lead to deformity.

The functions of bone are to form a framework about which the body is moulded; to give protection to the vital organs ; and to permit the body and limbs to be moved in various directions by the actions of the muscles.

CARTILAGE

Cartilage is a form of connective tissue closely related to bone. It is a hard pliant substance which helps to link up the skeleton. Cartilage

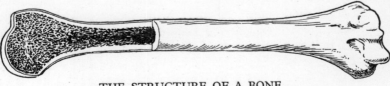

THE STRUCTURE OF A BONE
Showing the hard, ivory-like outer layer, and the spongy interior interlaced with blood vessels, nerves and lymphatics.

exists in two forms : when pervaded by fibres of connective tissue it is called "fibro-cartilage"; when clear and free of such tissue it is termed "hyaline cartilage." Fibro-cartilage is very tough and strong and is found in the inter-vertebral discs, epiglottis and cartilages of the knee joints. Hyaline cartilage is found in the nose, wind-pipe, rib cartilages and ends of bones (articular cartilage). Most bones are developed out of cartilaginous tissue. In long bones the band of cartilage which forms new bone is called the "epiphysis"; its activity persists until the age period of fifteen to twenty years.

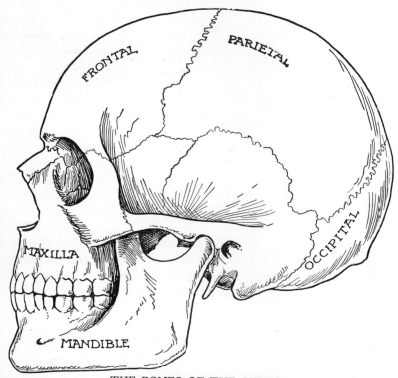

THE BONES OF THE SKULL

The skull bones are flat, and all, except the mandible or lower jaw bone, immovable.

THE SKELETON

The human skeleton is made up of over two hundred bones. It may be conveniently divided into an "axial" and an "appendicular" portion.

The axial skeleton consists of the skull, vertebral column, ribs and sternum.

The skull is composed of the cranium and the face. The cranium is the box-like protective covering of the brain. It consists of eight bones, viz., two parietals and temporals; the frontal, occipital, sphenoid and ethmoid. The face is formed by fourteen bones, viz., two upper jaw bones (maxillæ), two cheek bones (malar), two nasal, lacrymal, turbinal and palatal bones; one vomer and one lower jaw bone (mandible).

An abnormally small skull is found in certain cases of idiocy; enlargement of the skull occurs in acromegaly and in hydrocephalus. In rickets the skull tends to be square or box-shaped, and in congenital syphilis the forehead is vertical and the bridge of the nose depressed.

The skull bones are firmly united to each other by their dentated edges, and the resulting joint is known as a "suture."

The spinal column or back-bone supports the skull. It is made up of thirty-three small irregular bones called vertebræ which are linked together by discs of fibro-cartilage and by ligaments to form a flexible column. There are seven vertebræ in the neck or cervical region, twelve in the thoracic or dorsal region, five in the lumbar, five fused together as one bone called the sacrum, and four which form the coccyx or tail-bone.

Each vertebra consists of a body from which two processes of bone project backward to form a ring. These rings, one above the other, constitute a bony tube—the spinal canal. This transmits the spinal cord—the downward prolongation of the brain.

Normally the spinal column has four curves. These develop as soon as the child walks and they are instrumental in reducing shocks and jars, and give poise to the body. Marked abnormalities of spinal curvature occur notably in rickets and tuberculosis,

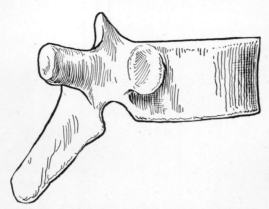

A SEGMENT OF THE BACK-BONE (i)

but slight degrees of it are common in debilitated children who are permitted to adopt faulty attitudes when at work in school. Unless corrected in the early stages such morbid changes become permanent.

The ribs form the greater part of the thoracic walls. There are twelve pairs of ribs which articulate behind with the thoracic vertebræ; in front the upper ten are joined to the breast bone (sternum) by strips of cartilage; the last two pairs of ribs have their ends free and are known as the " floating ribs."

The appendicular skeleton consists of the four limbs and their attachments to the axial skeleton.

The upper limb is joined to the thorax by means of the shoulder blade (scapula) and the collar bone (clavicle). The clavicle acts as a buttress to the shoulder and forms a protecting arch over certain large blood vessels and nerves. The humerus is the sole bone of the upper arm. Its upper rounded end fits into the glenoid cavity of the scapula and forms the shoulder joint. Its lower end is shaped to articulate with the two bones of the forearm, the radius and the ulna. Eight small bones make up the wrist (carpus); five bones are found in the palm (metacarpus), and fourteen bones in the fingers and thumbs (phalanges).

The hip bone includes three bones (ilium, ischium, pubis) which in early life are separate but in adult life are fused into one. The two hip bones are large flat expanded bones which spring from the sacrum behind and unite at the symphysis pubis. This girdle of bone forms a basin or pelvis. On the lower and outer aspect of the hip bone is a deep cup-shaped socket—the " acetabulum "—into which fits the head of the thigh bone or femur. This is the largest and strongest bone in the body. Its lower extremity rests on the upper end of the tibia and forms the knee joint. The fibula is a slender bone placed along the outer side of the leg parallel to the tibia. The knee-cap or patella is a small triangularly-shaped bone attached by strong ligaments to the tibia; it forms a protection for the knee-joint. Seven small bones make up the ankle or tarsus; five short bones form the sole or metatarsus, and fourteen are distributed amongst the toes or phalanges.*

JOINTS

The junction between two or more bones is termed a joint or articulation. Joints are classified as " movable " and " immovable." The latter occur where the bones are completely interlocked or fixed as in the skull and face; a layer of cartilage or fibrous tissue intervenes between the bones and firmly binds them together. The former occur where

* See section on The Feet.

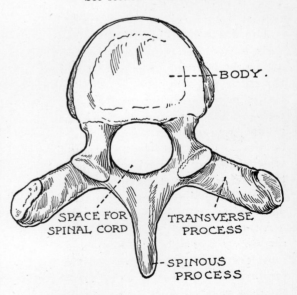

A SEGMENT OF THE BACK-BONE (ii)
A side view (i) and upper view (ii) of one of the 33 vertebrae which form the spinal column.

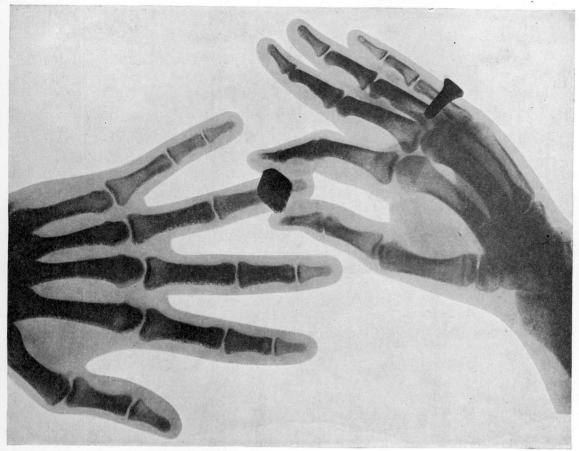

AN ENGAGEMENT UNDER THE X-RAY
A photograph showing clearly the bony skeleton of the hand.

[Keystone

very free movement is necessary and their structure is more complex and varied.

A typical movable joint is made up of the ends of two or more bones capped with articular cartilage in close apposition, enwrapped by a thin layer of connective tissue called the " synovial membrane." A natural joint lubricant, the synovial fluid, is produced by this membrane. The joint is also enclosed in a sheath of fibrous tissue, the capsule, which is strengthened and reinforced by ligaments—bands of tissue which stretch from bone to bone—and by the tendons of various muscles which act around the joint.

Several varieties of movable joints are described according to the nature of the movement they allow. The ball-and-socket joint gives a very wide range of movement in any direction and is found in the shoulder and hip. A to and fro movement taking place round one axis is found in the hinge-joint exemplified in the elbow and knee. Where the surfaces of the opposing bones merely glide over each other and there is very limited movement, as in the wrist and ankle, a gliding-joint is described.

MUSCLE.

Muscle constitutes what is popularly known as flesh. It is by virtue of its power of contractibility that movement is possible.

Muscles are divided into two classes— the " voluntary " and the " involuntary." The former act under control of the will ; the latter act independently.

Microscopically the voluntary muscles present a transversely striated appearance ; hence they are often termed the " striped muscles." Each muscle consists of a fleshy part known as

Voluntary Muscle.

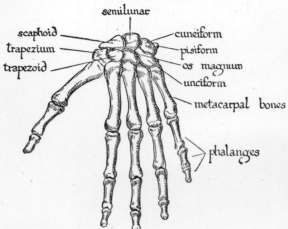

THE BONES OF THE HAND

and gentle massage will aid the circulating blood to remove the poisonous waste and to excrete it. Severe fatigue, however, may cause lasting damage to the body through its effects on the central nervous system. The psychological aspect of fatigue can be studied by means of an instrument known as the ergograph.*

The names and positions of certain of the important muscles can be studied from the diagram on page 551.

Rigor Mortis. After death a general stiffening of the muscles sets in, and this phenomenon is called "rigor mortis." It is caused by a coagulation of the muscle-plasma. The time of onset varies; it is seldom sooner than ten minutes or later than seven hours. The muscles of the neck and lower jaw are affected first; then there is a gradual spread downwards. The duration of rigor mortis is variable, but the average period is from sixteen to twenty-four hours.

Involuntary Muscles. Involuntary muscle (with the one exception of the heart muscle) is non-striated. It is composed of aggregations of fine elongated fusiform cells which are united together by a

* See section on The Mind.

the "belly"; this is enclosed in a fibrous sheath which terminates at each end in a sinew or tendon. The muscle acts over a joint and is said to "originate" from the fixed bone and to be "inserted" into the mobile bone.

Each voluntary muscle is made up of a number of bundles of fine fibres. These individual fibres are the muscle units, and each possesses the power of contraction and relaxation. In health, they act synchronously; the muscle shortens and movement is produced.

The voluntary muscles are also called the skeletal muscles, and there are over six hundred of them. They form the chief part of the bulk of the body. Each muscle has a special "motor nerve" which connects it with the spinal cord and brain. It can only function when this nerve is intact and healthy.

Living muscle is continually taking up oxygen from the blood and giving off carbonic acid. Carbohydrate (sugar) is the main source of muscular energy. When a muscle contracts more oxygen is taken up and the stored-up sugar is oxidised with the production of energy, heat and the waste products, carbonic and lactic acids.

Muscle fatigue sets in when muscles are made to work over a prolonged period. It is partly due to the consumption and reduction of available fuel but more particularly to the accumulation of the waste products of their activity. After moderate fatigue, rest

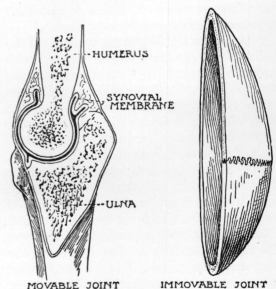

MOVABLE JOINT   IMMOVABLE JOINT

THE TWO KINDS OF JOINT

A contrast between the movable elbow joint and the immovable knee-cap.

cementing material. These cells are nucleated and have a delicate sheath.

Involuntary muscle forms the muscular coats of the digestive tract from the œsophagus to the inner sphincter of the anus. It is also found in the walls of the blood vessels, the ureters, and bladder ; in the uterus, skin, iris, trachea, and bronchi.

The muscle fibres of the heart, differing from other involuntary muscles, have faint transverse stripes. The fibres are short ; are united at intervals by short branches, and do not possess sheaths.

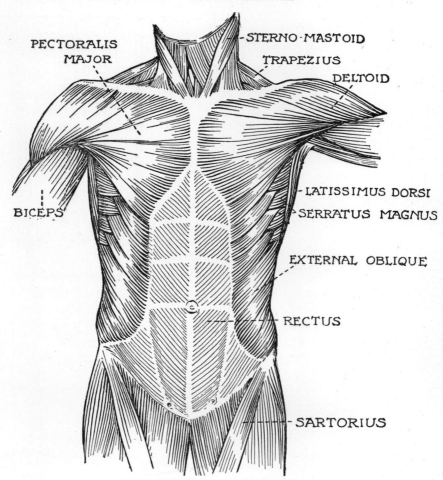

THE MUSCLES OF THE TRUNK
Showing the position and striped appearance of the chief voluntary muscles.

The involuntary muscles are controlled by the sympathetic nervous system.

DISEASES OF THE BONES

Osteitis, or inflammation of the bone, may be acute or chronic, and is generally the result of tubercular, syphilitic, or other organismal infection.

Inflammation. Acute inflammation is caused by micro-organisms (staphylococci or streptococci) which invade the bone either from an external wound or in consequence of some local focus of infection in the mouth, throat, or alimentary tract. Debility and lowered vitality are important predisposing factors ; injury from a fall or knock may act as the exciting cause.

The degree of inflammation varies in severity. A superficial inflammation of the bone and its enveloping membrane is called PERIOSTITIS. Extension of the disease process into the medullary cavity gives rise to OSTEOMYELITIS. *Acute* inflammation occurs, almost without exception, in the growing bones of children.

The earliest symptom of acute osteomyelitis is severe pain which comes on suddenly and is attended by extreme tenderness of the affected bone. This is associated with severe constitutional symptoms. Fever is marked ; the temperature rises to 104-105°F., and it may be associated with shivering fits and severe sweats. Delirium may occur at night. There is great physical prostration.

In the course of a day or two, as the inflammation makes its way to the surface, the limb becomes swollen, hot, red, and

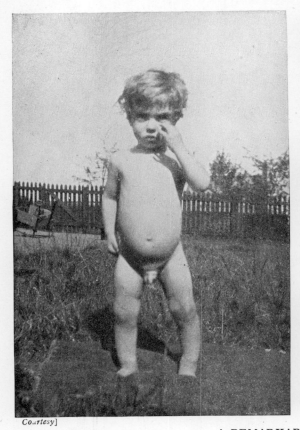
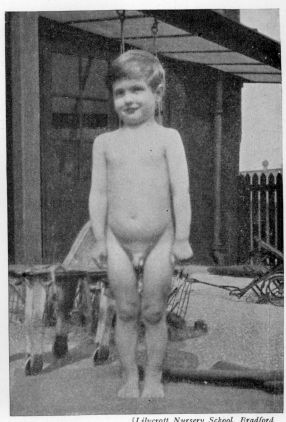

Courtesy]   *[Lilycroft Nursery School, Bradford*

A REMARKABLE RECOVERY

Left : a child of two showing rickets and arrested mental development due to malnutrition. *Right :* the same child after eighteen months on a suitable diet in healthy surroundings.

exquisitely tender to touch. Suppuration sets in and areas of bone are destroyed (necrosis). Abscess formation takes place, and there is danger of an extension of the suppuration to the neighbouring joints, or general blood-poisoning may result. At any stage death may occur from the severe constitutional disturbance.

Osteomyelitis most commonly commences in the articular end of a long bone—often the tibia—and there is some danger of its being confused with the joint inflammation of acute rheumatism.

The outlook in cases of osteomyelitis is always grave owing to the possible complications. The disease calls for immediate surgical operation—free incision and drainage—with the object of allowing the pus to escape and to remove any dead bone.

Convalescence is tedious and tardy. Nevertheless though large portions of bone are destroyed, ultimate repair by new bone formation gives an excellent functional result.

Closely related to osteomyelitis is EPIPHYSITIS, an inflammation which begins in the bone-forming cartilage and is met with in infancy. Suppuration, abscess formation, and invasion of the joint occur, but the constitutional symptoms are not so severe as in osteomyelitis. Chronic forms are always associated with syphilis or tuberculosis.

Chronic inflammation includes a number of tubercular, syphilitic, rheumatic and gouty conditions which lead to crumbling and destruction or to irregular thickening of the bone. As a rule these diseases manifest themselves insidiously.

Chronic Inflammation.

Tubercular disease of the bone usually occurs in youthful subjects. The favourite

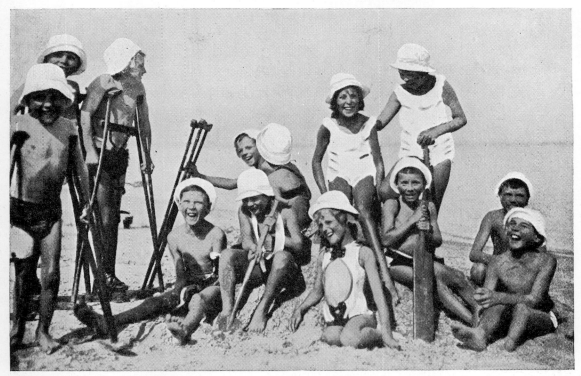

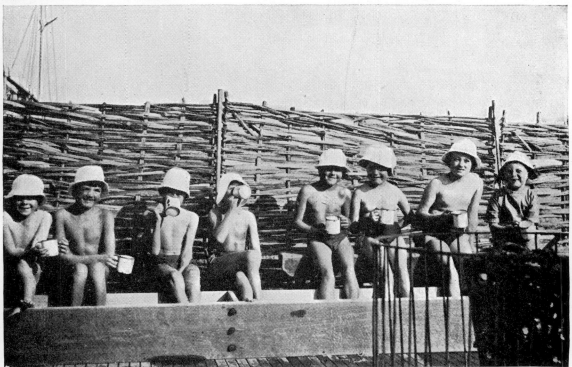

[*Photos by courtesy of Lord Mayor Treloar Cripples' Hospital, Alton and Hayling Island*]

CONVALESCENT FROM SURGICAL TUBERUCLOSIS

(*Above*) A happy group of children at Sandy Point; (*below*) after a bath.   The children are rubbed down before a brazier in specially prepared pens, after which they put their feet in warm water, have a hot drink and then a sun-bath.

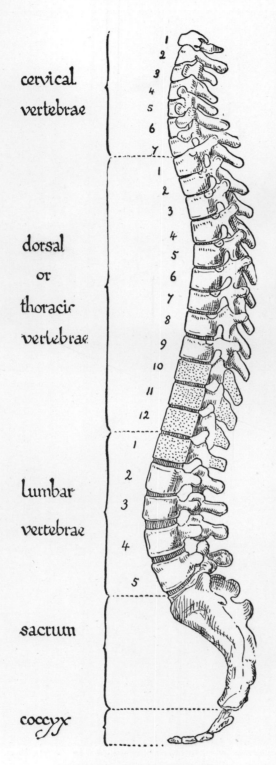

cervical
vertebrae

dorsal
or
thoracic
vertebrae

lumbar
vertebrae

sacrum

coccyx

THE NORMAL BACKBONE

Normally the spinal column has four curves, but in
such diseases as rickets and tuberculosis abnormal
curves may develop.

site of infection is the bone-forming
cartilage in the ends of the long bones,
and consequently disease in the
Tubercu- neighbouring joint (usually hip
losis. or knee) is liable to result. Involvement of the bodies of the vertebræ is
fairly common, and the collapse of the
diseased vertebræ leads to morbid curvature
of the spine (kyphosis).

The tubercular process leads to "caries"
or crumbling of the bone and to abscess
formation. The disease is very chronic;
there is an intermittent temperature and
there are often signs of tuberculosis elsewhere.

The course depends on the virulence of the
infection and the powers of resistance of the
patient. Treatment is directed to improving
the general health by rest, tonics, and a
nourishing diet. Operation may be necessary to evacuate abscesses or to remove
dead bone.

Syphilitic disease of bone is common both
in the acquired and the hereditary varieties.
In the secondary stage of ac-
Syphilis. quired syphilis localised inflammation of the periosteal membrane
produces swellings or "nodes"; in the
tertiary stage, large circumscribed areas of
caries (gummata) are of frequent occurrence
in the long bones, and sometimes in the skull.
Hereditary syphilis gives rise to much the
same conditions in childhood, and they are
apt to be mistaken for rickets.

The disease is recognised by the fleeting
pains which are characteristically worse at
night. There is usually evidence of syphilis
elsewhere.

The causal syphilis must be radically
treated.

Tumours of bone may be simple or malignant. Simple tumours are usually multiple
and only cause trouble by pressure
Tumours. or by their inconvenient size.
They are easily removed and as a
rule do not return.

Malignant tumours are either cancers or
sarcomas. Cancer is usually secondary to a
growth in some other organ—often the
breast; the sarcoma is primary in the bone.
Both produce rapid swelling, and there is a

tendency to spontaneous fracture. Treatment as a rule is of little avail.

Rickets. Rickets is a constitutional disorder of childhood associated with disturbance of nutrition, and attended with a softening of the bones. It is a disease commonly found among the children of the poorer classes who are indiscriminately fed and who are brought up in unhealthy surroundings. Imperfect oxygenation of the blood as a result of want of fresh

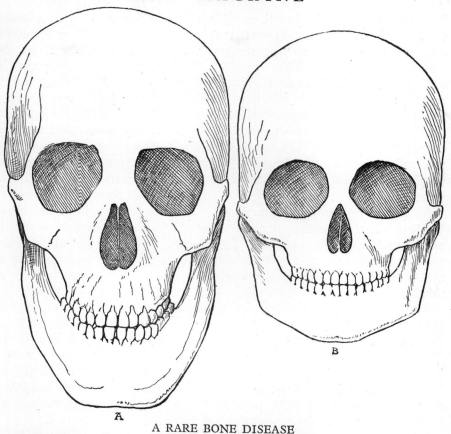

A RARE BONE DISEASE

A case of acromegaly (A) in which the bones of the hands, feet, and skull become enlarged, compared with a normal skull (B).

air and sunlight, and ill-health of the mother during pregnancy are contributory factors which favour the occurrence of this disease.

Insufficiency of fat with excess of starchy and sugary foods in the diet and a deficient intake of lime salts have long been held to have a causal relationship to rickets, but recent investigation has shown that the essence of the disease is an absence of certain vital substances only found in fresh foods— "vitamins." Rickets is now regarded as a "deficiency disease" and the absent vitamin is the one associated with animal fats—the so-called "fat soluble vitamin D."

It is important to note that a type of scurvy-rickets occurs amongst the children of the rich who are reared on proprietary food substitutes.

The most striking feature of rickets is the softness of the bones, due to an irregular process of bone formation. The cartilage of

the epiphysis proliferates in an active but aberrant manner, and the bone it produces is markedly deficient in lime salts. It gives rise to visible swellings which are best seen at the lower ends of the radius and tibia, and at the junctions of the ribs with their cartilages where an appearance of beading results—the "rickety rosary."

The symptoms are first manifest about the end of the first year of life. Disorders of the gastro-intestinal tract precede the outward signs of rickets. The child's appetite is poor ; vomiting and irregularity of the bowels occur. There is marked debility and wasting. The child is feverish, sweats freely, especially over the head, and is very restless at night. Eruption of the teeth is delayed, and bronchitis is a common symptom.

Later there is tenderness in the limbs, and the child becomes unable to walk or sit up. Changes in the bone then become visible. There are painful swellings at the ends of the long bones and at the junctions of the ribs with their cartilages. Should the child endeavour to walk a " bow-legged " or " knock-kneed " condition results. The cavity of the chest tends to become contracted ; the pelvis is distorted, and in females may in later years seriously handicap the process of childbirth ; morbid spinal curvature may occur. The bones of the skull are soft and the " fontanelle " remains unclosed long after the end of the second year.

As a rule rickets terminates in recovery, but leaves behind permanent deformities and malformations of the skeleton. During its course, however, certain intercurrent maladies—bronchitis, pneumonia, convulsions, or meningitis—may cause death.

Rickets is a disease which is eminently preventable. The fundamental causal factor indicates both the prevention and the cure. Treatment consists in regulating the diet by increasing the available fat-soluble vitamin, improving the surroundings, and preventing deformities. Children when possible should be breast-fed, for rickets seldom occurs in a child who has been nursed by its mother for six months. The carbohydrates of the diet should be decreased and the fats, in the form of milk and cream, should be judiciously increased. Cod-liver oil is the richest naturally occurring source of vitamin D., and its administration both protects infants against rickets and cures the disease. Abundance of fresh air and sunlight have a very beneficial effect in cases of rickets and recent experimental work has shown that exposure to ultra-violet rays mobilises the available vitamin D. in the body and hastens cure.

During the acute phase of the disease, the child must be prevented from walking lest permanent deformities result, otherwise operative measures may be necessary in later life.

It is obvious that if sound hygienic measures in relation to diet, sunlight, and fresh air were enforced in childhood, the occurrence of rickets would be a rare phenomenon.*

* See section on Vitamins.

Acromegaly is a rare disease associated with changes in the pituitary body. In the early stages there is marked enlargement of the bones of the hands, feet, and the skull. The lower jaw is especially increased and projects beyond the upper jaw. Later there is similar enlargement of the bones of the limbs, and thorax. It is associated with defect of vision.

Acromegaly.

The disease runs a very long course ; treatment is of little avail ; death results from some intercurrent malady.*

Osteomalacia (softening of the bones) is a progress disorder in which the bones become soft and yielding so that they are unduly liable to break or become distorted. It is due to the absorption of their lime salts by the blood so that the bones lose their rigidity and bend under the weight of the body.

Osteomalacia.

It occurs in women between twenty-five and thirty-five years of age, and is nearly always related to childbirth. The softening of the bone most commonly affects the pelvis and lumbar vertebræ, but the whole skeleton may be involved.

The actual cause of this malady is unknown but alleviation has resulted in some cases after removal of the ovaries, and it is presumed that it may be related to some disorder of the internal secretory glands.

DISEASES OF THE JOINTS

Joints are among the most susceptible parts of the body to infection. This would appear to be due to their exposed position, their subjection to minor injuries including wear and tear, and to their very rich blood supply.

SYNOVITIS is the term applied to any inflammatory process in the lining membrane of the joint cavity.

Inflammation.

Acute inflammations are a result of infection from an external wound or from some acute infectious disease such as scarlatina, typhoid, pneumonia, pyæmia, or rheumatic fever. The localisation of the infection in a particular joint is determined by injury, exposure to cold or previous disease of the joint.

* See section on The Ductless Glands.

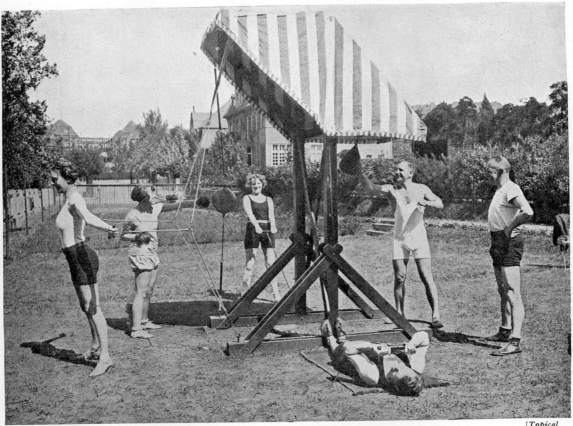

[Topical

EXERCISE ON SCIENTIFIC LINES
A compact training apparatus designed to provide exercise for all parts of the body.

In acute synovitis the joint becomes painful, red, swollen, hot, and is usually held rigidly in the flexed position. This may clear up in a few days or the inflammation may go on to suppuration and abscess formation with disorganisation of the joint. It is then termed ACUTE ARTHRITIS.

The terminations depend on the gravity of the causal infection and the success of treatment. In severe forms the joint may be permanently damaged by the formation of adhesions, or the joint may remain distended with fluid.

Treatment is surgical, and when convalescence is established, attention must be directed to the prevention of stiffness and deformity by movements, massage, and various baths.

Various inflammations of the joints may occur as a result of gonococcal urethritis.

Gonorrhœal rheumatism is a form of dry arthritis which tends to be persistent and progressive, and results in permanent crippling of the hands and fingers.

Gonococcal Affections.

A chronic synovitis is common ; the joint, usually the knee, becomes filled with fluid and movements are restricted. An acute synovitis, which may become suppurative, may also occur.

The presence of a gonorrhœal discharge is conclusive evidence of the origin of such joint infections.

Tuberculosis chiefly affects the synovial membrane though it may originate in the articular ends of the bones. Any joint may be involved but the commonest situations are the hip and knee-joints.

Tubercular Joint Disease.

It occurs mainly in children, and its insidious onset is generally revealed by slight pain, stiffness, and limping. Later the affected joint swells ; it is pale, and on palpation is doughy or pulpy. Gradually the use of the limb is lost and constitutional symptoms become prominent. There is intermittent fever, wasting, and great debility. In severe cases the tubercular process may completely destroy the joint ; abscesses form which may burst through the skin and the patient becomes gravely ill.

The disease may last for many years and the prospect of cure depends on the earliness of its detection and its prompt treatment.

SYPHILIS, GOUT, and RHEUMATOID ARTHRITIS are constitutional diseases which affect joints and all tend to produce chronic varieties of synovitis and arthritis.

In LOCOMOTOR ATAXIA (tabes dorsalis) a peculiar disintegration of the large joints without any acute inflammation sometimes occurs. Little pain or inconvenience is suffered. It is known as Charcot's joint disease.

HYSTERICAL AFFECTIONS of the joints in young women are not uncommon and may closely simulate true organic disease. Occasionally an early focus of disease may originate functional symptoms, and this hysterical mask may lead to an ignoring of the fundamental cause.

DISEASES OF THE MUSCLES

Definite diseases of the muscles are comparatively rare.

Inflammation (myositis) may result from a wound infection or may be associated with a certain parasitic infection. (Ingestion of " measly pork.")

Syphilis causes a gummatous myositis. A hard, almost painless swelling forms in the muscle and in time heals by the formation of scar tissue which may destroy the functional activity of the muscle.

Wasting of muscles occurs as a symptom of various degenerative diseases of the nervous system—such as infantile paralysis or progressive muscular atrophy. The muscles are deprived of the tonic influence of the nerve supply and consequently atrophy.

MUSCULAR RHEUMATISM (fibrositis) is one of the many manifestations of the rheumatic

diathesis which is conveniently described under the heading of " Chronic Rheumatism."

HYGIENE OF THE LOCOMOTORY SYSTEM

To maintain in health the various organs which constitute the locomotory system, *exercise* is a supreme necessity. This especially applies to the young, to those who practise sedentary occupations, and to the naturally indolent. The effects of exercise are not only beneficial to the muscles, joints, and bones, but are also essential to the healthy functioning of the vital organs. Muscle activity, by alternate contraction and relaxation, speeds up the circulation of the blood and lymph so that the useless and poisonous products of metabolism are more rapidly got rid of by the excretory organs. Consequently the natural processes of repair are also hastened on.

Want of exercise brings many evils. In early life the muscles and bones do not develop in the normal manner. Puny muscles are rapidly fatigued and lead to the habitual adoption of faulty attitudes which in time produce a permanent lateral curvature of the spine (adolescent scoliosis). This inevitably causes deformity of the thorax and abdomen so that distortion and displacement of the internal organs result and predispose them to disease.

Careful school hygiene will prevent these muscular weaknesses and skeletal deformities. The child must not be permitted to adopt awkward attitudes while reading, writing, or piano playing. Special care must be taken to prevent compression of the body by tight clothing. Short sight must be corrected and the general health must be maintained at its highest level.

The particular exercises prescribed must be selected to suit each special case. The movements are designed to strengthen the weak muscles and ligaments and to increase the flexibility of the spine. It is important that during the exercises the breathing should be regulated ; very deep breaths should be taken periodically. The exercises should be discontinued before the child feels fatigued ; massage is a useful adjuvant.

In the elderly, insufficient exercise leads to sluggish action of the various digestive organs. Dyspepsias, constipation, and obesity result. The heart muscle becomes flabby and atonic ; an impeded circulation with its attendant evils follows.

The locomotory organs must be made to function as regularly and efficiently as the digestive or excretory organs. This can only be attained through consistent physical training. Systematic exercises carried out at the commencement of the day's activity go a long way towards maintaining bodily and mental fitness.

The importance of dietetic hygiene in infancy as a means of preventing rickets has already been emphasised.

THE FEET

By ERIC GORDON FLEMING, D.C. (Universal Chiropract. Coll., U.S.A.), M.C.P.S. (Ont.), M.B. (Edin. and Toronto), formerly Honorary Physician to the British Hospital of Mental Disorders and Nervous Diseases, Camden Town.

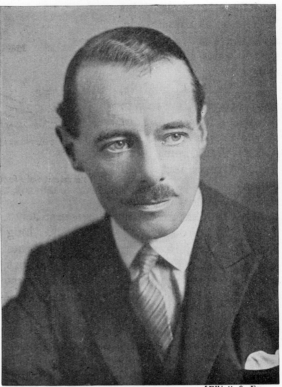

[Elliott & Fry
DR. ERIC GORDON FLEMING

THE bones of the foot, excluding the sesamoid bones,* are twenty-six in number, and for purposes of classification may be separated into three divisions. The hindermost division consists of the *tarsus* ; the middle is called the *metatarsus* ; and the foremost division the *phalanges*.

Bony Structure.

The bones of the tarsus are seven in number, and are called the calcaneus, astragalus, cuboid, scaphoid, internal, middle and external cunieform.

The calcaneus, os calcis, or heel bone is by far the largest bone of the foot, and is roughly cuboidal in shape. It is the only bone of the tarsus which normally touches the ground, and, when it does this, it serves to transmit the weight of the body to the

* These are small movable bones, usually two in number, which are developed in tendons to strengthen them where they exert the greatest pressure on the parts over which they glide.

ground. It forms a strong lever for the muscles of the calf.

The astragalus, talus, or ankle bone, is the second largest bone of the foot. It rests on top of the heel bone, and lies between it and the tibia, the larger of the two bones of the leg. The fibula, the smaller of the bones of the leg, joins or articulates with the ankle bone on the outer side. This part of the fibula which joins the astragalus is known as the external malleolus, and is the most prominent part of the ankle joint.

The scaphoid or navicular bone, so called from its resemblance to a boat, lies on the inner side of the foot immediately in front of the astragalus, and immediately behind the three cunieform bones. Its position can be recognised on most feet by the presence of a projection or tuberosity which can be felt just in front of the ankle itself.

The cuboid, named because of its shape, lies on the outer side of the scaphoid, and immediately in front of the anterior or foremost portion of the os calcis. The external cunieform bone also joins with it on the inner side, and the last two metatarsal bones lie in front of it.

The internal, middle, and external cunieform bones are situated in front of the scaphoid and between that bone and the first three metatarsal bones.

The metatarsal bones are five in number and are numbered from within outwards. They are long bones which join the tarsus to the bones of the toes. Each metatarsal bone has a base which articulates with the nearest or proximal phalanges. The first metatarsal bone is shorter but very much thicker than the rest. On many feet its base may be seen as a projection on the dorsum or upper part of the instep. Although this is not normal, it is by no means uncommon. The head of the first metatarsal appears to be very prominent in people who have bunions, or halux valgus.

The three middle metatarsal bones may

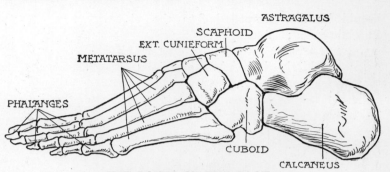

THE BONES OF THE FOOT
The twenty-six foot bones are separated into three groups; the tarsus, at the back, the metatarsus, and the phalanges or toe bones.

be felt as ridges in the middle part of the dorsum of the foot. The fifth metatarsal has a pronounced tubercle on the outer side of its base. These are recognisable on all reasonably slender feet, the prominence being both seen and felt with ease. This is perfectly normal.

There are two phalanges or segments for the great or big toe, and three for each of the other toes. Those of the great toe are known as the proximal and distal phalanges; those of the other toes as the proximal, middle and distal.

The ankle joint or tibiotarsal articulation is formed by the jointing of the astragalus

Joints of the Foot. with the lower extremity of the tibia above and the malleolus of the tibia on the inner side. On the outer side, it articulates with the external malleolus of the fibula. The joint is of the hinge type so that its movements are only those of flexion (bending upwards) and extension (bending downwards). It is supported by four strong ligaments.

The joints of the tarsus are of the gliding type, and are reinforced by a number of ligaments. Of these the plantar fascia and the plantar ligaments are the most important. The plantar fascia is a band of extraordinary strength which stretches from the tuberosities of the os calcis to the heads of the metatarsals and first phalanges. The plantar skin, that is, the skin of the sole of the foot, is attached to it. Layers of fibrous tissue pass upwards from the plantar fascia to form compartments for the muscles, blood vessels and nerves.

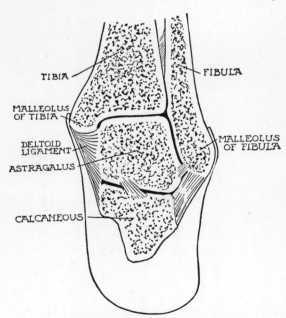

THE LEFT ANKLE IN SECTION
Drawn from the back to show how the leg bones—the tibia and fibula—fit on to the ankle bones.

The long and the short plantar ligaments extend from the os calcis to the cuboid, the long plantar ligament sending some fibres to the metatarsal bones. Another ligament of great importance is the calcaneo-scaphoid ligament which, as its name implies, joins the calcaneus to the scaphoid.

As the muscles of the leg are inserted into the foot they must be considered along with the muscles of the foot. The calf muscles are the gastrocnemius, the soleus, and the plantaris. All three of these muscles are inserted into the tendo-Achillis which is firmly attached to the back of the heel bone. Between the tendo-Achillis and the upper part of the calcaneus is a bursa, a little sac containing fluid, whose function is to prevent undue friction between the tendon and the bone. This bursa is subject to injury and sometimes to disease. From the point of view of foot health, perhaps the most important muscles are the tibialis posticus and tibialis anticus. The tibialis posticus arises from the tibia and the fibula, and its tendon passes beneath that of the flexor longus digitorum to the tuberosity of the scaphoid. This muscle gives way in flat foot.

Muscles and Tendons.

The tibialis anticus arises from the outer surface of the tibia and is inserted into the external cunieform bone and into the base of the first metatarsal. Weakness of this muscle is also a very important factor in the production of flat foot. Other muscles with which we are concerned are the flexors, which bend the toes downwards, and the extensors which bend them upwards. The flexor longus hallucis arises from the fibula and is inserted into the base of the second phalanx of the great toe. Its function is to bend the toe downward and enable it to get a firm grip of the ground whilst walking. It is a very important muscle so far as propulsion is concerned. The flexor longus digitorum and the flexor brevis digitorum bend the other toes downwards.

The nerve supply to the foot comes from the internal and the external popliteal nerves which are the two divisions of the sciatic nerve, the largest nerve cord in the body.

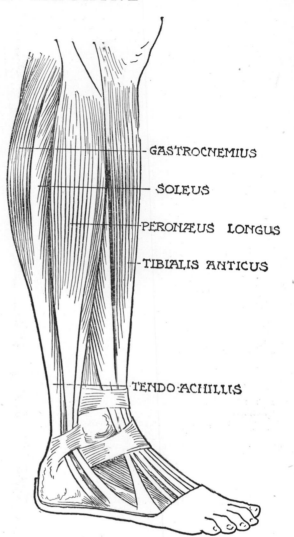

MUSCLES OF THE FOOT AND LEG
The three calf muscles are firmly attached to the heel bone by the tendo-Achillis. The tibialis anticus is an important muscle involved in flat foot.

MECHANICS OF THE FEET

The classification of the bones of the foot into three divisions, the tarsus, metatarsus, and the phalanges, is a purely anatomical one. The function of the foot will, perhaps, be understood best if it is described as being composed of two halves, an inner and an outer. The inner half is made up of the astragalus, scaphoid, the cunieform bones, the first and second metatarsals, and the phalanges of the great and second toes. This constitutes what may be called the *internal or spring arch* of the foot. The *external or*

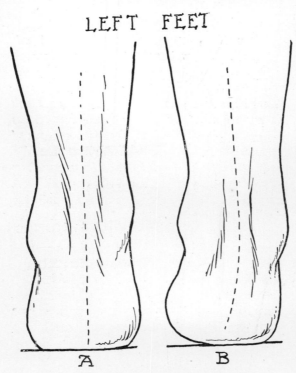

LEFT FEET

A   B

THE FIRST SIGN OF FLAT FOOT
In a normal foot (A) the tendo-Achillis is vertical;
when flat foot sets in it deviates to the outside, allowing
the heel bone to rotate inwards (B).

weight-bearing arch is composed of the other bones, namely, the calcaneus, cuboid, the last three metatarsals, and the phalanges of the third, fourth, and little toes. Another arch may also be described. This is the transverse arch and is formed by the five metatarsal bones.

The function of the foot is to support the body whilst standing and to propel the body in the act of walking or running. It has been shown already how complicated a member the foot actually is. Many people are inclined to think of it and to treat it as though it were jointed only at one place, the ankle, but twenty-six bones take part in its formation, and these bones articulate with one another in thirty-eight different places; that is to say, there are actually thirty-eight joints in the foot. The foot is constructed in this complicated manner for a very definite purpose; that is, to give it the maximum range of movement in any direction which is necessary and thus to enable it to perform its functions with the very highest degree of efficiency.

In aboriginal men feet are seen as Nature intended them to be. They have feet of definitely greater perfection and usefulness than those possessed by their more civilised brethren. Civilisation has made it necessary for us to clothe our feet. First this was done in order to protect them against jagged and uncomfortable surfaces, against the crawling things of the earth and the inclemencies of the weather. In its inception, clothing of the foot was probably a sound idea, but, as time went on, fashion began to take the place of common sense until one began to find that feet were being clothed with boots or shoes which were chosen primarily for their appearance, and secondarily only for any useful purpose.

Normally the weight of the body should be mainly carried on the ball of the foot, both in standing and in walking.

Poise. In this way a proper poise is maintained, the shoulders are thrown back, the chest forward, and the abdomen is drawn in. And as the weight of the body should be carried in this way the feet should be kept parallel both in standing and in walking, otherwise the balance of the body will be upset and the ankle and knee joints weakened. It has long been the custom of parents to criticise their children for walking on their toes and to endeavour to make them walk with their toes turned out. It is quite incorrect either to discourage the first or to encourage the second.

Apart from the times when one is engaged in athletic exercises or dancing it is usually deemed ungainly to walk so that the ball of the foot touches the ground before the heel; but this is the ideal method of propulsion. It is chiefly for this reason that it is advisable to have shoes which are fitted with heels of a requisite height, because they tend to throw the body forward on to the ball of the foot. If we were all taught from our babyhood to walk more or less on our toes and, when at rest, either to stand on the balls of our feet or to adopt the crouching attitude of the savage, heels would be unnecessary. But even though it is advisable for civilised people to wear heels, it is nevertheless inadvisable to allow the heel to meet the ground before the toe. The very function of the inner part of the foot, the spring arch, is to give that resilience which enables one to walk with the minimum of fatigue and without throwing any undue shock or strain on to any other part of the body. When the heel is brought into contact with the ground first, the body receives a jar with each step, and although each of these shocks is by itself only extremely light, their multiplication is bound to have an adverse effect upon the pelvis and spine of all but the most robust individuals.

DISEASES AND DEFORMITIES OF THE FEET

Weak Foot. Weak foot is commonly the precursor of flat foot and occurs chiefly in children and more especially in those of the rachitic type. In this condition the arches of the feet appear to be normal when the foot is at rest, and no

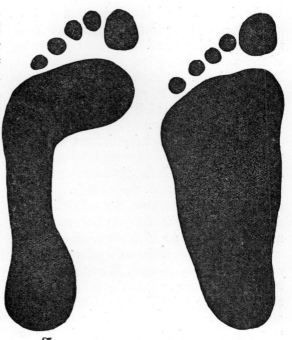

A   B
FLAT FOOT—THE DROPPED ARCH
(A) shows the print of a normal foot, with the arch well raised. In a severe case of flat foot (B) the whole sole rests upon the ground.

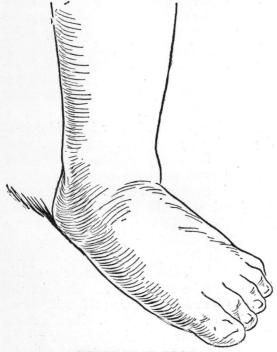

SEVERE FLAT FOOT
Showing how the arch drops completely in severe cases, giving an ungainly appearance to the foot.

weight is thrown on it ; but as soon as the foot bears the weight of the body the arches give way, and the foot has the appearance of being flat. This is due to a weakness of the muscles or ligaments, or both. If it is not corrected, permanent flat foot will be certain to develop. In the treatment of this condition it is essential to build up the bodily health and attention must be given to the diet. Vitamin—containing foodstuffs such as cod-liver oil, raw carrots, and oranges must form part of the daily dietary. In addition the feet must be massaged, and if the child is old enough it should be made to perform certain exercises.

The causes of flat foot are : (1) ill-fitting shoes ; (2) obesity ; (3) acute illnesses ; **Flat Foot.** (4) pregnancy ; (5) accidental injury, as in jumping from a height.

In flat foot one or more of the arches of the foot have given way permanently and changes have taken place in the position of the bones of the foot. There are two main varieties of flat foot, the *flexible* and the *rigid*.

In the former, the joints being still mobile, the bones can be brought back to their normal positions and the re-establishment of the correct formation of the foot may be brought about. In the other type, the rigid flat foot, changes have taken place in the bones and joints which render a return to normality impossible.

The first sign of flat foot is seen when the patient stands with his feet bare. The tendo-Achillis, instead of falling in its normal vertical plane, deviates to the outside. The os calcis is rotated inwards, the scaphoid faces downwards, and its tubercle becomes much more prominent ; and the cunieform bones, especially the internal one, are brought into contact with the ground. The heads of the metatarsal bones are usually also depressed, and, owing to the falling of the internal cunieform bone, the base of the first metatarsal is frequently seen to be in a most prominent position. This indicates that its head has fallen and the shaft has acquired an abnormally pronounced slant.

There is no adequate treatment for rigid flat foot. Manipulation is useless, and is only likely to initiate symptoms which were previously absent. Treatment. The patient with rigid flat foot is more often than not perfectly comfortable, as his feet have accommodated themselves to their abnormal state. Any type of arch support will cause continual discomfort, and in consequence this type of deformity should be left alone. Such, however, is not the case with the flexible type of flat foot. Here manipulation will be of the utmost benefit —in many cases a single adjustment of the internal cunieform bone bringing about complete relief from very distressing symptoms. It is frequently possible to depress the base of the first metatarsal and to restore the scaphoid and calcaneous to their normal positions by simple manipulative procedures. Many cases of flat foot require a number of manipulations to cure. This is particularly true in cases of long standing, because in these one frequently finds there is a tendency to the transition of a flexible flat foot into one of the osseus type.

Flexible flat foot usually gives rise to a considerable amount of pain. This is chiefly under the internal longitudinal arch, but may extend up the leg. When the transverse arch has fallen (and it will usually be found that it has), there will be a considerable degree of pain in the underneath of the fore part of the foot—a condition known as METATARSALGIA. This is caused by a falling of the metatarsal heads and can be corrected by manipulation and the wearing of properly fitted and supported shoes.

In discussing metatarsalgia it is well to remember the condition known as Morton's toe. In this condition, which is Morton's due to the depression of the head Toe. of the fourth metatarsal bone, there is a severe pain at the fourth metatarsophalangeal articulation, there being relatively little or no pain at the other corresponding joints. It has been included under this heading because its treatment is more or less the same as that which has been described, and will later be further discussed in connection with metatarsalgia.

Although manipulations are of the greatest benefit in the treatment of flat foot they will not suffice to cure these conditions unless other help is given. Massage tends to strengthen the muscles and ligaments. Exercises are of the greatest value, and lastly, but by no means least, the feet must be fitted with corrective shoes.

Excessive perspiration or hyperidrosis of the feet is very common, and occurs more frequently in males than females, Excessive and usually between the ages of Sweating. twenty and forty. It is frequently associated with flat feet. This excessive functioning of the sweat glands is due to a disturbance of the nerves which supply these glands. It is a symptom which must not be overlooked, and it is advisable to obtain medical advise regarding it. The diet will have to be attended to, as this will almost certain to be found at fault. Certain remedial measures may be used to cover up this unpleasant symptom. Dusting the insides of the socks and the feet themselves with a powder composed of equal parts of powdered

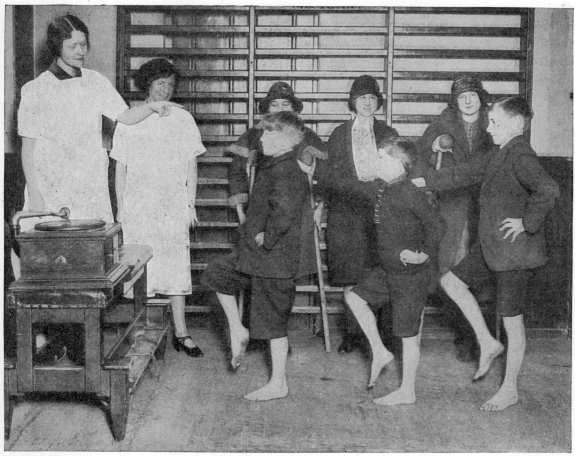

[Keystone

FOOT EXERCISES TO MUSIC

Exercises to the accompaniment of the gramophone are practised at St. Thomas's Hospital, London, to cure
flat foot and to strengthen the muscles of the feet and legs.

starch, boracic acid, and salicylic acid will frequently help. The socks must be of silk or wool. Cotton socks only tend to aggravate the condition. At night time and in the morning the feet should be plunged alternately into quite hot and very cold water. This should be repeated six or seven times, the last immersion being in cold water, after which the feet should be thoroughly dried with a coarse towel and dusted with the powder mentioned above. The footwear itself must receive attention as shoes which do not admit of the proper circulation of the blood and normal muscular movements will prolong the condition.

Hallux valgus is the term applied to the turning outwards of the great toe, *i.e.* when the great toe turns away from the mid-line and approximates the other toes too closely. Not infrequently it overrides the second toe,

Hallux Valgus. which gradually grows so that it is placed beneath the great toe. This is a very painful deformity and is almost invariably caused by badly fitting footwear. The friction on the inside of the joint causes a bursa to be formed. This is what is correctly called a BUNION, and it is extremely subject to irritation and inflammation.

In mild cases, that is, in cases where the metatarso-phalangeal joint is freely movable and the great toe itself can be forced without much pain into an almost straight line with the inner border of the foot, fitting of correct shoes is the first step to be taken. As flat foot and weak foot very often exist along with hallux valgus, it may be necessary to support the internal longitudinal arch. There are various applicances which may be worn both inside the shoe and in bed, but the majority of these are unsatisfactory.

Frequent manipulation of the toe joint in which the toe is forced inwards is of great value, but such manipulations must be done often and over a very considerable period of time. Many people believe that some deft manipulation by a bone-setter will cure their condition immediately. This is impossible. Inflammation of the bursa is best treated by hot applications such as linseed poultices, or better still by Anti-phlogistine.

Many cases of hallux valgus have advanced so far that such remedial measures as have been outlined will not bring about a cure. In these cases bony changes have taken place in and around the joint which make it impossible for the toe ever to assume a normal or even a nearly normal position. Surgical interference is necessary, and the advice of an orthopædic surgeon should be sought. The operation is relatively simple, and consists in cutting away a wedge-shaped piece of bone from the inside of the joint.

Corns are proliferations of the outermost or horny layer of the skin and are caused by the friction of badly-fitting shoes. **Corns.** There is usually a small process of this hardened epidermal tissue which has forced its way into the soft tissues of the foot. This is termed the root. In the treatment of corns we must again first look to the fitting of the shoes. The corns themselves should be attended to by a competent chiropodist.

For those who can do the operation themselves the following notes will be of assistance. The corn should be pared first with a very sharp knife. A one-edged razor blade in a safety holder answers the purpose extremely well. After paring, the feet should be soaked in hot water for about fifteen minutes, and an effort made to remove the root. If this is unsuccessful, a preparation containing salicylic acid should be applied to the corn morning and evening, and the root may then be removed after some four or five days. There is a variety of corn known as a soft corn which has no root and grows between the toes. Soft corns are generally very painful, and are due to constitutional disturbance more than to any other cause. A physician should be consulted and proper dietetic and hygienic measures prescribed.

Ingrowing toe nail is a common condition in which the nail, generally that of the great toe, grows into the flesh on the **Ingrowing Toe Nail.** one side or the other. It causes a very great deal of pain and is usually the result of badly-fitting shoes or cutting the toe nails in a wrong manner, or both. The toe nails should never be cut in a circular manner as is usually the practice with the finger nails, but they should be cut straight across and the sharp points at the sides finely clipped or filed off. If an ingrowing nail has occurred, the centre of the nail should be filed from top to bottom until it becomes very thin, and a V-shaped piece should be cut out of the middle at the top. In addition a small piece of cotton wool soaked in collodion should be placed between the toe nail and the flesh. If after two or three weeks of this treatment and the wearing of correct shoes, the toe is still troublesome, a surgeon should be consulted with a view to the removal of the nail.

When the foot at birth is fixed in a position in which it could not normally be placed if it were a healthy foot, the **Club Foot.** condition is known as congenital club foot. In medical terminology it is called *talipes*. There are four main varieties of this condition. Talipes equinus, in which the foot is held in a position with the toes pointing downwards ; talipes calcaneus, in which the foot is turned upwards ; talipes varus when it is turned in, and talipes valgus in which it is turned out. Parents whose children are afflicted in this manner must necessarily take a somewhat serious outlook as to their child's feet, but the condition is by no means incurable and can be readily

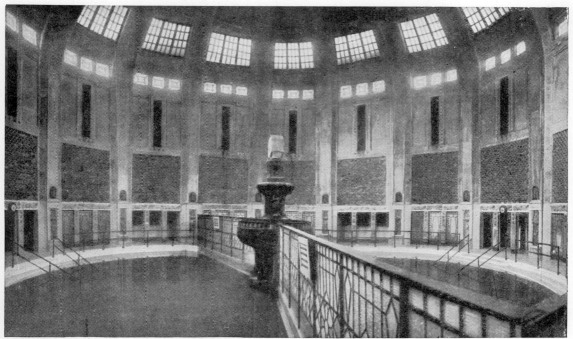

A MUD BATH FOR BONE DISEASES

The bath over the warm mud springs at Pistany, Czechoslovakia, where diseases of the bones and joints receive special treatment.

remedied if the correct procedures are adopted in time. In cases which are treated early, constant manipulation is of the greatest importance, the foot being gradually forced to go through the whole of its normal range of movement. It cannot be too strongly emphasised that the earlier the treatment the better will be the results. Delay means an operation which, although it may be successful in a great number of cases, is not always followed by the most satisfactory results.

Anterior poliomyelitis, or infantile paralysis, as it is commonly called, is a disease which occurs mostly in children, and is

Infantile Paralysis. one which not infrequently has a serious effect upon the feet. In its incipience this disease, which is marked by a rise in temperature to 102° and 104 °F., is usually looked upon by the parents as purely a severe chill or an attack of influenza. As its results may be extremely serious so far as the child's welfare is concerned it is most important that it should be recognised in its early stages. The foot troubles which

follow infantile paralysis are often of an intractable nature. The most common of these is called drop-foot and is characterised by a flaccidity and wasting of the muscles which cause the foot to drop down from the ankle. Once established, the only remedy for this condition is a shortening of certain tendons by operation—and this is very far from satisfactory. The main thing in this disease is to recognise the symptoms early—have the proper treatment immediately, and thus minimise, as far as possible, its disastrous consequences.

Little's disease, which is known medically as congenital spastic paraplegia, is one for

Little's Disease. which the medical profession has been unable to offer any hope of cure up to the present time. It is a disease which is present at birth but which is usually not recognised until some months later when the child is found to be unable to sit up or to kick its legs in the normal manner. As the child grows older the legs are found to be stiff and have a tendency to cross one another whilst the feet turn

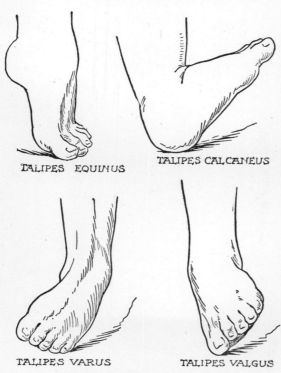

TALIPES EQUINUS   TALIPES CALCANEUS

TALIPES VARUS   TALIPES VALGUS

COMMON TYPES OF CLUB FOOT
Types of the deformity in which the foot is fixed
in an abnormal position at birth or from disease.

inwards. A surgical operation may give a certain amount of relief, but permanent improvement is very unlikely under any form of treatment.

A peculiar kind of sore called a perforating ulcer is sometimes seen on the sole of the foot. This ulcer is of unusual depth, and, on account of its painlessness may not be noticed until it has become well established. The advice of a physician should be sought immediately any ulcerous formation appears on the sole of the foot, as it may be a symptom of very serious consequence. As a matter of fact no ulcer, on any part of the foot, should be treated by home remedies, whether the ulcers have apparently been caused by injury or not; a physician should be consulted in every case.

Perforating Ulcer.

FOOTWEAR

By FREDERICK G. PAGE, Footwear Specialist to D. Neal & Sons, author of "Foot Health," etc.

SEVENTY per cent. of our people have foot trouble of one kind or another, and it is, in fact, very rarely that a perfectly normal adult foot is seen. The large majority of these troubles are directly traceable to incorrectly fitting shoes and are, therefore, avoidable. Shoes as articles of fashion are naturally sold as such and with little consideration of the effect they may have upon the wearer's feet, or whether they may be harmful or helpful. Shoe sellers are usually lacking in any knowledge of foot-anatomy, are, in fact, shoe sellers only, and it is, therefore, not really surprising that seven out of ten people suffer needless pain.

With painful feet the ability to take sufficient outdoor exercise is diminished and the general health suffers in consequence. Where a foot becomes malformed or is so weak that its normal position is lost, there are strains thrown upon the entire bony superstructure and the supporting muscles and ligaments. The body is thrown out of alignment, often with disastrous results. Pains, frequently mistaken for rheumatism, lumbago, sciatica, etc., are often due to unnatural strains caused by misshapen feet —faulty foundations.

The feet are the most complicated bony structures in the human body, the twenty-six bones in each forming a series of arches with weight-bearing points. They not only have to support the body's weight with whatever load may be added to it—and think what this may mean in the case of such workers as railway porters—but must be able to function freely if we are to move with grace and freedom.

For an arch of the foot to fall—and an arch falling elongates—there is at once a strain on the supporting muscles and ligaments which is immediately felt, but it must be remembered that in most cases there *would* be no falling and elongating if the muscles had been sufficiently strong to maintain the normal position. The question naturally follows, " What caused the muscle to become weak ? " Malnutrition, illness, pregnancy, rapidly increased weight, too rapid growth in children—each may predispose to the trouble, but it is safe to assert that in the majority of cases ill-fitting shoes are the main causal factor.

It is common knowledge that muscles exercised become strong, whilst those that are *not* exercised or are restricted in their functioning become weak. It is by restricting the functioning of the muscles of the foot and the leg that shoes cause so much trouble.

From the heel to the ball of the foot and below the ankle there is very little movement, and this part of the foot should be **Weakened Muscles.** fitted closely, but from the ball of the foot forward there must be such freedom as will allow for unrestricted movement in every joint, in each toe, and room, too, for each to lie perfectly straight in the shoe without side pressure.

It is observed that foot troubles are much more prevalent in women than in men, and this is accounted for by reason of the fact that women's shoes have higher heels and are usually made with a strap across the instep.

The higher heel creates a greater incline from the heel to the ball, down which the foot moves—as the light strap is not sufficient to prevent it—the toes are forced into the end of the shoe, restricted in their move-

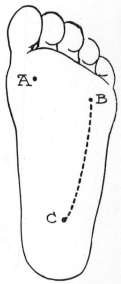

WHERE THE WEIGHT RESTS

The weight of the body is borne on the ball of the big toe (A), the ball of the little toe (B), and all along the outer edge of the foot to the heel (C).

ments, and often forced into an unnatural position.

Bunions and hammer toes are both caused in this way, whilst weakened muscles following the restriction of movement result in a weak foot that will develop into flat foot unless the proper precautions are taken.

Metatarsalgia—a falling of the transverse arch (the arch between the ball of the great toe and the base of the little toe)—is also caused by the backward pressure on the ends of the toes when coming into contact with the end of the shoe, and is, of course, aggravated by the atrophying or wasting of the foot muscles owing to their lack of free usage.

Men's shoes have lower heels, so there is less slope and, therefore, less inclination to move forward, whilst they are invariably of the laced variety, forming a bandage or support to the instep and arch and preventing the foot from moving forward in the shoe.

In the question of the height of heels, **Heels.** as in other matters relating to fashion or custom, it is well to ask what Nature intended.

Nature, the perfect builder, gives us an example in the baby, who, with feet unspoilt by custom or convention, when first he begins to " toddle," walks upon the ball of his foot, with the heel raised from the ground, and immediately the heel is lowered he sits down. It may be argued that this is because the baby has not learned to walk, but consideration of the grown-up baby, the primæval savage, the North American Indian, Samoan, or the African native, reveals that these unspoilt sons of

FITTING THE TOE JOINT

The inner arch should be well supported, and there should be no space between the shoe and the foot behind the big toe joint. (*Above*) an ill-fitting, and (*below*) a perfectly fitting shoe.

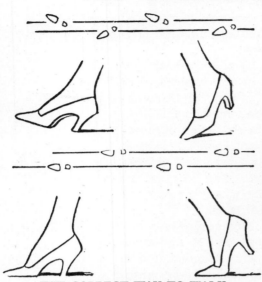

THE CORRECT WAY TO WALK

The human frame is in the position intended by Nature when it is erect, with heels raised and the feet parallel (*below*)—never with the toes turned out (*above*).

Nature walk in exactly the same way, and that when they wish to come to rest, they squat upon their haunches, the heels being well raised from the ground.

When walking is done on the balls of the feet, and with heel raised, there is no jarring, because elastic muscles are holding the heels in an elevated position with the front parts of the feet depressed to receive the force of each impact against the ground, muscular elasticity absorbing all jarring effects very perfectly. On the other hand, when walking is done completely on the heels there must be a slight jar throughout the entire body at each step in this unnatural posture.

Erect and with heels raised, the human frame is in the position that Nature intended, and it is in this position, and in this position alone, that the muscles of the feet, of the legs and of the lumbar regions are exercised and properly employed, thereby gaining strength. It is, of course, well known that all physical culture exercises are done upon the toes, for in this position there is the natural inclination for the chest to be thrown out, and the abdomen drawn inwards : the poise of the vigorous and athletic.

The question now arises exactly how high the heel bone should be elevated from the ground, and by observation it has been found that the normal distance in the adult is approximately one and half inches, so that to go above or below this height is against the rule of Nature.

In further considering the correct way to fit feet if they are to be kept strong and healthy (in addition to the remarks regarding the necessity of firmly supporting the instep by a close fitting from the heel to the ball of the foot) it will be well to study briefly the normal weight-bearing points.

We see that the weight is borne on the base of the heel, the ball of the great toe, the ball of the little toe and *all along the outer edge of the foot.*

With shoes with heels being worn there is a bridge formed from the heel to the base of the little toe and little or no support given by the shoe. It is essential that there should be, particularly when the foot muscles are weak and the arches likely to fall, so that weak feet should be fitted with shoes that are made with metal plates inserted between the inner and outer soles. Loose metal plates should not be worn unless they have been prescribed, *and fitted* by an orthopædic surgeon. It is believed that in time they will be entirely discarded for they are heavy and unsuited to fitting into shoes which have not been specially constructed to take them and which, in consequence, are thrown out of shape.

Metal Plates.

The inner arch of the foot needs to be carefully fitted, and when selecting shoes great care should be taken to see that the ball of the great toe is in the exact position it should occupy. There is a place for this joint in every shoe and it will be found to be very slightly behind the widest part of the sole. If on trying on shoes there is any space between the foot and the shoe behind the joint, it is almost certain the shoe is too short.

The sketches at the foot of page 569 will show what is happening.

In the upper sketch the arch of the foot and the arch of the shoe do not synchronise, and the foot is unsupported at this point

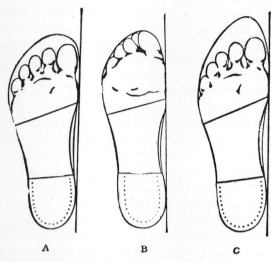

HOW THE TOES SHOULD LIE
(A) is a correct wide-fitting shoe with the big toe lying straight. In (B) the shoe, though wide enough, is too short. (C) shows a pointed shoe which still allows the toes to lie correctly.

whereas it should be supported. If the shoe were longer in the waist, as a larger shoe would be, this would not be the case, and in addition, the foot would be farther back in the shoe and greater freedom for the toes would follow. In the lower sketch the arch is correctly fitted and supported.

The shoes constructed with reinforced waists for weak feet are usually made with a special support for the transverse arch too, for it is found that in weak feet with a tendency to falling of the longitudinal arch there is nearly always a falling of the transverse arch. Across the ball of the foot and behind the joint, the inner-soles are not flat in such shoes, but are slightly moulded upward, so that the arch is restored and the pressure taken off the metatarso-phalangeal heads. Callous skin at this point is nearly always present where there is metatarsalgia, and the callous is, of course, due to pressure at a point that nature had intended *not* to receive pressure. The correction afforded by such shoes usually results in the disappearance of the callous.

It is unfortunate that mere mention of remedial or corrective footwear will conjure up visions of square-toed, squat-heeled unsightly shoes, but square toes are *not* necessary whilst the height of heel has already been

dealt with. Pointed or round toes *will* be worn as long as they are fashionable and they may be if they are long enough.

Figure A shows a foot correctly fitted with a wide-toed shoe, and it will be noticed that the great toe is allowed to lie perfectly straight and thus canno⁺ be malformed. The next (B) shows how a shoe with a *wide* toe *fitted too short* can malform the great toe and force it into an incorrect position, with the result that a bunion will form.

In the third illustration (C) it will be noticed that although the toe of the shoe is pointed, the great toe lies in straight lines with the inner border of the foot, and all the other toes are free from backward pressure and will not be forced into the unnatural positions which cause "hammer-toes." The small amount of extra length given with a narrow-toed shoe can have no bad effects, but is merely a concession to fashion made to meet the demands of those who prefer such styles, and consider it enhances the appearance.

Morton's Toe can often be relieved by fixing to the inner sole of the shoe an oval piece of sponge rubber or cork that will correct the unnatural depression. It will, however, be apparent that this pad will need to be fitted in exactly the right spot by an expert, or the condition may be made worse.

Where hyperidrosis (excessive perspiration) exists care must be exercised in the selection of shoes and hose. The Excessive Sweating. excessive warmth of the foot, together with the acid excretions, will often cause the leather to perish so

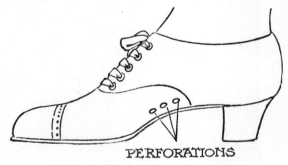

PERFORATIONS

A METHOD OF FOOT VENTILATION
Holes punched through the inside arch of the shoe admit cool air and relieve excessive warmth.

badly that the soles or heels of shoes completely break away from the uppers, whilst the upper leather will crack and break long before it would do with a normal foot. The upper leather should be selected for its porosity, glacé kid being the most porous, calf skin less so, and patent leather should on no account be worn. Considerable relief may be obtained—cool air allowed to percolate through to the foot at each step—by having three or more holes punched right through the shoe uppers at the highest

FOR DAILY EXERCISE
The correct posture of the body for foot exercises performed in the standing position.

point of the inside arch of the shoe. These are not seen and are not likely to allow wet to enter as they will be at least an inch from the ground. Pure wool or pure silk hosiery alone should be worn, since they absorb moisture more readily than cotton or Lisle thread.

BUNIONS are essentially a result of ill-fitting shoes, and usually originate in childhood. It should be remembered that to malform the great toe of an adult so badly as to cause a bunion would be such a painful process that it would not be tolerated, but in childhood, when the bones are in the process of formation and are of a cartilaginous nature, they can be malformed with comparatively little pain. In passing, it should be noted that because a child does not complain that the shoes being worn are hurting is not conclusive proof that they are not *harming* the foot.

When the bunion has reached a stage where there is no mobility (hallux rigidus), nothing but a surgical operation will correct the deformity, but if the joint is still flexible relief can often be obtained. Naturally the first step is to secure footwear that has sufficient room along the side of the great toe to permit it to assume the natural straight position. There are various appliances made to bring the toe back to the normal, one in particular, " Rectopede," has been found quite successful, and as it is made entirely of elastic fabric, it is gentle in its action and can be worn without discomfort. Placing a rubber pad between the great toe and the next one is not to be recommended, for as the smaller toes are the weaker they are apt to be deflected, whilst the great toe remains in its malformed position.

CORNS, with the exception of the soft variety between the toes, are directly caused by pressure, so, here again, the correct fitting of the shoes worn must receive attention if the cause is to be removed. If this is not done, any treatment, chiropodial or otherwise, will only afford temporary relief, for the trouble will recur.

INGROWING TOE NAILS are another result

of ill-fitting shoes. The attention of a qualified chiropodist and correct footwear will eliminate the trouble.

CHILBLAINS are not caused by, but may be aggravated by, tight shoes, for it is essential that there should be nothing to impede the normal circulation of the blood, and small shoes certainly do so, particularly by retarding free movement of the toes which is essential to healthy circulation.

Foot exercises can be of great assistance where there

Foot Exercises. is a weak foot or tendency to metatarsalgia, and those illustrated have been proved to be of great benefit.

If in place of counting one, two, three, four, five, etc., the patient will take a series of short inhalations through the nose sufficient entirely to fill the lungs with the final one, and then exhale rapidly and completely through the nose, it will be found to be of benefit to the entire system.

The exercises should be done by an open window whilst loosely clad, the body being held erect, the chin up, chest out, and abdomen held in. To sponge down at the conclusion and briskly rub with a fairly coarse towel is a further help.

When walking is done on the balls of the feet, and with heels raised, there is no jarring,

Correct Way to Walk. because elastic muscles are holding the heels in an elevated position with the front parts of the feet depressed to receive the force of each impact against the ground, muscular elasticity absorbing all jarring effects very perfectly. On the other hand, when walking is done completely on the heels, a slight jar must be felt throughout the entire body at each step in this unnatural posture. Erect, with heels raised and the feet parallel —never with the toes turned out—the human frame is in the position intended by Nature, and it is in this position alone that the muscles of the feet, or the legs, and of the

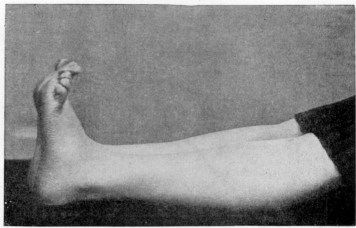

AN EXERCISE FOR SUPPLE FEET
Sitting on the ground, turn the foot (1) as far upward and backward, and (2) as far downward and forward as possible. Repeat six times.

lumbar region are exercised and properly employed, thereby gaining strength and healthy tone.

ARTIFICIAL HEELS—THEIR USE AND ABUSE
By Sir W. ARBUTHNOT LANE, Bart., C.B., M.S., F.R.C.S.

SINCE there is much confusion in the minds of the public concerning the part played by artificial heels in the mechanics of posture and movement, I think I cannot do better than briefly revise the important features of the structure of the foot and demonstrate, in as simple a manner as possible, the nature of their function.

The astragalus or ankle bone rests on top of the os calcis or heel bone, lying between it and the tibia and fibula—the stout and slender bones of the leg—to which it is secured by powerful ligaments. In this way is formed the ankle joint which is a perfect example of the hinge type of articulation, allowing movement only in an upward and downward direction. The ankle bone is firmly attached to the upper surface of the heel bone by a strong ligament which permits a certain amount of rotation or gliding movement.

In front of the heel bone lie the cuboid, named because of its shape, and the scaphoid, so called from its resemblance to a boat. A strong ligament extends from the under surface of the heel bone to the under surface of the cuboid, making a joint and also helping in the formation of an unyielding arch which supports the entire weight of the body. The scaphoid is connected to the heel bone by means of a powerful ligament whose fibres are arranged in a spiral or corkscrew-like manner as illustrated on page 575; it also articulates with the rounded head of the ankle bone.

Attached to the prominent tuberosity of the scaphoid is the tendon of an important muscle, the "tibialis posticus," **Spiral Ligament.** which exerts a traction in an upward and backward direction. When this muscle contracts, it raises the outer end of the scaphoid and causes this bone to rotate upon the rounded head of the ankle bone. In so doing, it winds up the corkscrew ligament and diminishes the angular interval between the scaphoid and the heel bone. It also forces the head of the ankle bone outwards upon the upper surface of the heel bone, and, in this way, the pressure transmitted through the heel is taken off the spiral ligament and is transferred to the inelastic, unyielding but powerful arch of the foot. By so reducing this angular interval, the inner margin of the foot is made to form an angle open inwards and the length of this margin is consequently at its shortest. If, on the contrary, the tibialis posticus muscle is relaxed and ceases to exert traction upon the scaphoid, the outer end of this bone drops and the spiral ligament unwinds. Thus, the angular interval between the scaphoid and the heel

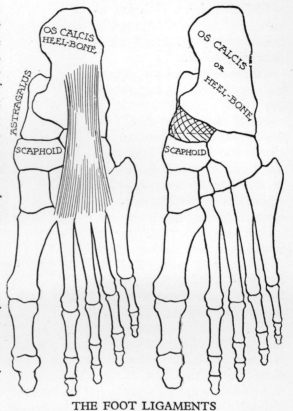

THE FOOT LIGAMENTS

The under surface of the foot, showing (*left*) the supporting ligament, and (*right*) the spiral, corkscrew-like ligament which connects the scaphoid to the heel bone.

bone is increased and it becomes occupied by the head of the ankle bone which moves inward to fill the space. In this state of muscular relaxation, the inner margin of the foot is elongated and forms an angle open outwards.

Much confusion has arisen from the mistaken supposition that the foot bears the body weight solely through bony arches supported by elastic ligaments, and this view was held until 1886 when I demonstrated the structure and function of the spiral ligament which is the pivotal mechanical device essential to the proper functioning of the foot.

It is clear that in a position of activity, as assumed in running, the feet are turned inwards, their inner

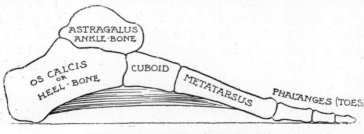

THE STRUCTURE OF THE FOOT

Showing the bones on the outer side of the foot, and the strong ligament which supports the arch.

margins making with one another an angle open backwards and being at their shortest ;

Activity and Rest. while, in the position of rest, the feet are turned out, the angle formed between their inner margins being open forwards and the length of the foot being at its greatest.

In labourers who carry heavy loads on their backs, the attitude of activity of the foot is, of necessity, assumed so habitually that the head of the ankle bone, being constantly displaced outward upon the upper surface of the heel bone, forms a new and definite joint with it. This displacement of the head of the ankle bone (and incidentally of the superjacent body weight) on to the rigid arch leads to an economy of nerve and muscle energy which is the purpose of all devices induced to meet the demands made by labour upon the body. When the condition is fully developed, the feet of such a labourer are fixed permanently in a state of activity and cannot assume that of rest.

If, however, because of constant standing, the tibialis posticus muscle becomes exhausted and so allows the corkscrew ligament to unwind to its extreme limit, the head of the ankle bone is displaced inwards and the foot becomes flattened. Such a condition, when fixed by the permanent contraction of the muscles on the outer side of the foot, is spoken of as " flatfoot." It is seen frequently in postmen and in others who have to stand or walk most of the day.

In order that the foot shall function normally, it is essential

Economisers of Energy. that it shall habitually perform a suitable alternation of periods of activity and of rest with the necessary sequence of attitudes. Since civilisation compels most of us to be constantly on our feet, in

proportion as we combine attitudes of activity with those of rest, so are our feet normal, structurally and functionally ; but, if circumstances necessitate much standing or walking, there is a great waste of energy involved. To meet this, the individual employs artificial means by which the attitude of activity can be assumed as much as possible without voluntary effort, which end is effected by the wearing of heels. In proportion as the height of the heel is increased and the attitude of rest obviated, to that extent is the attitude of activity assumed of necessity. By raising the heel sufficiently for very many hours, however, the foot may become fixed in a position of activity, so that, in an extreme case, the owner cannot assume the attitude of rest and finds it difficult or even impossible to place the heel on the ground. This is seen frequently in the feet of women who wear very high heels.

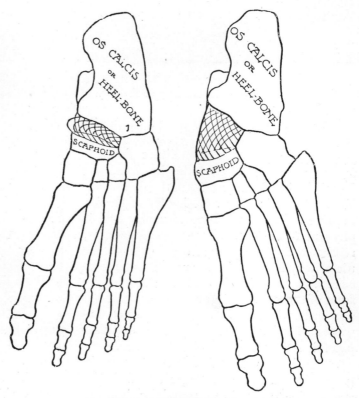

THE SPIRAL LIGAMENT AT WORK
When the tibialis posticus muscle contracts, the corkscrew ligament winds up and draws the scaphoid close to the heel bone. When it relaxes, the ligament unwinds and the inner margin of the foot lengthens.

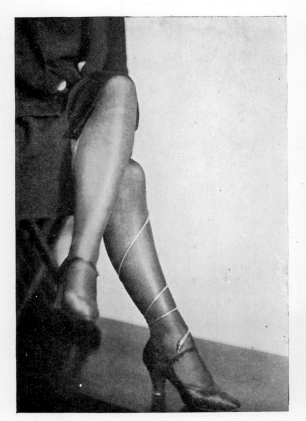 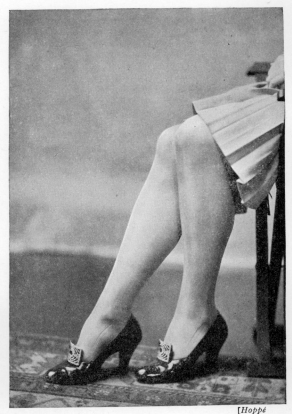

[*Hoppé*

TYPICAL MODERN HEELS
Showing the tendency to distortion of the foot with heels which are too high.

In women who stand constantly, the use of the heel is obviously advantageous in reducing the expenditure of muscle energy, in obviating flat foot, and in the shortening of the foot which has an æsthetic value. It is also of service because it gratifies a natural vanity and is pleasant to look at. Much harm, however, results to the fore part of the foot from the use of very high heels, because it is made to occupy a constricted pointed space in the front of the shoe—the great toe being forced outwards while the others are driven inwards. Bunions, hammer-toes, and other painful troubles ensue in consequence.

High-heel Dangers.

While the wearing of heels is beneficial in proportion to the advantages afforded, the evil results to the fore part of the foot can be materially obviated if shoe makers will insist on making the inner margin of the shoe *straight*, allowing sufficient space for the accommodation of the toes, and also if women will consent to such trifling modification as will, if skilfully effected, make little change in the graceful and smart appearance of the shoe.

To condemn without qualification the use of heels is obviously absurd, since their absence would reduce the usefulness of a very large proportion of the community who are compelled to stand or walk constantly for their livelihood. As is usually the case, the use of heels in moderation is decidedly beneficial, though, when they are too high, serious and painful changes distort the form and hinder the function of the foot.

In this study of the foot, we see yet another illustration of the fundamental law that " we bear a simple mechanical relationship to our surroundings. If that relationship is altered in any particular, our anatomy is modified in a corresponding manner."

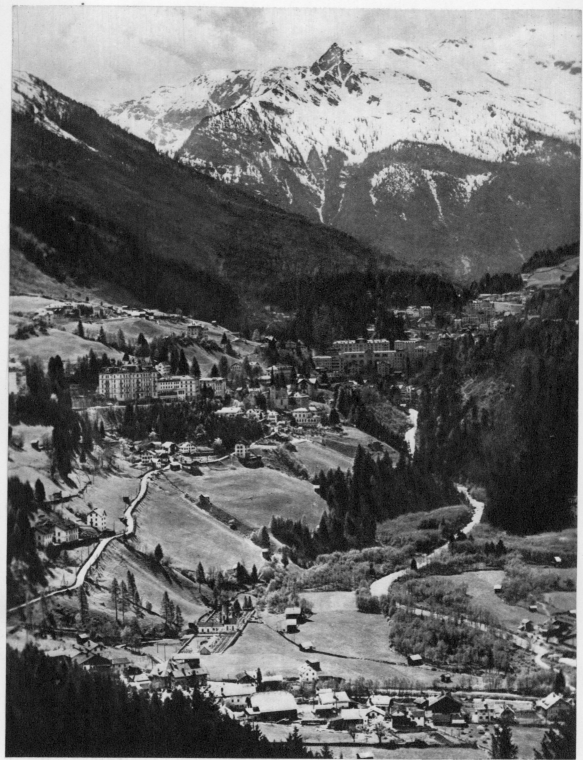

[Zechmeister

A HEALTH RESORT FOR NERVE DISEASES

Austria's most celebrated spa, Bad Gastein, where nervous diseases, especially tabes and nervous exhaustion, are treated.

THE HUMAN MACHINE
THE NERVOUS SYSTEM

By MACPHERSON LAWRIE, M.A., M.B., B.Ch., Clinical Assistant Physician to St. Luke's Hospital for Mental and Nervous Diseases.

THE SYSTEM AT WORK

THE nervous system is fundamentally a mechanism by which rapid communication can be attained throughout the organism. The circulating blood also forms a means of bringing the body tissues into close relationship, yet it is the nervous system which is responsible for the co-ordinated activity of the body as a whole. Though, for many people, thinking, feeling, willing and memorising are mysterious properties of the brain which science will never be able to elucidate, experiment and observation in bio-chemistry, psychology and comparative anatomy are gradually leading towards a complete knowledge of nervous activity.

The cell unit of the nervous system is called the neuron. It consists of a nucleated body with branching protoplasmic processes (dendrites) —small fine filaments intermingling with those of neighbouring cells, and one long branch, the axon. Through the outer communications of the dendrites impulses pass from one cell to another ; their junction is called a synapse, and the exact mechanism by which a nerve impulse passes a synapse is uncertain since there is no direct anatomical connection between the dendrites. The axon becomes a nerve fibre and transmits impulses to distant parts of the body, its length varying according to the distance. It may end in some tissue, such as a muscle fibre or a gland cell, which it excites to activity, or it may arborize round the receiving cell of a sense organ, carrying an impulse from it to the central neuron, or it may terminate by branching filaments which surround another nerve-cell, causing the transmission of the impulse to be relayed.

Dr. MACPHERSON LAWRIE

Three kinds of neurons are thus described : *receptor* or *sensory* nerve-cells, which are specialised to receive specific stimuli and convey them to the *motor* or *efferent* neurons, which in turn send out appropriate responses —commands to the muscles to contract, to the glands to pour out secretions, etc. Finally there are the *adjustors* or intermediate neurons which co-ordinate the various commands, storing impressions and registering experiences. Man has more adjustors than any other animal because he has the most highly evolved nervous system. It is one of the secrets of his superiority, enabling him to give a considered " intelligent " response to new situations.

The Reflex.

When a receptor cell is stimulated by some condition in its environment, a nervous impulse passes to the central nervous system along the axon of a sensory neuron ; it is transferred by an intermediate neuron to the cell body of a motor neuron, and thence proceeds along its axon to stimulate those particular cells from which some response is required. Such is a " reflex action," which may be defined as a motor response to a sensory stimulus. The central nervous system converts an incoming impulse into an outgoing one, directing its course appropriately.

The impulse which enters the central nervous system can influence many neurons. It may evoke the *whole* body to immediate action. A simple reflex does not occur in the human body, some distribution of the impulse to neighbouring neurons must take place as there are many intermediate or adjustor neurons. Resistance at a synapse may be lessened by repeating similar stimulation. Habit lessens resistance, opening

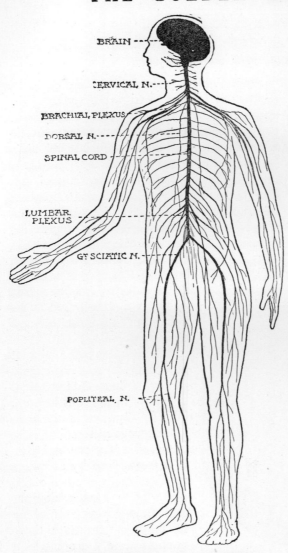

BRAIN

CERVICAL N.

BRACHIAL PLEXUS

DORSAL N.

SPINAL CORD

LUMBAR PLEXUS

Gt SCIATIC N.

POPLITEAL. N.

THE CHIEF NERVES OF THE BODY
Rapid communication is obtained throughout the body by means of the intricate network of nerves, connecting the various tissues with the brain and spinal cord.

afterwards pain may cause the brain to send additional messages. A particle of grit in the eye causes an instant blink, followed perhaps by an attempt to wash away the foreign body by tears. If this device is ineffective the brain takes the matter in hand and applies a more sophisticated remedy. Reflex actions need no reflection. There is an instant response or sending back of messages to muscles or glands, for the matter is urgent. It is clear that such instinctive responses have a very important survival value in evolution, since they save time, effort, and energy. Each animal species possesses a set of reflex actions as part of its hereditary equipment. Man's repertoire is poor compared with that of a chicken or a bee, whose instinctive capabilities are well-developed at birth. A baby can suck when it is born, blink at three months, shed tears at four months, and acquire other reflexes during its early development. This capacity of reflex action involves three organs ; first a receptor appropriately stimulated, then a long or short path for transmitting the message, and finally an effector organ, which, in man, is always a muscle or gland. Moreover, the message is marked " urgent." What counts most in human behaviour is the way in which reflex actions are conditioned, or educated. Reflex actions arise in course of evolution in response to fundamental organic needs ; and development implies the acquisition of new dexterities or adjustments to supplement those which are hereditary. It is the business of the educator to foster these.

The axons of nerve-cells, when collected into bundles, form nerve trunks which con-

Peripheral Nerves. nect the various tissues of the body with the central nervous system (the spinal cord and the brain). They carry the axons of both sensory and motor neurons and constitute the " peripheral nerves." According as they emerge from the brain or spinal cord they are called respectively cranial and spinal nerves.

There are twelve pairs of cranial nerves.

accustomed paths for the conduction of the impulse. The synapsal junction limits the spread of conduction and directs its course.

Reflex action is a type of response which is of supreme importance for all kinds of animals. Most of the body is run by reflex activities, which involve response without conscious effort. Breathing, thinking, trembling, coughing, swallowing, crying, mouth-watering are all reflex actions. Long before pain is felt a reflex response has been made ;

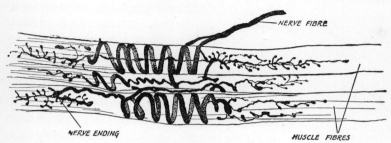

NERVE-ENDING IN MUSCLE

Each nerve-cell or " neuron " has one long branch, the " axon," which, continuing as the " nerve fibre," transmits impulses to and from different parts of the body.

They are attached to the brain and their fibres pass from the cranial cavity through formina (apertures) in the skull bones. Within the brain their origins, terminations, and connections with each other are complex, so that active co-ordination may occur.

Cranial Nerves.

The first pair are the nerves of smell, the olfactory nerves. These sensory nerves arise from cells situated in the mucous membrane lining the upper part of the nasal cavity. They pass directly upwards and are collected into bundles which pierce a thin perforated sheet of bone called the ethmoid, to enter the olfactory bulbs.

The second pair, the optic nerves, are concerned with vision. They have a complicated path and are described under the special senses.

The third pair are called the oculo-motor nerves. They supply all the muscles which govern the movements of the eyeball, except the superior oblique and lateral rectus muscles. Through a connection with a ganglion they supply the intrinsic muscles of the eye, the ciliary muscle and the sphincter pupillæ. They arise from extensive nuclei (bunches of cells) in the brain whose stimulation causes the eyeball to look upwards and inwards and the pupil to be contracted.

The fourth pair, the trochlear nerves, arise from nuclei situated in the brain close to those of the third nerves. They are the smallest of the cranial nerves and are directed forwards to enter the orbits through fissures in their bony wall, the superior orbital fissures. They supply the superior oblique muscles of the eyeballs, and when stimulated cause the eyeballs to look downwards and inwards. The remaining ocular muscles, the external recti, are supplied by the sixth cranial nerves, the abducent. They arise from cells in the brain which lie posterior to those which give rise to the third and fourth. Their fibres enter the orbits through the superior orbital fissures. On stimulation they cause the eyeballs to look directly outwards.

The three nuclei of the third, fourth, and sixth nerves lie in close proximity. They all receive association branches and connections which enable co-ordinated movements of the eyeball to be performed.

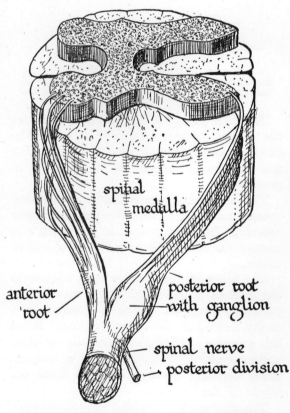

SPINAL CORD WITH A SPINAL NERVE

Impulses are conveyed *to* the spinal cord by fibres within the posterior root of the nerve, and *from* the spinal cord to the body by the anterior root.

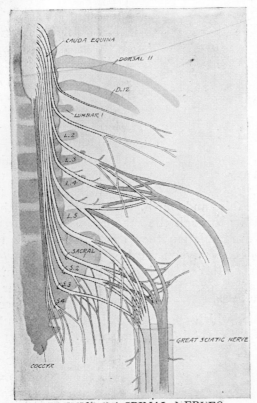

A PLEXUS OF SPINAL NERVES

This diagram shows how the spinal nerves leave the backbone through apertures on each side to unite to form a network from which emerge the peripheral nerves.

The fifth pair, the trigeminal nerves, are the largest cranial nerves. They are the chief sensory nerves to the head and face and the motor nerves to the muscles of mastication.

The trigeminal nerve has a motor and sensory root. The fibres forming the motor root arise from two nuclei in the brain and control the muscular movements of mastication.

The fibres of the sensory root arise from the cells of a ganglion, the semi-lunar or gasserian ganglion, which is situated in a cavity formed in the temporal bone. From this ganglion axons pass centrally to their various cerebral destinations. To it come axons carrying nervous impulses from the whole of the face.

The fifth nerve is divided into three main branches, viz., the ophthalmic nerve, the maxillary nerve, and the mandibular nerve.

The ophthalmic and maxillary are composed of sensory fibres, but the mandibular nerve contains the fibres from the motor root.

The nerves contain sensory branches from the corneæ of the eyes, from the conjunctivæ, the lacrymal glands, and from the skin covering the forehead, the eyelids, the nose, chin, cheeks, lips, the mucous membrane lining the mouth, the lower nasal cavity and the teeth.

The seventh pair or facial nerves, are mainly motor nerves supplying the muscles of the face, the ear, and the scalp. Their nuclei lie deep in the floor of the fourth ventricle in the brain. They carry some sensory fibres associated with taste and general sensation.

The eighth pair are the nerves of hearing and are distributed to the innermost compartment of the ear. They are composed of two sets of fibres both carrying impulses from the internal ear to the brain. The destination of each group differs, one group being concerned with balance and the other group transmitting those impulses which give rise to the sensation of sound.

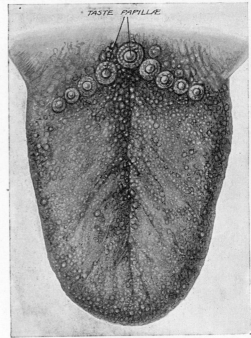

THE ORGAN OF TASTE

The tongue, showing the papillæ, which contain " taste-buds " and are the real detectors of taste qualities.

The ninth pair, the glosso-pharyngeal nerves, contain both sensory and motor fibres. The motor fibres supply certain muscles of the pharynx and the base of the tongue and also secretory fibres to the parotid salivary gland. The sensory fibres of the glosso-pharyngeal nerve convey impulses of ordinary sensation from the mucous membrane lining the pharynx, the mouth, and the

accessory, these fibres running in branches of the vagus. Therefore these two nerves can be considered together.

The nerve runs down the neck in close association with the large blood vessels, it descends through the chest cavity beside the trachea to the root of the lung, and proceeds through the diaphragm into the abdominal cavity to branch around the stomach. Along

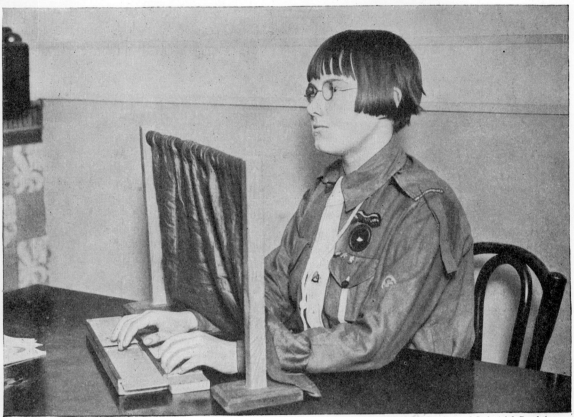

[*National Institute of Industrial Psychology*

TESTING THE SENSE OF TOUCH
Selecting grades of glasspaper with the right hand to correspond with those under the left. The skin of the finger-tips is especially sensitive to touch and pressure.

palatine tonsil, and impulses from that portion of the tongue which is associated with taste.

The tenth pair, or vagi nerves, have a very extensive distribution, sending branches into the thorax and abdomen. The filaments of the nerve emerge from the lower part of the brain and are collected into a flat cord which leaves the cranium through the jugular foramen. It is joined by the accessory part of the eleventh cranial nerve, the spinal

its course it gives off branches, in the neck, in the thorax, and in the abdomen. The nerve is composed of both sensory and motor fibres. It is sensory to the mucous membrane lining the larynx. It carries motor fibres to the muscles of the larynx, to certain muscles of the pharynx, to the muscle contained in the walls of the œsophagus, stomach, and small intestine, to the bronchial tubes and to the secretory digestive glands in the stomach walls. Through it the heart

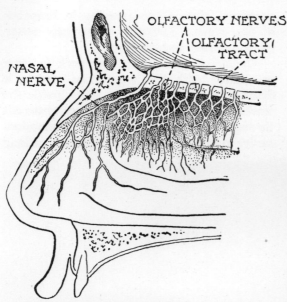

NASAL NERVE

OLFACTORY NERVES

OLFACTORY TRACT

THE SEAT OF THE SENSE OF SMELL
A section through the nose showing the nerves in the mucous membrane which convey smell impressions to the brain, via the olfactory tract.

may be inhibited and respiration regulated.

The spinal portion of the eleventh spinal accessory nerve is motor and supplies fibres to the sternomastoid and trapezius muscles of the neck.

The last and twelfth pair of cranial nerves are the hypoglossals, which are motor nerves, sending their fibres to the muscles of the tongue and to some of the muscles of the larynx.

THE SPINAL CORD AND SPINAL NERVES

The spinal cord is a prolongation of the lower part or medulla of the brain, and occupies the upper two-thirds of the bony canal formed by the arches of successive spinal vertebræ. Through apertures on each side of this canal emerge thirty-one pairs of spinal nerves which are distributed to each side of the body. Each nerve has two roots, an anterior, from which pass motor axons carrying impulses to different parts of the body, and a posterior, by which impulses received from the body enter the spinal cord. Upon the posterior root there is a collection of nerve-cells called a ganglion.

The spinal cord consists of an outer layer of white matter, an inner portion of grey matter and of supporting connective tissue. The white matter is composed of axons, running longitudinally, ascending or descending ; the grey matter of nerve-cells and connective tissue. The nerve-cells situated in the anterior horn of grey matter send out motor axons to join the anterior nerve root, while other cells form points of relay, where terminal filaments of the axon of one cell arborize and intermingle with the dendrites of other neurons which then continue and direct the impulse.

The mixed spinal nerves correspond to segments of the cord divided into levels according to the number of vertebræ. There are eight pairs in the cervical or neck region, twelve in the thoracic, five in the lumbar, five in the sacral, and one in the coccygeal. The spinal mixed nerves unite to form plexuses. These are :—

1. The cervical—formed by nerves from the first, second, third, and fourth cervical segments. Its branches are distributed to the neck, the back of the head, and the diaphragm.

2. The brachial—formed by nerves from the fifth, sixth, seventh and eighth cervical segments and the first thoracic. Its branches supply the upper limb and the shoulder.

3. The lumbar—formed by nerves from the upper four lumbar segments. Its branches supply the genital organs and the pelvis.

4. The sacral—formed by nerves from the fifth lumbar and upper four sacral segments. Its branches supply the lower limb and the buttock, and from it arises the largest nerve in the body, the great sciatic, which runs down the back of the thigh, dividing above the knee into two main branches.

In the thorax the spinal nerves run separately, as intercostal nerves, round the chest along the ribs.

The nerves from the lowest segments which do not join the sacral plexus supply the region around the anus.

All these spinal nerves are composed of both motor and sensory fibres. The motor *emerge* from the cord by the anterior root. The sensory *enter* via the posterior root, having the cell bodies of their axons situated in the ganglion upon that root. They convey impulses which arouse sensations of pain, of heat and cold and deep pressure, and sensations which enable us to locate a spot touched. They also carry fibres of muscle and joint sense which enable us to know the position of our limbs and thus to know, without looking at our limbs, if our involuntary movements have been carried out. By impressions received from muscles and tendons we judge weights and resistances which, together with tactile and visual sensations, help us to understand by our past experiences various qualities of an object. These deep and undefined impulses arise from many different end-organs in the muscles, tendons, joints, and in the soft tissues around them. They may or may not

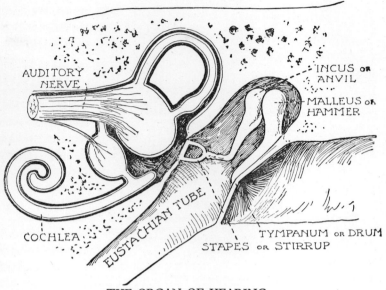

THE ORGAN OF HEARING

The passage from the outer ear is closed by the tympanic membrane or drum; the Eustachian tube leads to the pharynx; the hammer, anvil, and stirrup bones convey sound vibrations from the drum to the inner ear.

arouse consciousness, but they enable us to appreciate our position, to regulate our posture, and to co-ordinate our movements.

THE ORGANS OF SENSE

In lowly creatures all parts of the body are equally sensitive and can respond to stimulations of touch, light, sound, taste, heat, etc. In more advanced types, patches of the animal become particularly susceptible to specific stimulations—the worm has no eyes, but small areas of the skin in its foremost segments can respond to light rays. Other areas probably receive sound vibrations. In man and the higher animals elaborate and specific organs of sense have been developed, responding to chemical, mechanical, and radiant stimuli. Since by them we are " put in touch " with the world they are naturally among the most interesting of man's bodily structures.

The skin is one of the oldest and vaguest of the sense organs; it is distributed over the whole surface of the body. **The Skin.** Just beneath are myriads of nerve-endings which receive messages for conveyance to the great nerve-centres. Many of these " nerve bulbs " are valuable pain indicators—danger signals which, by

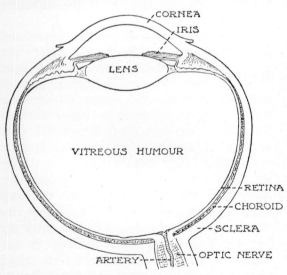

THE HUMAN CAMERA

A diagram of the eye, showing the iris, which concentrates light rays, the lens which focuses them, and the retina which receives them as an image upon its surface.

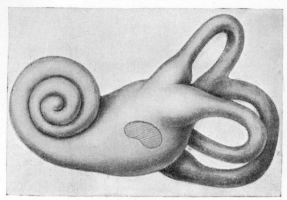

THE INNER EAR

The bony labyrinth consists of the cochlea, shaped like a snail's shell, which is the organ of hearing, and the semicircular canals which are concerned with balance.

their insistence, may even cause the sleeper to wake in self-protection. The skin is not equally sensitive in every part, the tongue and finger-tips can distinguish as separate two points one twenty-fourth of an inch apart ; the skin on the back cannot make this distinction until the space is two and a half inches. The finger-tips are better judges of pressure than the tongue or lips. Another division of the sense of touch—temperature—is localised in a curious way. The thicker skin of the hands and feet is notoriously insensitive, but other parts of the skin seem to be divided into tiny areas, some of which are sensitive to cold and some to heat, but not to both.

Taste. The sense of taste lies in the mouth, principally in the tongue, but also on the surface of the palate, epiglottis, and throat. There are eight or ten small papillæ or epithelialel evations across the base of the tongue, and others, of a slightly different form, on the sides and tip ; these contain taste-buds and are the real organs of taste. The substance to be tasted must be in solution before it is effective, and then it is found that sweet tastes are perceived best by the tip of the tongue, acids by the sides, and bitter by the back ; salty tastes are perceived more quickly than the others. The sensation of taste stimulates the production of saliva.

Allied to the sense of taste is that of smell. When we say we smell with our

Smell. noses, we mean that one of the functions of the nose is smelling. The mucous membrane of the upper and back part of the nose contains the delicate terminations of the olfactory nerves which lead to the olfactory tract—an outgrowth of the brain. In lower animals this tract is hollow and of a considerable size ; in man it is smaller and comparatively more solid, except in the embryonic stage. Thus man has reduced the effective area, with the consequence that the sense of smell is, compared with that of lower animals, almost negligible and, although not necessarily degenerating, is certainly becoming desensitised. The cells themselves are only sensitive to gaseous or vaporous particles, and, if the nose is filled with water containing eau-de-cologne, there will be no smell. This is practically what occurs when an excess of mucus is present : we complain, rightly, that with a cold in our heads we cannot smell ; taste also is impaired, but this is due, primarily, to lack of smell. If the membrane is too dry, also, smell is seriously impaired. A vigorous " sniff," however, will often produce a sense of smell which quiet breathing has failed to detect—for by this process the odoriferous particles are drawn into close contact with the surface of the olfactory membrane.

Hearing. The ear is a very complicated organ and may be considered in three parts : the outer, the middle, and the inner ear. The outer fleshy part is reduced in man, and seems to serve no useful purpose, whereas in other animals the greater size and flexibility of this part appears to make for a greater acuteness of hearing. The middle ear is a cavity in the bone, closed by membranes—the tympanic—leading to the outer ear and —the fenestra ovalis—to the inner ear which is also connected with the outer air by the Eustachian tube leading to the pharynx. In this chamber are three small bones, the hammer, anvil, and stirrup bones, the first of which attaches to the tympanic membrane and the last to the fenestra ovalis. Sound vibrations, on reaching the tympanum which is fairly loose and unevenly stretched across the orifice, cause it to vibrate. These vibrations are carried via the small bones, or ossicles, to the inner ear. The Eustachian tube keeps the air pressure properly adjusted in this chamber. Temporary deafness can be caused by too great or too small a pressure, and can be relieved by opening the tube in a kind of swallowing movement.

Actual hearing takes place in the inner ear—a bony labyrinth enclosing a loosely-fitting membranous lining. The spaces between the bone and membrane, and also in the membrane itself, are filled with two liquids : the movements of the stirrup-bone are conveyed to the membrane and from that to the auditory nerve-endings through these liquids. This process occurs in the vestibule and cochlea ; the semicircular canals, which also form a part of the labyrinth, are balancing organs. Thus, finally, a vigorous change of pressure in the air is passed on, first as a mechanical movement, and then as a pressure-change on a membrane in a liquid medium.

The range of hearing is approximately between forty and forty thousand vibrations per second. This range, especially at its upper end, is considerably curtailed in old age. It is interesting to notice that vibrations can be conveyed directly to the middle and inner ear through the teeth and forehead.

Compared with the ear, the structure of the eye is simpler but more adaptive, consisting of an apparatus sensitive to light which is reflected from an object upon which light has fallen. The eye may be looked upon as a delicate form of camera, in which the light rays from an object are concentrated by means of a contractile diaphragm, the iris, focused by the lens, and received as an inverted image upon a sensitive surface, the retina.

Vision.

The whole eyeball, protected by the eyelids, and by its position in a bony cavity lined with fat, is enclosed in a tough covering, the sclerotic, which is continued in front as a transparent membrane, the cornea. Within this covering is another membrane, the choroid, which is continued across the front of the eyeball, behind the cornea, as a circular curtain, the iris, with a central aperture, the pupil. Between the iris and the cornea is a space containing a fluid called the aqueous humour. The lens lies immediately behind the iris, a solid substance of concentric layers of cells, whose curvature can be altered for the purpose of focusing by the action upon it of muscles attached to it. The space between the lens and the retina, which lines the posterior portion of the eye, is filled with a substance of jelly-like consistency known as the vitreous humour. The retina contains the fibres of the optic nerve which are spread out over it, decreasing in sensitiveness from the centre towards the edges. The sensitive element of the retina is a layer of cells called the rods and cones, containing pigment which is affected by the action of light so that impressions are transmitted by the fibres of the optic nerve and registered in the brain as the sensation of sight.

Through the sense of sight we can interpret certain sensations and appreciate not only light, but colour, and shape, and the relative positions and distances of objects which surround us. When we see an object and appreciate its qualities and its distance, it is not merely by registering a vision upon the retina, but by associating with this sensation experiences due to many other sensations.

SYMPATHETIC NERVOUS SYSTEM

The sympathetic nervous system is concerned with the internal organs of the body. It distributes fibres to plain involuntary muscle, such as exists in the walls of the blood vessels, and through its innervation, mechanical processes over which we have no voluntary control, and of which we are not usually conscious, are carried on continuously within the body.

The sympathetic system of nerves is intimately associated and connected with the cerebro-spinal system. Its fibres run mostly in the spinal and cranial nerve trunks and are thus distributed throughout the body.

Along the course of its fibres are cell relay stations or ganglia. Both fibres and ganglia are collected into great plexuses which are situated in the thorax around the heart, in the abdominal cavity behind the stomach, and in the pelvis behind the pelvic organs.

Vaso-dilator and vaso-constrictor fibres pass to the muscle in the walls of the blood vessels, causing the finer terminals to dilate and constrict, thereby regulating the flow of blood through a tissue. In this way the blood-flow through the skin is influenced, and the loss of heat from the body regulated. When the surrounding air is cold the vessels contract, thus conserving heat within the body; when the surrounding air is hot they dilate, and heat is given off.

The fibres of the sympathetic also control the activity of the sweat glands. The body is cooled by the evaporation of sweat, which cannot occur so easily when the air is moist, so that the effects of heat are felt at a much lower temperature when the air is moist than when it is dry.

Sympathetic fibres to the heart control the rhythm of its activity, and the calibre of the bronchial tubes and their branches is influenced by the fibres supplying the plain muscle which they contain.

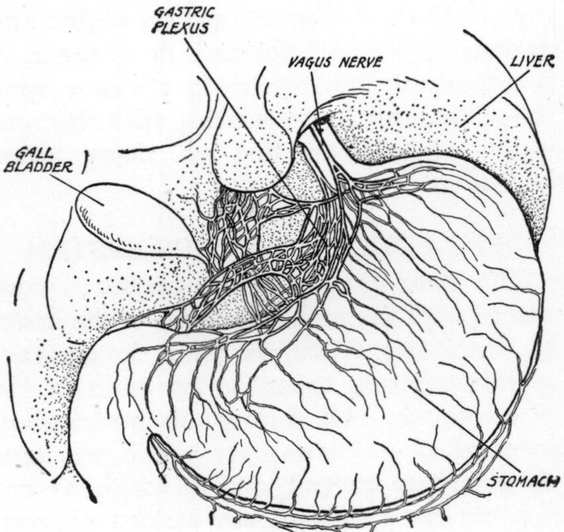

Fibres run to the eye, controlling the dilatation and contraction of the pupil, and to the digestive glands in the mouth and stomach. They regulate the movements of the stomach and intestine, send motor and inhibitory fibres to the urinary bladder, and control the reflex mechanism of the genital organs.

Most of the internal organs of the body are insensitive to ordinary stimulation; handling the intestine gives rise to no sensation of pain. Stimulations arising in the viscera, however, from stretching, from pressure, and from disease, may cause impulses which create conscious feeling and also acute pain, as for instance intestinal colic, and spasm of the ureter from the presence of a stone.

THE BRAIN

The central nervous system is composed of the spinal cord, which lies within the bony spinal canal, and that upper, greatly expanded portion, the brain, which lies within the cranium.

The brain is covered with membranes, an outer layer, the dura mater, and an inner, the arachnoid, while a delicate vascular membrane called the pia mater invests the entire surface of the brain. Arterial blood is carried to the brain by the internal carotid and vertebral arteries which form a complicated anastomising circle, the circle of Willis. From this circle vessels enter the brain substance. The venous blood is collected into large sinuses which are drained by the internal jugular vein, and passes via the heart to the lungs for purification.

The tissues of the brain are bathed with a clear fluid, the cerebro-spinal fluid, which also runs down the spinal cord through a small central canal. Changes occur in this fluid in certain diseases of the brain and spinal cord, and it can be extracted by spinal lumbar pucture and examined. The brain consists of white matter—conducting fibres; of grey matter—nerve-cells, both supported by connective tissue.

SYMPATHETIC NERVES OF THE ABDOMEN

The sympathetic nerves regulate the various vital processes which go on inside the body and of which we are normally unconscious. The diagram shows one of the great plexuses into which the nerve fibres collect.

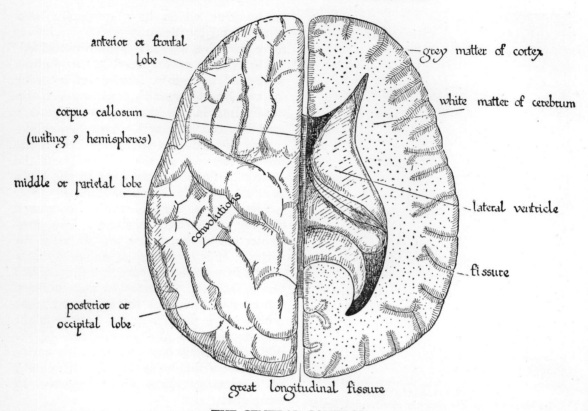

anterior or frontal lobe

grey matter of cortex

corpus callosum

(uniting 2 hemispheres)

white matter of cerebrum

middle or parietal lobe

convolutions

lateral ventricle

fissure

posterior or occipital lobe

great longitudinal fissure

THE CENTRAL CONTROL

The cerebrum, consisting of two massive hemispheres, forms about nine-tenths of man's brain. It controls the more primitive nervous system, the different lobes being associated with different functions.

The lowest portion of the brain is called the medulla oblongata. It is the proximate upward continuation of the spinal cord. It forms the connecting link between the higher brain and the spinal cord. Upon the integrity of this part depend the reflex mechanisms associated with the most vital bodily functions. Within it are the centres of those nervous connections which control respiration, circulation, and digestion. It receives impulses from all the important organs of the body. From it, motor fibres pass which serve the acts of swallowing, coughing, and talking. From the medulla motor fibres pass to the stomach and intestine and inhibitory fibres go to the heart. Injury to the medulla means paralysis of vital functions and death.

The medulla transmits downwards motor impulses from the brain cortex and upwards sensory impulses continued from the spinal cord.

The pons lies above the medulla. It is composed of fibres which connect the two cerebellar hemispheres. Transverse fibres form a path of conduction connecting the cerebral hemispheres of one side with the cerebellar hemispheres of the opposite side. The pons also transmits down-going motor fibres and the up-going sensory fibres.

The Pons.

The cerebellum lies behind the medulla and pons. It is oval in shape, occupying the lower occipital region of the cranial cavity. It consists of two lateral hemispheres and a median constricted portion, the vermis. It is divided into a series of leaves by fine fissures, into lobes by larger fissures, all of which extend deeply into its substance. The cerebellum is attached to and linked up with the other divisions of the brain by bands of fibres.

The Cere-bellum.

Both white and grey matters are found. The white matter is composed of afferent

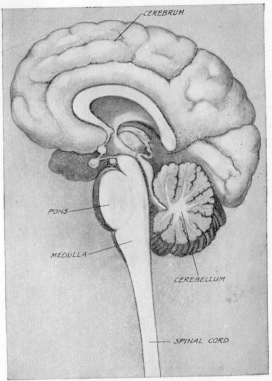

THE THINKING MACHINE
The human brain, showing the relative position of
the various parts.

brain tissue which have gradually been evolved and by means of which the lower, more primitive, nervous system is controlled.

The surface of the cerebral hemisphere is divided up into a number of irregular folds or convolutions by fissures which dip deeply into it. By this means the surface area is much increased. Each hemisphere is also divided into four *main* lobes : the frontal, the parietal, the temporal, and the occipital. Hidden away deep in the brain is a fifth lobe, the island of Reil.

The cerebral hemispheres are composed of grey and white substance. The grey matter covers the surface and is called the cortex. It is composed of nerve-cells supported by a mass of connective tissue called neuroglia. Its thickness is not uniform, some areas having a thinner cortex than others ; it is thinner at the bottom of the fissures than at the prominence of the folds. Its microscopic structure also varies. The white substance is composed of bundles of conducting fibres also supported by neuroglia.

Some areas have been found to be associated with definite function. The frontal lobe is separated from the parietal lobe by the central sulcus or fissure of Rolando, and the convolution forming the anterior or frontal wall of this fissure controls muscular movements. Stimulation of this convolution from above downwards produces muscular movements in the toes, ankle, knee, hip, shoulder, elbow, wrist, fingers and neck and face. Sensation from these parts reaches the cortex in that convolution of the parietal lobe which forms the posterior or parietal wall of the central sulcus. The extreme front of the frontal lobe is believed to be related to the highest function of the brain —that of mind.

Impressions from the eyes are directed to the lower visual centres and from them towards the cortex of the occipital lobes. Impulses received from the ear which give rise to sensations of sound are carried by nerve fibres which radiate towards the cortex of the highest convolution of the temporal lobe.

and efferent fibres. It consists of a central stem which branches like a tree. The grey substance is found upon the surface, fringing the white areas, and extending over all the fissured cortex. Masses of grey matter are found also in the interior forming nuclei or cell stations.

The cerebellum receives impulses from the deep tissue of muscles, joints and tendons. It receives impulses via the vestibular division of the auditory nerve from the semi-circular canals. These impulses are concerned with regulating movement and balance. When disturbed, ataxia or muscular inco-ordination results, and normal muscle tone is diminished.

The Cerebrum. The cerebrum consists of two massive hemispheres separated by a long deep fissure. They are connected below by a band of fibres named the corpus callosum. These two hemispheres together constitute about nine-tenths of the whole weight of the brain in man. They are enormous outgrowths of

When we consider the central nervous system as a whole with its complicated neuron association, we realise that excitation of the sensory apparatus will give rise to impulses which pass in many directions. The cell matter in the brain cortex is linked up so that the brain reacts as a whole, enabling us to appreciate, for instance, the many qualities of any object which stimulates our sense of sight. Again, when we hear a spoken word, it creates in our minds an impression possessing many different properties. Speech involves not only putting into action the muscles controlling its mechanism, but it involves the associated combined activity of almost every part of the brain. We may be unable to speak although our muscular mechanism for utterance is undamaged.

With the growth of the cerebral hemispheres has come increased intelligence. The reaction to stimuli is guided by these higher centres and is influenced by the experiences of the individual. He is able to recall to memory varied sensory impressions of the past and his responses to them are in accordance with his knowledge.

The axon of a sensory nerve-cell ends by branching around cells which have been specialised in such a manner that they are thrown into activity by changes which occur in their environment. They are adapted to receive some special form of stimulation and the impressions caused by their excitation are specific according to their specialised function.

Sensation.

The sensory neurons conduct impulses towards the central nervous system, and they may or may not be registered upon the consciousness. Those which rise to consciousness cause us to become aware of environmental change.

Forms of energy exist which we have no reception apparatus adapted to receive, but there are many conditions in our environment which are continuously stimulating the sense organs which we possess.

From the skin we appreciate touch and temperature. From our special sense organs, the eye, the ear, the tongue, and the nose, we receive impulses which give rise to sensations of sight, of sound, of taste, and of smell. Our muscles, joints, tendons, and the soft tissues around them are endowed with end organs which are excited by pressure and tension ; these, associated with impressions received from the internal ear, inform us of our posture and help us to maintain the equilibrium of our body and to co-ordinate our movements.

A constant stream of afferent impulses from our internal organs flows towards the spinal cord and brain. They are concerned with internal mechanisms. They cause organic reflexes by which the active function of our internal organs is maintained. In health they give rise to no conscious feelings, but in disease they warn us of disorder. Increased tension or pressure, internal irritation or inflammation, will register through these nerves the disturbance upon the mind.

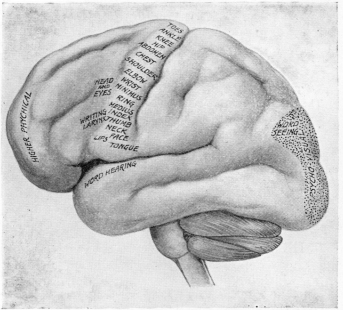

THE HEADQUARTERS OF THE NERVOUS SYSTEM
Indicating the areas in the surface of the brain which are associated with definite functions. Stimulation of the motor area (from " toes " to " tongue ") produces corresponding muscular movements.

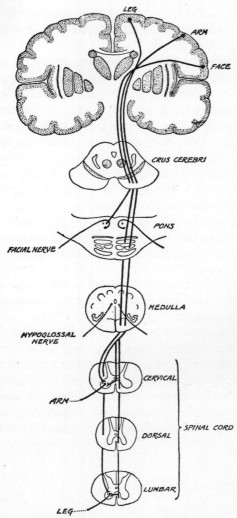

THE PATH OF NERVE-MESSAGES
The telegraph system along which impulses are conveyed from the brain to the leg, arm, face and tongue muscles.

Our array of sense organs is varied and immense. They are stimulated by varied forms of energy. From them nervous impulses are conducted to our spinal cord and brain ; they are sorted, relayed, and associated, *consciousness* depending upon the sensations to which they give rise.

Nervous tissue is essential for the manifestations of conscious states and should it be diseased, malformed, or under the influence of drugs, such as chloroform or alcohol, some alteration in the course of conscious processes is the inevitable result. Consciousness is the elemental function of the mind upon which all mental life is dependent. Its essential features are its never-ending changes and its intimate relation to past and future consciousness. It is easiest to visualise consciousness as a stream which is constantly flowing. This simile is of value in so far as it allows us to represent different levels of conscious states. "At any moment there is always part which is in the focus or full glare of consciousness, and part of which we are dimly conscious or wholly unconscious, but of which we may at any moment become conscious—for example, the ticking of a clock in the room. We may imagine that as the stream of consciousness flows on, different portions come to the surface at different times and under different conditions, while others fall below, often to such a depth that they pass beyond the margin of consciousness." (*Halliburton.*)

DISEASES OF THE NERVOUS SYSTEM

By MACPHERSON LAWRIE, M.A., M.B., B.Ch., Clinical Assistant Physician to St. Luke's Hospital for Mental and Nervous Diseases.

AFFECTIONS OF THE CRANIAL NERVES

THE normal function of a cranial nerve may be disturbed by some lesion which implicates it in its course, or it may be affected by some poison which may be circulating in the blood. The local lesion may be inflammatory in nature ; it may be a tumour growth ; it may be syphilitic in origin or it may be due to some vascular disorder which interferes with its blood supply. Cranial nerves may also be affected by the sclerotic or degenerated patches which occur in disseminated sclerosis. As the nerves pass from the brain substance and from the skull they are liable to become involved in inflammation of the membranes, in inflammation of the periosteum of the bone, and in fracture of the skull.

Loss of the sense of smell (ANOSMIA) occurs

following lesions which involve the tract of the olfactory nerves ; especially may this be so when the loss is confined to one side. Most cases of anosmia, however, are due to disease of the mucous membrane of the nose.

The optic nerve is liable to inflammation and to atrophy. OPTIC NEURITIS may result in partial or total blindness. It may be due to inflammatory septic conditions occurring in surrounding structure such as in the nasal cavities, the frontal sinuses, the antrum, and perhaps even in the teeth. Syphilis and disseminated sclerosis are frequent causes ; the former type may recover with early treatment, the latter always leaves some degree of atrophy. In diabetes a progressive form occurs. It causes failing sight which advances to blindness. Optic neuritis is a cardinal sign in brain tumours.

OPTIC ATROPHY means a degeneration of nerve fibres in the optic nerve which causes diminution of vision. Optic atrophy may follow neuritis, especially when the inflammation has persisted for a long time, or where scars have formed which embrace and crush the nerve fibres. It may arise from injury and also primarily owing to degeneration of the nerve-cells in the retina.

Interference with the motor nerves of the eyes (third, fourth, and sixth cranial nerves) occasions inco-ordinated and limited movements of the eyeballs with squint, and results in double vision. Difficulty in judging the exact position of objects in space may arise from loss of muscle sense.

The most common pathological agent is syphilis. The harmonious

functioning of the oculo-motor nerve may be disturbed by inflammation of brain tissue, by tumours within the brain or by patches of disseminated sclerosis.

The fifth cranial nerve is the nerve of NEURALGIA. Any branch may be affected. Irritating foci occurring anywhere throughout its peripheral distribution tend to give rise to pain. Following destruction of nerve fibres, loss of sensation may result which may lead to ulceration of the cornea of the eye owing to the protective mechanism failing to function.

TRIGEMINAL NEURALGIA or " TIC " is usually unilateral and confined to one branch of the nerve. As attacks recur the region affected becomes more extensive. Cold draught or facial movements sometimes appear to start an attack. The pain

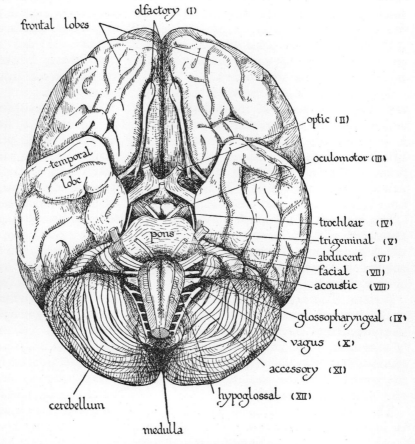

THE CRANIAL NERVES
The twelve pairs of nerves which leave the brain through apertures in the skull and are involved in many well known nervous diseases.

is sharp and piercing and sudden in onset. It may be followed by a boring sensation, but usually ends as suddenly as it begins, or the attack may be more prolonged and dull in character throughout. The skin covering the nerve is tender. The attacks are often crippling and exhausting. Every effort must be made to find local sources of irritation. Severe and persistent cases require surgical treatment.

The facial nerve is commonly paralysed. It may be involved in any part of its course by inflammation, tumour, or vascular lesions. Frequently affected at its exit from the skull, it gives rise to BELL'S PARALYSIS. This occurs usually after exposure of the face to cold. The onset is sudden, perhaps preceded by slight pain behind the ear. The side of the face affected cannot be moved ; the eye cannot be closed. Articulation is often embarrassed and fluids may dribble from the mouth. The facial expression varies with the degree of paralysis. These cases recover, although the condition may require weeks or many months to do so.

The eighth cranial nerve is concerned with two functions. It transmits impulses which give rise to sensations of sound and it is concerned with the maintenance of balance. Irritating lesions give rise to tinnitus (ringing sounds in the ears)—destructive ones to deafness. Giddiness follows interference with the vestibular portion.

Involvement of the ninth nerve is usually associated with a lesion, often a tumour, which causes loss of taste over the posterior portion of the tongue with some paralysis of the pharynx.

Lesions affecting the tenth cranial nerve or its central nuclei show themselves in pharyngeal and laryngeal paralysis with loss of sensation. The palate may be low and immovable ; the voice nasal. Paralysis of the larynx alters the tone of the voice and may give rise to stridor.

The eleventh spinal accessory nerve may be injured by accidents or operations which involve the neck. It supplies the sterno-mastoid muscle and the trapezius. Paralysis of the latter causes difficulty in raising the arm above the level of the shoulder. Paralysis of the sterno-mastoid muscle is usually compensated for by the surrounding neck muscles.

The twelfth nerve is usually affected together with other nerves. Paralysis and wasting of the tongue muscles follow producing difficulties in articulation and swallowing. The lesion may be unilateral or bilateral.

AFFECTIONS OF THE BRAIN AND SPINAL CORD

ANY condition tending to produce degenerative changes in the walls of the blood vessels of the brain tends to result in hæmorrhage. The tendency is specially marked in people who suffer from progressive kidney disease and cardiac hypertrophy, while over-eating, over-indulgence in alcohol, and syphilis tend to produce arterio-sclerosis with subsequent rupture of the affected vessels. Other contributing factors are old age, heredity, and persistent intoxication resulting from constipation.

Cerebral Hæmorrhage.

The degenerated vessel may bleed directly, or an aneurism, formed on account of its weakened wall, may rupture. The blood escapes into the surrounding nervous tissue, resulting in its destruction ; death does not immediately ensue, the damaged area is gradually encapsuled by scar tissue. A cerebral hæmorrhage is called an APOPLEXY.

The typical apoplectic stroke is of sudden onset. The patient becomes suddenly unconscious and falls. He cannot be roused, his breathing is slow and possibly stertorous, his face blue, and urine and fæces are commonly passed unknowingly. In other cases the onset differs. Unconsciousness develops more slowly and may be preceded by slight disturbances of speech or by giddiness.

Death occurs in some cases. Others recover consciousness but are usually left with some obvious paralysis. According to the tissue in the brain which has been involved, so will the disorder vary.

The cortical motor area or the motor tract on one side is commonly implicated, producing paralysis of the opposite side of the body (hemiplegia) which may be limited to the face, the arm, or the leg. If the lesion has been slight complete recovery may occur. Usually, however, some degree of permanent paralysis, revealed in the dragging of a foot, remains. Loss of sensation is usually slight except in deeper hæmorrhages.

The most common cause of Cerebral Embolism is valvular disease of the heart.

Cerebral Embolism. A particle separated from one of the damaged valves circulates in the blood stream and blocks a vessel in the brain. The symptoms are sudden in onset and vary according to the area cut off from its blood supply. A state resembling apoplexy may occur following the lodgement of a large embolus.

Cerebral Thrombosis. Cerebral Thrombosis is usually slower in onset. It is due to a sluggish circulation through a diseased blood vessel. Syphilis is a frequent factor in its causation. Recurring weaknesses in an arm or leg and disturbances of speech are signs of its occurrence. The signs and symptoms of the condition vary with the areas temporarily or permanently involved.

Progressive vascular changes occurring in the brain commonly give rise to a slowly advancing impairment of mental power associated with failing memory.*

Aphasia. The commonest causes of Aphasia, or loss of speech, are cerebral hæmorrhage, embolism, thrombosis, and tumours. The condition depends upon interference with those paths and areas of the brain, situated in the left cerebral hemisphere, which are associated with speech. Its onset and course vary according to its cause, and the type and degree of disturbance and the permanency of the damage depend upon the area affected and the amount of its destruction. Aphasia may be motor, or sensory, or both, in varying degrees. In motor aphasia the patient may be unable to speak at all, or while he may not be able to speak spontaneously, he may retain the power of repeating what he hears. He may, or may not, be able to write.

*See Senile Dementia : Section on Mental Diseases.

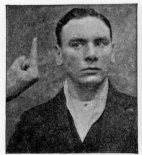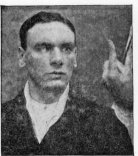

Courtesy]　　　[" *Diagnosis of Nervous Diseases*,"
Sir J. Purves-Stewart (Arnold & Co.)

PARALYSIS OF A MOTOR NERVE OF THE EYE

A case in which movement of the eyeballs is restricted owing to paralysis of the left sixth cranial nerve. The eyes are normal on looking right, but on looking left the left eye stays in mid-position.

In complete sensory aphasia the patient can understand neither the spoken nor the written word, but if the destruction is not complete, he may retain the power of speaking, reading, and writing, suffering only from word deafness. In other cases he is able to read aloud, repeat what he hears, and even write to dictation without understanding the words which he reads or writes.

Encephalitis. Acute inflammation of the brain substance gives rise to symptoms such as headache, with drowsiness passing on to coma, signs of irritability associated with convulsions, vomiting, and fever. The inflammation may arise during the course of acute specific fevers such as measles and scarlet fever. It may occur primarily from infection with the virus of polio-myelitis. It may follow wounds of the skull or result from the spread of some inflammatory process existing in surrounding structures. The onset varies. It is often sudden with a fatal termination. In cases which recover some impairment of cerebral function usually remains.

Brain Abscess. Abscesses in the brain may be single, large, and surrounded by a protective wall, or they may be multiple and show a more diffuse character. A single circumscribed abscess causes signs and symptoms which resemble those associated with intracranial tumour, and its localisation presents similar difficulties. Paralysis, signs of irritation, and inco-ordinated movements with drowsiness and coma, are common symptoms. Other cases are sudden in onset and may pass rapidly to a fatal termination with vomiting, fever, and delirium. Some abscesses remain latent, giving rise to little inconvenience, or they may expand slowly until surgical interference becomes absolutely necessary. Suppuration in the brain substance follows infection elsewhere. The infection may be carried to the brain by the blood stream from distant parts of the body. It is more commonly due to the extension of some disease existing in the vicinity, of which infective conditions in the middle ear, the frontal and other sinuses in the skull, are examples. Intracranial suppuration may also follow injuries which admit infection.

The name Encephalitis Lethargica is given to a disease (" sleepy sickness ") which **"Sleepy Sickness."** is characterised by drowsiness and general intoxication. Isolated cases of the disease have been recognised in many parts of the world, and it has also occurred in epidemics. The onset may be sudden in general. The symptoms vary widely according to the area of the brain involved. There appears to be a vascular congestion with some local cellular degeneration. The onset of the illness is associated with general toxic symptoms, fever, headache, gastro-intestinal disturbances, aching pains, and general uneasiness.

Mental lethargy gradually supervenes and may become very deep, the sufferer taking no notice of his surroundings. He may remain apparently unconscious for a period which varies greatly in different cases. Involvement of cranial nerves may occur. Cases seldom recover completely : impaired mental function remains which shows itself in a change of personality often associated with a depressed apathetic state. Improvement may proceed over years, making it difficult to estimate what degree of permanent damage will remain.*

Tumours may arise in the brain from proliferation of some nervous structure, or **Tumours.** they may arise in the supporting and connecting elements. The tumour may be tubercular or syphilitic in origin. Hæmorrhagic, inflammatory, or degenerative changes in or around a tumour which has been latent for years suddenly may cause acute symptoms. As a general rule, tumours in the brain occasion certain general symptoms which are due to increased intracranial pressure or local symptoms due to interference with nerve-cells and paths.

The general symptoms are (1) optic neuritis ; (2) headache, seldom localised except when the skull is involved : the headache is due to stretching and pressure which irritate nerve-endings in the membranes covering the brain substance which itself is insensitive to pain ; (3) vomiting.

Local symptoms do not always appear. Many tumours existing in the brain give rise to no signs which enable their position to be located. There are some areas, however, which are known to be associated with definite function. Interference with these will give

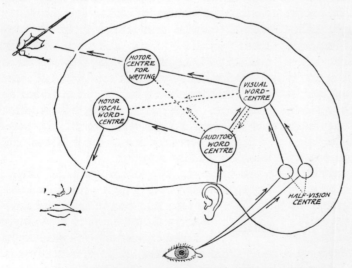

THE MECHANISM OF SPEECH AND WRITING

A diagram (after Bramwell) showing how the various brain-centres concerned in speech and writing are co-ordinated. The dotted lines denote possible but less usual paths for the impulses.

* See Section on Mental Disease.

rise to definite disorder which indicates the position of the tumour.

A tumour in the motor area may cause definite paralysis which, according to the position, affects a whole side, or an arm, a leg or the face. Destruction of the occipital lobe affects the field of vision, and of the temporal lobe on the left side the function of speech. Cerebellar tumours diminish the unconscious maintenance of balance, the movements becoming slow and clumsy. Mental changes may follow tumours growing in the frontal lobes.

The membranes, or meninges, which cover the brain may become infected by Meningitis. micro-organisms from extension of infection from neighbouring parts, as in injury to the skull and middle ear disease. Acute inflammation of the meninges occurs in cerebro-spinal fever,* and in goconoccal, pneumococcal, streptococcal, and staphylococcal infections.

TUBERCULAR INFECTION of the membranes, most commonly seen in children, is usually carried by the blood stream from a distant tubercular gland or bone.

The early symptoms are restlessness, general malaise, headache and fretfulness, followed in a few days by mental dulness, deepening into stupor. The patient lies in a cramped position with the head stiffly drawn back. This head retraction and a typical high-pitched cry are most characteristic symptoms. A squint, due to paralysis of some of the eye muscles, may be present. The stupor passes to deep coma, followed by death in about three weeks from the date of definite onset.

The membranes investing the base of the brain are most commonly inflamed in SYPHILITIC MENINGITIS. The disease takes the form of a chronic, diffuse inflammation involving the blood vessels, with a consequent softening of the brain tissue which they supply. Owing to the patchy, diffuse character of the disease, a great variety of symptoms is produced. Involvement of the cranial nerves supplying the eye muscles is common, one of its typical effects appearing

* See Specific Infectious Fevers.

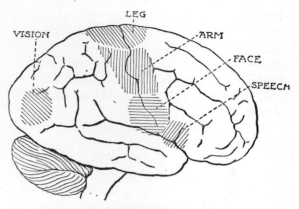

SPECIAL REGIONS OF THE BRAIN
Some areas of the brain are associated with definite functions, so that disorder of a bodily function will often indicate the exact position of a local brain disease.

as " ptosis," or dropping of the eyelid. Other symptoms are headache, worse at night, local spasms due to cortical irritation, and general impairment of mental function, showing itself in irritability, lack of concentration, and a depressed, lethargic mental outlook.

In Disseminated Sclerosis there are found distributed irregularly throughout the central nervous system small areas of Disseminated Sclerosis. inflammation which affect grey and white matter alike, and which are eventually replaced by scar tissue. Inflammatory patches may occur in any region. The axons of nerve-cells are early pressed upon by the products of inflammatory reaction, and their powers of conduction thereby lessened, but they may not be permanently destroyed. As the inflammation subsides they again begin to function, except those which have been obliterated by scar formation.

The symptoms of the disease therefore fluctuate and change and combine in varied forms according to the appearance of new patches and the subsidence of others, and according to individual cases. Early manifestations may be transient, and the mode of onset therefore overlooked. Certain symptoms occur which are common to many cases.

A feeling of heaviness in the legs associated with stiffness and followed by weakness is often the first complaint. It may recover, but often recurs, and may end in spastic paralysis. Nystagmus, in which the eyes oscillate when the patient tries to fix them in a lateral direction, and disturbance of articulation, speech becoming slow and "scanning" in character, are later symptoms.

A characteristic tremor occurs in the arm when voluntary movement is attempted. It has therefore been called "intention tremor." When the patient is asked to touch the tip of his nose with the tip of a finger, jerky movements of his arm take place as his finger approaches his nose, and he is often unable to locate the nose. This tremor may eventually render him unable to carry out any delicate voluntary movement with his hands. Mental symptoms such as failing memory and impaired intellect arise. Emotional reaction is more easily evoked.

The prognosis of the disease varies. Remissions and recurrences are common, and

A SYMPTOM OF TABES
Perforating ulcers sometimes occur on the soles of the feet in tabes dorsalis, a disease of the spinal cord affecting the gait and causing disorders in many parts of the body.

years may elapse between the appearance of symptoms, the patient enjoying good health during the interval. On the whole, the outlook is bad, the patient gradually becoming ataxic and bedridden, and suffering from the involuntary passage of fæces and urine.

Syphilis is a very common cause of organic nervous disease. It attacks chiefly the nervous tissue of the brain and spinal cord. Usually both are affected at the same time in varying proportions. The membranes, the supporting structures, and the blood vessels are frequently involved, causing more remote degenerations of nervous tissue. Some disorders of the central nervous system may commence early in the disease, other affections appear perhaps thirty years after syphilis has been contracted.

*Effects of Syphilis.**

The symptoms present great variety according to the nervous structure involved. Amongst them are spasms and fits, due to irritation ; paralysis, weakness, and disorders of sensation ; affections of the cranial nerves, especially squint ; dimness of vision ; disturbances of speech and swallowing ; headache and giddiness ; mental dulness and altered personality ; and attacks of unconsciousness.

The chief forms in which the disease attacks the brain are softening of the brain tissue following deficient blood supply, infection of brain tissue and membranes by extension from disease of the skull bones, and gummatous tumours. In the spinal cord similar changes occur. They may commence in the blood vessels, in the membranes, in the bones or supporting structures. As in the brain, parts cut off from their blood supply suffer from interference with the nervous structure. Pains in the arms and legs, a sensation of tightness round the trunk, numbness and other cutaneous sensory disturbances are common symptoms, and difficulty in starting micturition is an early complaint. Paralysis, associated with stiffness, varies in degree and distribution.

* See also section on Mental Disease : General Paralysis.

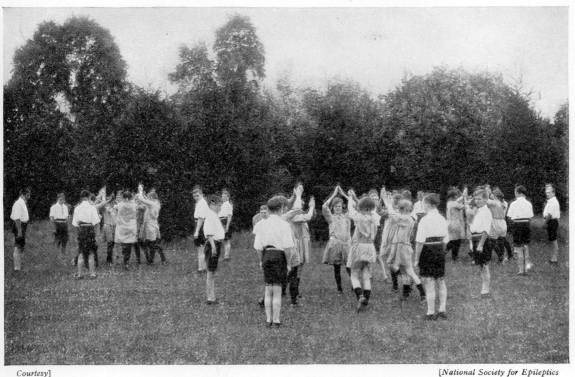

Courtesy]   [National Society for Epileptics

A SCHOOL FOR EPILEPTIC CHILDREN
A dancing class in the open at Chalfont Colony School.

Tabes Dorsalis (Locomotor Ataxy) is one of the most common of spinal cord diseases, and is of syphilitic origin. It usually appears about ten to twelve years after the original syphilitic infection. The period, however, varies.

Locomotor Ataxy.

The nervous tracts carrying sensory impulses up the spinal cord towards the brain are principally affected, and also the cranial nerves, especially the oculo-motor nerves, causing squint and double vision. Disorders of sensation are very numerous. Numbness, "pins and needles" sensations and tingling commonly occur in the hands and feet. Dull aching pains in the limbs are often varied by sharp, stabbing, so-called "lightning pain" affecting both limbs and trunk. Loss of sensation, particularly loss of deep pressure sensation and muscle and joint sensation, leads to unsteady gait. The patient has to maintain his position and guide the movements of his limbs mainly by his eyes. He is forced to watch his limbs. In the darkness he stumbles, and he may become so ataxic as to be bed-ridden. The mechanism of micturition is disturbed early with incontinence or attacks of intense desire to pass water and an inability to do so. Such crises commonly affect the various organs, causing severe gastric pain and vomiting, but as the disease progresses these crises tend to become less frequent. Painless destruction of joints occurs, especially those of the lower limbs, with accumulation of fluid and resulting deformity. A less common form of the disease affects chiefly the upper limbs (Charcot's Joints).

The duration of the illness varies, some cases remaining stationary for years. The brain may be involved, but more commonly the mind remains clear, the patient becoming bedridden and dying from some intercurrent infection.

Paralysis Agitans (Parkinson's disease, shaking palsy) is a disease usually commencing in late middle life which progresses slowly to a degree of muscular stiffness and weakness which eventually

Shaking Palsy.

597

condemns the sufferer to a bedridden existence.

The cause of the illness remains unknown. Its onset is insidious, stiffness of the muscles being the first sign. It affects early the muscles of the face, the neck, and the trunk. The face becomes " mask like " owing to the immobility of the facial muscles. The body leans forward, the position is stooping, the trunk, on account of the rigidity of the neck, is moved with the head. The patient's centre of gravity tends to be displaced. He attempts to maintain it by taking short steps. Given a push, he may break into a run. He tries to recover his centre of gravity but owing to his stiffened attitude is compelled to chase it.

As the disease advances weakness and tremors become marked and general. There is a continuous rubbing movement of the thumb and fingers resembling the movements made in rolling a cigarette. Walking becomes difficult ; the body fixed ; weakness advances, until after many years the patient is forced to take to his bed, death occurring most frequently from some other intercurrent disease such as pneumonia.

Epilepsy.* Epilepsy is a disorder of the nervous system associated with sudden loss of consciousness. The disease commences most often in childhood. Consciousness may be lost for only a fraction of a second and may be regained so rapidly that the occurrence passes unobserved. This fleeting attack is spoken of as " petit mal." In other cases the loss of consciousness is conspicuous and is accompanied by a fit. Unaccountable behaviour may follow either type, the patient remembering nothing of it. He may suddenly undress, injure somebody— apparently on purpose, and suffer from maniacal excitement, or may remain for hours restless and deluded. The name post-epileptic automatism has been given to this condition.

An epileptic attack is in many cases preceded by some disturbance which is immediately followed by loss of consciousness. The disturbance is called the " aura." The same aura usually appears in the same individual and after several attacks serves as a warning to him that a seizure is about to occur. Auræ vary with different people. They may be psychical, giving rise to a feeling of fear or unaccountable anxiety ; motor, with twitchings and movements ; or sensory, associated with peculiar sensations referred to the skin, the internal organs, or the special senses, of taste, light, sound, or smell.

Following the aura comes loss of consciousness. Except in those minor cases which may not even appear noticeable, the patient suddenly collapses.

If he has received and recognised a warning signal, he may place himself out of harm's way. The fit is at first tonic in character, the whole body being possessed by muscular spasm. The patient's face becomes congested and blue, his lips livid. Asphyxia appears imminent. The tonic spasm gives way to one which is clonic in character. Twitchings arise in various parts of the body, increase and spread, throwing the whole body into a violent jerking convulsion. During a fit the tongue is often bitten by the convulsive movements of the jaw, blood-stained saliva appearing. Urine is commonly passed.

The condition subsides gradually and is usually followed by deep sleep. When consciousness is regained the patient may have no recollection of the matter. Seizures vary in severity. In many cases they are slight. Sometimes a patient will pass from one attack into another without regaining consciousness. This condition is called " status epilepticus," and when severe is associated with high mortality.

Several independent seizures may occur in a day or there may be an interval of months between the attacks. An attack may occasion accident including severe injury or death, owing to the patient becoming unconscious in dangerous surroundings.

The mental capacity of an epileptic follows no rule. It may be poor and deficient or high mental qualities may be present.

* See sections on Mental Disease and First Aid.

Eventually some deterioration usually appears. Temper and memory become affected and may be followed by apathy and progressive dementia.

Migraine. Headache, sickness, and giddiness are the characteristic features of an attack of migraine. The headache is often severe, usually commencing in the morning, gradually increasing in intensity throughout the day, exhausting the patient. Often vomiting occurs. An attack lasts many hours and is followed by sleep. It is a disease of early and middle life, tending to disappear with advancing years. Migraine is a common disorder. Knowledge regarding its pathology is small.

Chorea (" St. Vitus' Dance ") is a nervous disorder rheumatic in origin. It occurs most frequently in young children, and **"St. Vitus' Dance."** more commonly in girls. The child is often restless and irritable and emotionally unstable and easily tired for some months before movements are observed. Upsetting her glass at meal time may be the first sign of the disorder. Chastisement aggravates the condition. The movements are not under control of the will and are irregular.

The face is commonly involved, the child grimacing frequently. The hands are constantly moving and twitching, the legs jerking. The condition increases in severity. At times movement may become so forcible as to shake the whole body. Swallowing and talking may be difficult. Inadequate nourishment and sleeplessness sometimes exhaust the patient.

Cases vary widely. Most cases improve in two or three months, the movements

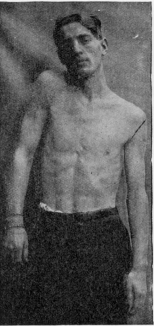 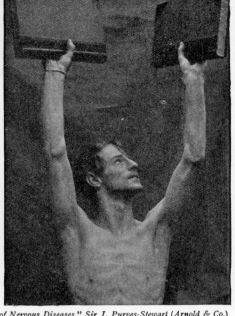

Courtesy] [" *Diagnosis of Nervous Diseases,*" *Sir J. Purves-Stewart (Arnold & Co.)*

A CASE OF HYSTERICAL PARALYSIS

A type of nervous disease extremely obscure in origin. *Left :* a patient suffering from hysterical paralysis and loss of sensation in the left arm tries to shrug his shoulders. *Right :* the same patient after cure.

ceasing. Attacks are liable to recur. Owing to its rheumatic origin, chorea is often associated with heart disorder. The valves are commonly attacked, chronic heart disease following.

Neurasthenia. The name, Neurasthenia, has been applied to many states of ill-health which rightly should never come under this heading. The term neurasthenia is applied frequently to pathological conditions which we do not understand and whose cause often remains obscure. The patient undoubtedly suffers, although to locate the seat of disorder is sometimes impossible to the doctor. Cases of insanity may, in their early stages, give rise to so-called neurasthenic symptoms, and many nervous manifestations which are considered due to psychical causes alone arise from the exhaustion, the starvation, or the poisoning of bodily organs.

The patient complains of various subjective symptoms which he tends definitely to associate with some particular organ. Examination of the organ reveals no

599

pathological condition. The body is obviously disturbed and function disordered. The patient is unwell, usually unhappy, easily tired, restless, and irritable. Many complain of pains in the head indefinite in character. A feeling of pressure or weight or a sensation of " emptiness " is common. Dimness of vision occurring with or without a heavy feeling behind the eyes is often present. Other patients locate their discomfort in the stomach, complaining of vague dyspepsias, constipation, and apprehension owing to sexual irritability or supposed weaknesses. Aching pains in the limbs and back are usual. The patient is very open to suggestion, and his complaints are often directed to his heart or to any other organ by morbid reading or by discussions with his friends.

The nervous symptoms may appear more definitely in the mental sphere, the main characteristic being instability of the mind. The patient becomes hypersensitive and particularly nervous of meeting people or of performing some act in the presence of others. He feels that his friends are critical and observe clearly his failings. His power of paying attention is lessened ; he cannot concentrate his mind for long upon one thing. Ordinary work becomes a labour. Marked restlessness often appears early, the patient moving from one momentary occupation to another. No environment satisfies him for long or gives him rest. Sleep becomes disturbed, and he may suffer from dreams of a distressing, perhaps frightening character. The sleeplessness aggravates the condition. Slight worries develop into anxieties. Emotional reaction is easily evoked and prevents him from being at his ease even amongst his closest friends. Failing self-confidence is common to all cases. Clear judgment cannot be expected, decisions cannot be made, the patient being obsessed with various doubts and fears. Other cases follow a more depressed and miserable course associated with vague ideas of unworthiness and with introspective hypochondriacal obsessions.

Nerve exhaustion may create a mental attitude which alters the whole outlook of the patient towards life. There is perhaps nothing more distressing than mental suffering, particularly when clear insight remains. The condition may become more crippling to the individual than many a disease of more definite character.

The pathology is difficult to demonstrate. Some disturbance of the harmonious interacting activities of the endocrine glands appears in many cases. The influence of heredity is sometimes clear. A weakened organism may be transmitted which breaks down easily under strain.

Improper nutrition stands out as a contributory cause of nervous exhaustion. Most especially is this so when it has occurred during the periods of growth and adolescence. There is probably no one factor which contributes more largely to nervous instability in later life than poor nutrition during that chapter of life when the body is establishing sexual maturity. The stress and strain of these years is very great. Physical changes perplex and disturb the emotional equilibrium of the mind. It is a phase of life often misunderstood and misguided. The child requires every care if it is to emerge stable and mature from adolescence. Auto-intoxication is a factor in some cases. Septic foci in the teeth or other localities may pass toxins into the blood.

Nerve exhaustion is often considered to be due to worry, sometimes to alcohol. Excessive worrying and "taking to alcohol" are more often early symptoms of a nervous breakdown, the preceding signs of which are usually restlessness, sleeplessness, and irritability of temper.

It must also be remembered that the sympathetic nervous system, which in health does not arouse consciousness, can in pathological organic disease occasion feelings and sensations, nagging and wearing in type, whose persistence may exhaust the nervous system of a patient.

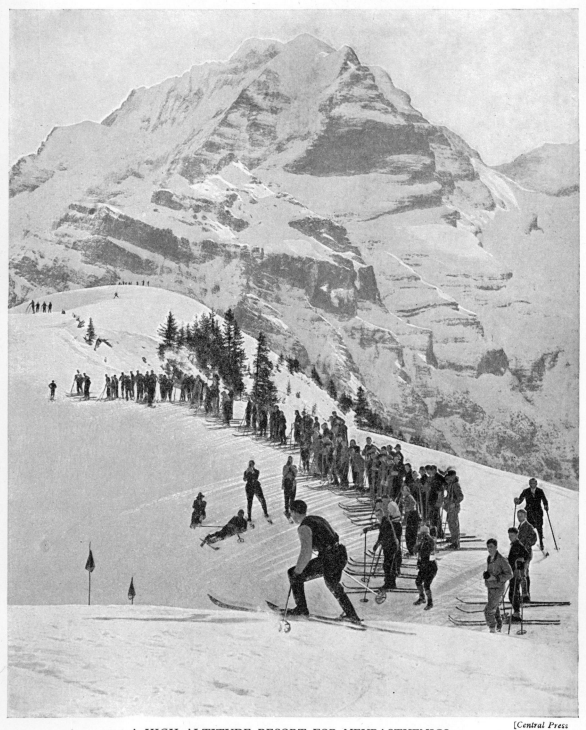

[*Central Press*

A HIGH ALTITUDE RESORT FOR NEURASTHENICS
The start of a ski-race at Mürren, Switzerland, a well-known resort for the milder
forms of nerve trouble.

601

DISEASES OF THE SPINAL CORD

The signs following compression of the spinal cord depend upon the segment affected. Pain, which radiates along the nerves whose roots are involved, is usually the first symptom. Muscular weakness in the region supplied follows and is associated with increasing stiffness. Paralysis of spastic type gradually develops. The sphincter mechanisms are commonly disordered. The patient may find difficulty in commencing micturition. Later retention may occur, with overflow. The rectal sphincter may be unable to control defecation, when the motions are loose.

Compression.

Tumours may either compress the cord or actually invade its substance. An aneurism of the aorta may slowly erode the bones of the spinal column and press upon the cord. Tubercle bacilli commonly attack the bones of the spinal canal and constitute a common cause of compression, especially in children. Inflammatory conditions may not give rise to progressive symptoms. Temporary inflammatory congestion may subside, relieving the pressure.

The formation of cavities in the substance of the spinal cord is the conspicuous lesion in Syringo-myelia, which is a disease of early adult life. The characteristic symptom is a loss of sensation to painful and thermal stimuli. Sensibility to other forms of stimulation such as touch remains normal.

Syringo-myelia.

For example, a patient will be able to hold and smoke a cigarette with full awareness, but may burn his fingers with the lighted end and remains unconscious of the pain.

The area involved varies according to the position of the lesion.

Apart from injury, hæmorrhage into the substance of the spinal cord (Hæmato-myelia) is rare. The symptoms appear suddenly and consist of sensory disturbances with paralysis or weakness which tend gradually to pass off. Some permanent disability may remain. Distribution of the symptoms depends upon the site and extension of the hæmorrhage.

Hæmato-myelia.

The lesion in progressive muscular atrophy is a degeneration of the motor nerve-cells of the anterior horns of the spinal cord, and of certain motor nuclei, or collections of nerve-cells in the medulla of the brain. The degeneration may be more marked either in the brain or in the spinal cord. In either situation it is followed by wasting of the muscles which derive their nerve supply from the affected nuclei. The upper limb is usually the first to be involved and the wasting begins in the muscles of the hand, particularly the thumb, extending up the arm until it attacks the shoulder. The muscles of the lower limb and the trunk are less commonly affected than the upper limb.

Muscular Atrophy.

When the nuclei of the medulla are affected, the muscles of the tongue are early involved, causing disturbance of articulation; also the muscles of mastication and of swallowing are affected. The mouth may remain open, with saliva dribbling from it, the lips waste, and weakness of the facial muscles produce lack of expression. If the nuclei supplying the nerves to the larynx are affected, phonation becomes altered. The disease is progressive and

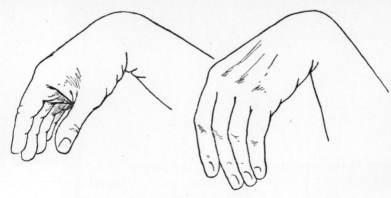

WRIST DROP
Poisoning by lead, arsenic, or alcohol may lead to this condition, affecting the muscles of the wrist and fingers and producing wasting.

recovery does not take place ; its duration is variable, bulbar cases being especially rapid. Pulmonary disease is a common cause of death.

AFFECTIONS OF THE PERIPHERAL NERVES

Peripheral nerves and nerve plexuses may be damaged or torn by accidental injuries. They may be involved in dislocation or fractures or pressed upon by a new growth. The signs and symptoms which follow depend upon the nerve affected and its sensory and motor function.

INTERSTITIAL INFLAMMATION may attack any peripheral nerve trunk, but more commonly is found associated with the larger nerve trunks or the plexuses from which they arise. It is regarded as being of rheumatic origin. The connective tissue which holds together the nerve fibres suffers, the inflammation usually being diffuse. It gives rise to pain which radiates along the course of the nerve. The pain is boring in character with sharp exacerbations. The muscles supplied show wasting. The area affected is tender to pressure, movement and stretching often causing acute pain. Disorders of sensation are sometimes present such as numbness and tingling. Fibrositis in adjacent tissue is common.*

MULTIPLE NEURITIS can arise from varied causes. In some cases no cause can be discovered. It consists of inflammatory changes which involve
Neuritis. the fibres of peripheral nerves. It usually arises from poisons such as alcohol, arsenic, and lead. ALCOHOLIC NEURITIS is becoming less common. It follows persistent drinking, usually of spirits. The inflammation involves most frequently the smaller branches and affects chiefly the lower limbs. The initial symptoms are disorders of sensation such as tingling and cramps. Loss of sensation to light touch is found associated with increased and sometimes severe pain on deep pressure. Weakness and wasting of the affected muscles follow. A common symptom is dropping of the foot, giving rise to a high stepping walk.

* See section on Chronic Rheumatism.

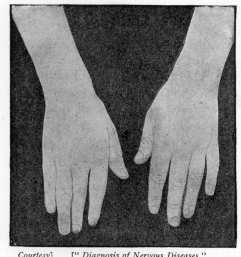

Courtesy]   [" *Diagnosis of Nervous Diseases,"*
Sir J. Purves-Stewart (Arnold & Co.)

NEURITIS AFFECTING THE HAND

An example of disease of the peripheral nerves as a result of which the skin has become glossy and the finger-tips wasted and tapering.

ARSENICAL NEURITIS may arise from beer contaminated by arsenic, or from the use of arsenic as a drug. The disease resembles alcoholic neuritis, but tenderness may be a more prominent symptom and the paralysis more often attacks all the limbs.

Neuritis due to lead poisoning is found most commonly amongst those people, such as painters and plumbers, who work with materials which contain lead. It differs from alcoholic and arsenical neuritis in that sensory disturbances only rarely occur. The motor disability is usually confined to the upper limbs, affecting the extensor muscles of the wrist and fingers and producing wrist drop with muscular wasting.

The toxins produced in diphtheria appear to be specially damaging to nerve tissue. One of the great dangers of diphtheria is the frequency with which it is followed by some form of paralysis. The local signs of diphtheria may be very slight, yet serious paralysis may occur as a complication. Paralysis of the part affected is due to the toxins travelling up to the nerve-cells whose axons supply the region.

In paralysis of the soft palate there is difficulty in swallowing ; fluids tend to regurgitate through the nose ; and the voice becomes nasal. Multiple peripheral neuritis follows the general circulation of the toxins and appears usually during convalescence. Its description will be found under the complications of diphtheria.

Peripheral neuritis may also be found associated with other diseases such as dysentery, typhoid fever and malaria, and occurs in disorders such as diabetes and beri-beri.

HEADACHES

By ROBERT M. MACFARLANE, M.B., Ch.B., D.P.M., Assistant Medical Officer at the West Ham Mental Hospital.

HEADACHE represents one of the most disabling of the minor ailments of civilisation, and for this reason deserves the attention of the practitioner of preventive medicine. Since it is such a universal experience it is only natural to expect that it should take origin not in one or two causes, but in many. Such, indeed, is the case ; headache is not a disease but a symptom. That is to say, it is merely the outward sign of some less obvious and perhaps hidden derangement of health. The disorder responsible may be purely trivial and one which is readily amended ; on the other hand, the headache may be a manifestation of very severe disease of the neighbouring or remote structures. Although relief from pain or discomfort is the main if not the sole result expected at the hands of the doctor, nevertheless it is clear that symptomatic treatment without knowledge of the cause of the pain savours of " a shot in the dark " and falls very short of the ideal. The doctor's first concern is therefore with *diagnosis*.

In the process of correctly ascertaining the cause of a particular type of headache, a certain amount of information can be obtained from a careful inquiry into the *character* of the pain. Thus the physician will inquire into such important points as to the time relations ; whether the headaches are of daily occurrence or only occasional ; if present on waking ; whether they tend to improve or become worse as the day advances. The site of the pain—whether frontal, bi-temporal, or ocular ; whether situated on the summit or at the back of the head—is to be noted. Attention must be paid to the type of pain—slight or severe ; whether dull, throbbing, boring or darting. Lastly, one must take into account the factors which tend to aggravate the pain and take special note of the influence of reading and close work, of noise, worry, mental and physical exertion, stooping, bending, and so on.

Some of the more important varieties of headache may be considered in greater detail.

As representing one of the most common types, the headache of *eyestrain* may be dealt with. This is a pain—usually dull in character—which tends to come on after needlework or reading—particularly in bad illumination. The pain is most commonly situated in the frontal region or may be referred to the back of the eyes, but pain in the occiput (back of head) is not common. In addition the eyes themselves may smart and the lids become sore, heavy, and reddened.

Fatigue headaches are very similar to those of eyestrain ; they usually appear towards the middle of the day and tend to grow more severe. They are accompanied by a sensation of sleepiness which renders difficult, if it does not even preclude, any attempt at study or mental effort.

In cases of prolonged mental exertion or overwork the characters of the headache may resemble those of *neurasthenia* or mental exhaustion. The pain in such cases alters somewhat in character, it partakes less of the nature of an actual ache, more of a sense of weight and of constriction. Patients liken the sensation to that of a " weight pressing on top of the head ," or " to a tight band around the forehead." The former complaint used to be described by the older physicians as the " clavus " or " hysterical nail."

In this country *rheumatism* is responsible for a large number of our headaches. Infiltration of the muscles at the back of the neck with rheumatic thickenings is a responsible agent. The pain in such cases is situated at the back of the head and neck

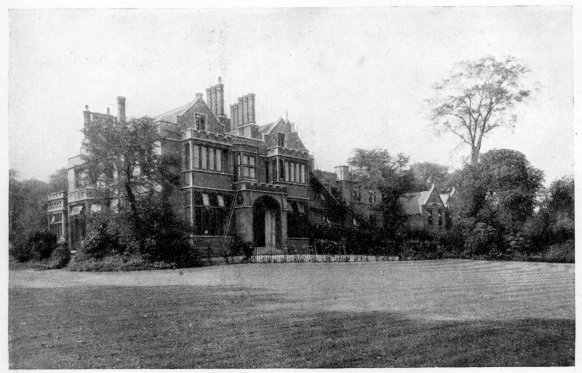

A HOSPITAL FOR NERVOUS DISEASES.
The In-Patients' Department of the West End Hospital for Nervous Diseases, Regent's Park, London.

and is accompanied by an uncomfortable feeling of tiredness and general malaise. On pressing deeply in the painful muscles the fingers will discover areas of exquisite tenderness, which represent the formation of the typical "rheumatic nodules."

Another type of headache which is of common occurrence is that due to *constipation*. Every one is familiar with the dull, early-morning headache accompanied by an out-of-sorts feeling and a distaste for food which usually coincides with an omission from the regular habit of bowel activity. Of similar, though more severe nature, is the headache occurring after an evening of unwisdom in the matter of food and (more especially) drink.

Of especial interest are those peculiar "sick-headaches" which so often prove a disabling factor in the efficiency of the young student or brain worker. They are known also by the names, "bilious headaches," "hemicrania," or "migraine." Although variable in type according to the individual, certain

Sick-Headache.

general characteristics stand out so as to make the diagnosis clear. These common features may be considered more closely.

(1) They are essentially paroxysmal, successive attacks being separated by an interval of, say, a week, a month, or even longer.

(2) The attack is usually precipitated by some factor such as excessive study, emotional anxiety, or temporary gastro-intestinal upset.

(3) Each attack starts (in a typical case) with some peculiarity in the vision, such as lights dancing before the eyes, coloured spots, or specks, or mistiness of vision. There may even be a transitory blindness for central vision or for objects situated to the right or to the left.

(4) Next in order of appearance is the headache, which is of great severity, and is strictly limited to one-half of the head. Brushing or combing the hair may be a most unpleasant procedure.

(5) While the headache is in process the victim suffers from intense malaise and prostration ; he becomes nauseated and giddy.

Work of any description is usually out of the question, and the patient feels impelled to remain at absolute quiet.

(6) The attack usually terminates by the patient vomiting. Afterwards comes a sensation of fatigue, and the patient usually falls asleep.

There are headaches which are of nasal origin, and are due to an acute or chronic inflammation of the accessory sinuses of the nose. Pain of this origin is dull and throbbing in character and is situated either in the cheek-bones or in the region immediately over the eyes. The pain is altered by changes in posture ; for example, the act of bending forward usually aggravates the discomfort. In acute cases the pain is like a bursting sensation in the face or head. Headaches may also arise in conditions of chronic turgescence of the nasal mucous membrane, with defective air entry.

Varied Origin.

In elderly subjects, and in individuals with arterial hardening, headache is not an uncommon complaint. The pain is usually dull in character and is aggravated by fatigue and especially by physical exertion ; it tends to get worse towards evening. As a rule it is accompanied by a sensation of giddiness. Headaches of similar type occur in individuals suffering from chronic kidney disease and from gout, whatever the age of the subject.

A particularly intractable variety of headache may come on after concussion or severe head injuries. There may be an intervening period of freedom shortly after the actual accident and then at the later date the pain makes its first appearance. It gradually becomes constant and tends progressively to become worse. Other symptoms may co-exist such as forgetfulness, inability to concentrate, and a sensation of fatigue and general malaise. Any exertion—physical or mental—aggravates the pain.

The headaches which result from increased tension within the intracranial cavity are most important from the standpoint of the physician. They occur as important symptoms in such conditions as brain tumour, brain abscess, and meningitis. In the earlier stages the pain may be slight in intensity and dull in character. Any part of the skull may be the seat of the pain. Usually the pain is present on waking in the morning and tends to wear off as the day progresses. Any exertion like bending, straining, coughing, or lifting will aggravate the symptoms. A most common feature in this type of headache is that vomiting is usually present. In the later stages the headaches may be of the utmost severity so that the subject is forced to lie motionless and in absolute quiet. Every now and again—particularly in cases of meningitis—a peculiarly intense exacerbation may cause a sensation of pain to dart through the head.

There are various types of neuralgias which may be referred to the head or skull, some of them of temporary nature, others being permanent and more severe in degree. Thus one meets with cases of OCCIPITAL NEURALGIA, where the pain shoots from the head, over the back of the head to the crown ; SUPRA-ORBITAL NEURALGIA, which arises from the region of one eyebrow and darts over the forehead to the top of the head, remaining, however, always strictly unilateral. A rare variety—spoken of as SHIDER'S NEURALGIA—has its chief situation at the root of the nose. Paroxysms of sharp pain localised to one eyeball may sometimes be the result of the so-called CILIARY NEURALGIA.

Neuralgias.

Syphilitic subjects are particularly prone to headaches whether the nervous system is directly attacked or not. The most characteristic feature of the syphilitic headache is its tendency to get worse at night-time, and hence frequently to prevent sleep.

An important type of headache—located particularly in the eyeball—occurs in acute glaucoma. Vomiting is a frequent accompaniment and unless particular inquiry is directed towards the state of the vision, the real nature of the complaint may be missed.

Lastly we may take note of the multitudinous types of headache which are of *hypochondriacal* nature. In such instances the patient's description of the symptoms are lengthy and the patient dilates upon his symptoms ad nauseam. Similes of the bizarre and incongruous variety are thrown out with complete disregard of all the canons of physiology or anatomy—" my skull is on fire " ; " insects are darting beneath my scalp " ; " my brains are being eaten away and corroded as though with acid "—these are typical of the statements of the hypochondriac.

PREVENTION AND TREATMENT OF HEADACHES

Although preventive measures are of no avail to avert some of the more especial types of headache, yet there are certain cardinal rules which if followed out will insure against the onset of some of the minor and yet most common types of headache.

(1) Avoidance of eyestrain is the first rule ; this is to be carried out by precluding reading, writing, or close work in bad illumination ; small print upon cheap paper is best avoided ; do not read in trains, buses, or trams ; the cheap seats in cinemas are extremely trying. At the first hint of eye-strain, an ophthalmic surgeon should be consulted, and his advice conscientiously followed.

(2) Overwork, worry, and insufficient sleep are potent and often avoidable sources of chronic headache.

(3) Anæmia and debility can be cured by attention to proper intervals of rest and an adequate dietary. In a large proportion of such cases there is discernible a smouldering nidus of infection—whether in the tonsils, the teeth, ears, or appendix. Amongst women, the genital tract is a fertile source of such sepsis. Treatment must first be directed along these avenues.

(4) Attention to the dietary is occasionally necessary. While little harm is to be found in the mixed dietary of the average person, nevertheless a bread and butter and tea regime, which is often the staple food of a section of the community, is a potent source of headache. Excessive meat eating—as also excessive smoking or drinking—may at times be demonstrable as a factor in the production of headaches.

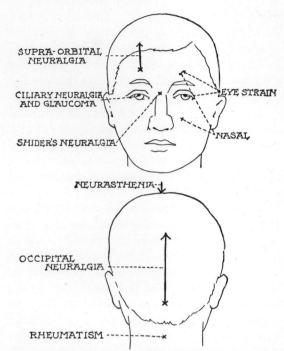

THE DIAGNOSIS OF HEADACHES
Showing how the site of the pain in the various forms of headache may help to establish the cause.

The treatment and prevention of headaches—as indeed with any other similar bodily complaint—is intimately bound up with the question of diagnosis. In the absence of accurate knowledge as to the disease factors at work any efforts at treatment must be purely palliative in nature, and hold no place in the realm of preventive medicine. The curative measures therefore will comprise first those efforts directed against the underlying disorder (such will also constitute the preventive efforts), and secondly measures which are purely symptomatic and aim at nothing beyond immediate though temporary relief. One may consider the latter class of measure first.

Headaches, of any severity, will require the sufferer to rest, and no other measure can be considered as having had *Immediate Treatment.* a fair trial if the patient is continuing his mental and bodily exertions. If the headache is intense then the patient must lie down in a quiet and preferably darkened room. Caffeine, in the form of tea or coffee, is often of itself successful in relieving the headache, and, in any case, it enhances the action of other measures. A mild aperient is sometimes of avail in cutting short the course of a headache, and in this connection nothing is so good as a draught of one of the many effervescing preparations which are available. Application of cold evaporating lotions to the head are helpful—and among such preparations cold water, eau de cologne, vinegar, or menthol may be mentioned. While resting, the patient should be forbidden reading and conversation.

There are numerous drugs upon the market—good and bad—which are employed

Drugs. for the relief of headache. Some of the proprietary preparations of unproclaimed composition are efficacious but dangerous. But amongst the better known varieties which can be recommended are aspirin (gr. 5-10), phenacetin (gr. 5-7), amidopyrin (or pyramidon) (gr. 5-10), antipyrin (gr. 5). Of these the first named is perhaps of most general utility. There exists, however, an individual peculiarity with regard to these drugs, one person finding benefit from one example and none at all from another. Furthermore, with continual use the patient tends to become tolerant to the drug, which then appears to lose its former efficacy ; in such cases the patient should switch over to another drug of that class.

Certain rules should be observed when taking these preparations :—

(1) The drug should be taken on an empty stomach, i.e. immediately before a meal.

(2) The tablet should be crushed into powder and placed on the tongue. (These two rules make the action of the preparation quicker and more certain).

(3) The powdered drug should be washed down with a little water, and followed by a cup of tea or black coffee.

(4) The patient should then lie down for half an hour afterwards.

If these rules are disregarded then the drug is not given favourable circumstances for its action, and may fail to relieve.

There exists in certain circles a prejudice against taking these types of drugs as a palliative measure. This spirit of caution—commendable no doubt—is rather exaggerated. The drugs are not harmful in the doses stated, cases in which harm has accrued have been due either to impurities contained in cheap preparations, or—much more commonly—to overdosage. There is an especial proclivity towards habit formation, and those rare instances of aspirin addiction occur in unstable persons who are liable to excess of all kinds. Indeed aspirin over-indulgence is often a symptom of morphinomania or cocainism.

Besides these general efforts towards alleviation which are of value in all types, there exist special measures for dealing with particular varieties of headaches.

For example, experience teaches that the neurasthenic headache does not show the

Special Measures. same response to aspirin and other pain-lessening drugs, but, on the other hand, it is relieved by general nerve sedative mixtures, containing bromides and valerian. In obstinate cases various local electrotherapeutic measures—such as Le Duc Faradism, high frequency " static breeze "—often help. The rheumatic type of headache finds especial relief in aspirin as well as other derivatives of salicylic acid. In addition, relief is obtained by deep massage of the neck muscles with iodex and wintergreen oil liniment. Local applications of heat—whether in the form of radiant heat, or of simple hot flannels or thermogene—afford relief.

Constipation headaches are curable by remedies directed to the intestines rather than by the administration of anodyne drugs. The headaches following alcoholic over-indulgence can often be avoided and frequently relieved by calcium ; thus sixty grains of calcium lactate taken immediately before the anticipated banquet—repeated later if necessary—often serves to avert any unpleasant after-effects.

The treatment of migraine stands in a special category ; treatment must mainly be directed in the inter-paroyxsmal periods towards the avoidance of subsequent attacks. For this purpose the eyes must be most carefully tested and small errors of refraction will require to be corrected. In those rare cases in which particular foodstuffs seem to be responsible for each migrainous bout, the offending article must obviously be avoided. Mental overstrain and prolonged study must be forbidden, and the patient may require a temporary holiday with abstention from bookwork and a course of iron, strychnine, and arsenic. Of the many drugs which have been employed, luminal (in small doses) to-day holds the position of favourite. For the relief of the attack itself, absolute rest is necessary and a moderately large dose of pyramidon (or aspirin) combined with bromide, caffein and benzil benzoate is required.

Headaches of renal or arterio-sclerotic origin are often resistant to ordinary therapeutic measures. The maximum relief is to be expected from that treatment which tends to bring back to normal the intra-cerebral circulation. In many cases—probably the majority—the headaches are the expression of a deficient blood supply to the cerebrum, and in such, tonics of the strychnine type are of most value. When it is clear that the headaches are congestive in origin, i.e. due to a plethora, then depressant drugs must be exhibited; of these, three preparations stand out as being of especial merit—sodium nitrate, potassium iodide, and vinum antimoniale.

Treatment of the severer types of headache —such as result from cerebral syphilis, increased intracranial pressure, post-concussional states, and the neuralgias—require the immediate attention of the physician.

TREATMENT OF ORGANIC NERVOUS DISORDERS

By ROBERT M. MACFARLANE, M.B., Ch.B., D.P.M., Assistant Medical Officer at the West Ham Mental Hospital.

IT is a reproach commonly levelled at the nerve specialist that his attainments in curative treatment fall very short of his diagnostic and scientific abilities. Some even assert that, surgical interference apart, syphilis of the nervous system is the only neurological disorder amenable to treatment. The entire incorrectness of such a dictum is, of course, obvious even though the neurologist may be often slow to defend himself.

Once highly developed cellular tissues are destroyed, anatomical and functional restoration are rarely to be expected. This statement is especially true of nervous disease; the dead nerve-cells can never be replaced, and regeneration of the nerve fibre is only to be hoped for in the case of the body nerves. This fundamental principle does not, however, secure the doctor from withholding any curative or palliative measure which will relieve symptoms, and, in short, make the best of what nerve tissue remains.

Patients suffering from chronic—and what are virtually incurable maladies of the nervous system—can be made comfortable to a degree beyond the hopes of the chronic arthritic, or of the renal, cardiac, pulmonary, or dyspeptic patient. Much, then, is possible in the way of symptomatic treatment for the relief of pain, the control of spasticity, the improvement of sphincter control, and so on.

The principal therapeutic avenues may be mentioned as they apply to the various types of nervous disease.

There are numerous disorders in neurology which result from the action of microbic invasion (of known or unknown nature) or from the actions of poisons of diverse kinds. Such are exemplified by meningitis, the various types of encephalitis, infantile paralysis, syphilis of the nervous system, disseminated sclerosis, and polyneuritis.

Treatment in such diseases aims at—
(1) The destruction and removal of the causative organism or poison.
(2) The repair of the damaged tissue caused by the noxious processes.
(3) The prevention of subsequent re-invasion by increasing the patient's resistance; and
(4) The education of the patient's crippled nervous system so as to minimise the disabling efforts of permanently damaged nerve tissue.

Thus, in meningitis one endeavours to remove the responsible agencies by drawing off the spinal fluid by repeated lumbar punctures, and secondly by the administration of appropriate neutralising serums.

In neurosyphilis one aims at attacking the causative organism by introducing into the body such powerful antagonising drugs as arsenic, bismuth, or mercury, and by hastening the absorption of scar tissue with iodide of potassium. Recently it has been noted that cases of brain syphilis often improve to some degree after prolonged fever; this observation has been utilised by actually giving these patients malaria, which is maintained just so long as the physician chooses. Under this method of artificial pyrexia, numerous beneficial results have been recorded.

Only too often, however, by the time the patient seeks advice, the damage has been done; nerve-cells have been damaged beyond the hope of repair, and dense scar tissue has been laid down. In such cases, palliative treatment alone can be carried out. But with re-educational exercises the patient trains other sense avenues, and so learns to overcome in some measure the disability caused by his recalcitrant limbs. Massage will help in the reduction of spasticity or stiffness, and will maintain the nutrition of the affected muscles. Other agencies too lie at the physician's disposal for the relief of pain and discomfort, of defective bladder control, of cramps and the numerous other incidental symptoms which add to the patient's burden.

The modern scourge of epidemic encephalitis still rages amongst us, and is responsible for a tremendous amount of chronic nerve disease. An especial difficulty lies in respect of this particular disease; in the early stages—when treatment would hold out its greatest promise of a cure—symptoms may be so slight or indefinite as to cause the sufferer no alarm. A passing sleeplessness, a light delirium, a fleeting blurring of the eyesight or transient double vision, an unusual sleepiness—such may be the sole indications of an encephalitis, and the patient may well hesitate to consult a doctor or even to lie up. Unfortunately the disease does not disappear at this stage; it dies down—apparently altogether—but we know that it lies smouldering within the brain, and slowly—insidiously but inevitably—it progresses and produces a characteristic disability. We know of no treatment as yet which will stop the march of the disease at this stage, and the resources of the doctor are taxed to the utmost to relieve the more outstanding symptoms. Hyoscine, belladonna, stramonium—these will be the chief measures indicated.

Although to-day we are equally in ignorance as to the nature and the specific treatment of disseminated sclerosis, it is fairly safe to predict that this disorder will yield its secrets to the researches of the future. In this disorder, the nervous system is attacked periodically, each bout of illness causing a temporary disability which later clears up to a large extent. The improvement is not complete, however; a permanent residuum usually remains which increases with each fresh attack. As a final result the patient may be rendered paralysed and bedridden.

Until the perfection of an adequate serum or vaccine therapy we are at present forced to rely upon the administration by the vein of arsenic, particularly in combination with silver. This is often reinforced by iodides, mercury, and arsenic given by mouth. For a time a mode of treatment was in favour—in an aim to increase the resistance of the patient—by the production of fever and stimulation of the immune substances of the blood by means of injections of protein, milk, or typhoid vaccine. In the late stages of the malady, the greater part of the treatment will comprise careful nursing, the avoidance of bedsores, and contractures, and the relief of incidental symptoms.

Polio-myelitis and polio-encephalitis (infantile paralysis) are nowadays treated during the acute phase by the intravenous or intrathecal administration of convalescent-serum.

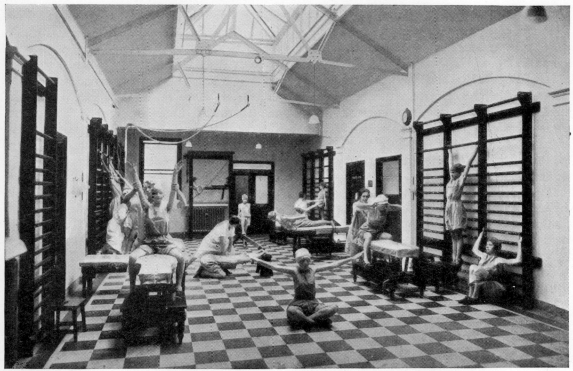

Courtesy]   [Royal National Orthopædic Hospital, Gt. Portland Street, London.

RE-EDUCATING CRIPPLED LIMBS
An exercise class in the gymnasium of the Royal National Orthopædic Hospital.

Skilful nursing is essential at this stage if subsequent deformities are to be avoided. During the post-acute or paralytic stage, treatment is directed towards the care and stimulation of the affected muscles ; for this purpose prolonged massage and active movements are required ; electricity, too, is given—though with doubtful results. Should certain muscle groups be damaged beyond hope of repair, the ingenuity of the orthopædic surgeon will be required to utilise to the best advantage what muscles are spared, by the fitting of appliances or by judicious tendon transplantations.

Tumours. Treatment of tumour formations in the brain and spinal cord lie ultimately within the province of the surgeon. The whole success of an operation will depend primarily, however, upon the skill of the physician in determining beforehand the exact site of the growth. There are two main objects in cases of operation for brain tumours. In the first place, the mere act of removing a portion of the

skull bones has a decompressive effect, and relieves the increased intracranial tension. This measure immediately obviates the distressing symptoms of headache, vomiting, and drowsiness, and in most cases also (except when the disease is too far advanced) averts the threatening blindness. The second object in advising operation is the hope of successfully removing the growth itself.

In a proportion of cases it is possible to remove the growth completely, with little or no damage to the brain itself. Such cases are comparatively rare, however, because most brain tumours are either seated or else are of such a malignant nature as to destroy the brain tissue in which they lie. Attempts at removal in such cases may do more harm than the tumour itself, which should therefore be left alone. Unfortunately we have not yet arrived at that diagnostic level whereby we can foretell before operation which tumours are removable and which are not ; research along these lines is being carried out all over the world, and it is probably not too rash a speculation to predict that in future the physician will be able to diagnose the nature of the growth before operation.

The scope of radium and of deep X-ray therapy for the treatment of inoperable brain tumours is not yet known. Here, again, the work of contemporary investigations holds out a promise of hope in the treatment of what is now usually a fatal malady.

Tumours of the spinal cord can usually be localised with a high degree of accuracy, so that operation can be undertaken directly over the site of the disease. In a large number of cases—provided the operation is undertaken early—the patient is restored to his former strength. No other form of treatment is of avail.

The brain disorders which depend upon degenerative changes in the brain blood
Disease of Brain Vessels. vessels occupy an important part in neurological practice. Cerebral arterio-sclerosis is responsible for many of the nervous disabilities of late middle life and old age. In some cases the effects are shown by obvious paralytic signs—resulting from hæmorrhage or softening within the brain. At other times the effects are less dramatic but more insidious,

and a gradual decline in the intellectual level may be the clue to a progressive cerebral arterio-sclerosis. The treatment of such cases is purely palliative, but none the less is important and often conspicuously successful. Here, again, our general methods of treatment have undergone a change during the past generation. Hitherto it was customary to recommend depressant drugs or measures with the object of relieving cerebral plethora or congestion. We are now inclined to regard the symptoms of cerebral arterio-sclerosis as usually the result of an *insufficient* blood supply to the brain, even in those cases in which the blood pressure is notably increased. One, therefore, endeavours to increase the cerebral circulation and to enrich the quality of the blood by the administration of mild stimulants and by tonics rather than by drugs which lower the blood pressure.

The paralytic manifestations are best treated by massage and passive manipulations of the affected limbs. Electricity usually aggravates rather than relieves the symptoms.

Another group of neurological disorders which demands therapeutic interference
Injuries. comprises the effects of injuries. Brain concussion, fractured skull, fracture-dislocation of the spine, injuries of the body nerves and plexuses constitute an important chapter. In all cases correct treatment depends upon an accurate diagnosis made in the early stages—particularly is this true when the possibility of operation arises. It must be borne in mind, moreover, that the ill effects of injury do not always appear soon after the accident, but—as in the case of damage to the head—may develop months afterwards, at a time when the patient has made an apparent recovery.

It is vitally important to stress the necessity for rest ; the patient should remain in bed for three weeks after concussion, however short the period of unconsciousness. Failure to observe this precautionary measure may occasion months or years of subsequent suffering. Other procedures in treatment include the lowering of intracranial tension

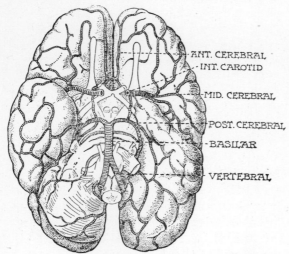

ANT. CEREBRAL
INT. CAROTID
MID. CEREBRAL
POST. CEREBRAL
BASILAR
VERTEBRAL

THE BLOOD VESSELS OF THE BRAIN
Many nervous diseases can be directly traced to changes in the brain blood vessels and an insufficient blood supply is responsible for many symptoms, especially in later life.

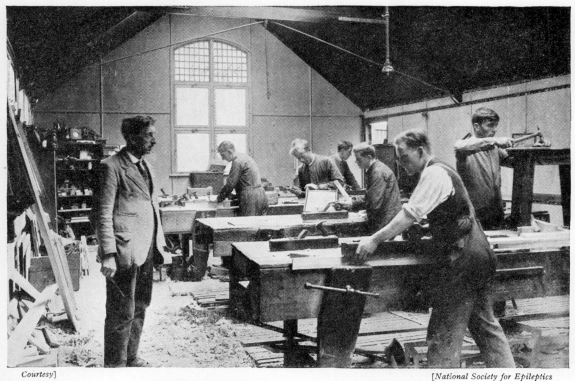

Courtesy]   [National Society for Epileptics

EPILEPTICS AT WORK AT CHALFONT COLONY
The colonists have the choice of many useful occupations; this photograph was taken in the
carpenter's shop.

by purges, lumbar puncture, or the administration of concentrated solutions of salt.
Operation will be indicated when there is
evidence of bleeding from a single large
vessel.

The majority of patients attending a
neurological clinic is composed of epileptics.

Epilepsy.   Herein lies an interesting and
satisfactory problem in therapeutics. It will scarcely be doubted that
to-day the treatment of epilepsy is more
hopeful than ever before, and we now
realise that the possibility of a " cure " of
genuine epilepsy is no longer beyond one's
aspirations. Satisfactory treatment, however, necessitates patience; each case is a
problem in itself; the finding of the drug
most suited to the individual; the assess-
ment of the optimum dosage are matters
which cannot be determined in a month or
two. Moreover, after a satisfactory prescription has been compiled, the patient must
continue treatment for a prolonged period.
" Two years after the last fit " used to be

the rule as the length of time over which
the drug must be continued. We now know
that this is not long enough, and the patient
is well advised to continue medicine for
several years after the apparent cessation of
fits.

The main features in the treatment and
certain other general considerations may be
worth mentioning. First, the most powerful
agents we possess against epilepsy comprise
certain drugs, particularly bromides, borax,
and belladonna. To those one adds the
latest—and probably the most efficacious—
namely, luminal. These drugs are usually
given in combination.

A point of utmost importance lies in the
correct estimation of the time factor—the
object of medicinal treatment is to anticipate
and so avert a threatening attack. Therefore,
the medicine should be taken about one hour
before the usual time of the fit. It is useless
to give medicine thrice daily to a patient
when fits occur always in the middle of the
night. Again, many epileptics can foretell an

approaching fit by diverse premonitory symptoms which may appear several hours or even a day or two beforehand. In such cases, the individual should take an extra dose of his medicine at these times.

Advice is usually sought as to the mode of life which should be adopted by the epileptic patient. What occupation should he follow? What should be his recreations? Here, again, the correct reply will depend upon the particular case, but in general terms it may be stated that any occupations can be pursued except those which may entail a possible source of danger to the patient or to others. Thus the epileptic should under no circumstances be allowed to drive a motor-car; it is usually unsafe for him to work near revolving machinery into which he might fall or be entangled. He should not be allowed to scale ladders or scaffolding. Most sports and recreations are within the patient's competence, with the possible exception of swimming, which might prove a source of danger.

In general terms it may be said that the epileptic patient is best suited when at work. Enforced idleness has a deleterious effect on the individual, and mental boredom is almost as potent a precipitating factor as intellectual or emotional excitement. In the same way the epileptic child should not be allowed to stay away from school. If the intellect is too inferior for ordinary classes then a special school will be necessary; it is not in the best interests of the child to keep him at home.

Certain general rules as to the conduct of medicinal treatment are important; thus the patient must be made to realise the vital importance of taking his medicine regularly and conscientiously, exactly as prescribed.

This rule is, of course, necessary in all types of disease, but in the case of epilepsy it is of paramount importance. Omission of antispasmodic drugs — particularly luminal — often leads to the sudden appearance of a large number of severe fits which may prove fatal.

An additional necessity for regularity of treatment depends upon the fact that every epileptic fit increases the epileptic tendency and facilitates subsequent attacks. It has been stated succinctly that " the best way to cure oneself of fits is not to have them."

The patient should never omit the treatment during an intermittent illness. Thus, the patient is sometimes very wrongly advised to leave off the medicine during an attack of bronchitis, influenza, or any other disability or during the course of pregnancy. This practice is entirely wrong, and may have most serious consequences.

The psychological aspect of the treatment of epilepsy is most important. One is only too often inclined to " molly coddle " the epileptic and to deal with him as an individual apart; the patient soon realises this and is apt to regard himself as a social outcast or pariah; in this way a very definite neurosis may develop and seriously hinder all efforts at restoring the patient to physical and mental health. The epileptic should— as much as is humanly possible—be treated as a normal individual. If the rules mentioned are carried out, there is no necessity to impress upon the epileptic the risks he runs in crossing streets; it is doubtful, indeed, if the epileptic stands in any appreciable degree in greater danger than the normal individual.

Questions as to diet will always arise with regard to epileptics. Here again a vast amount of unwarrantable interference, based upon uncertain and incorrect knowledge, has arisen. Within the past half century the epileptic has had his dietary attacked on all sides. Salt, protein, carbohydrates, alcohol, tea, coffee, tobacco, have all been restricted in turns. To-day, actual starvation is carried out as a therapeutic measure. One form of therapy forbids meat; another claims success from a diet rich in fats and cream. A common-sense view of the problem, however, reveals that the importance of diet has been greatly overrated. There are, however, two main dietetic aspects which are of importance in the treatment of epilepsy; in the first place the patient should not be allowed to indulge in any particular foodstuffs which are known as a matter of experience to be unsuitable. Secondly, the patient is perhaps best suited on an alcohol-free regime as well as on a diet moderate in red meat, strong tea and coffee.

If these provisos are followed out, further interference with the diet is unnecessary in the average case.

THE DUCTLESS GLANDS

By GEORGE SOMERVILLE, M.D., D.P.M., Deputy Medical Superintendent at the West Ham Mental Hospital.

RECENT investigation into the functions of the ductless glands has revolutionised scientific opinion concerning the constitution and working of the human mind and body. Anomalies of development, idiosyncrasies of the personality and certain disorders of mental functioning have been found to be definitely related to variations in the secretory activity of these glands. Consequently understanding of the motives of human behaviour has been increased. Though man cannot be regarded as a mere victim of chemical reactions, these secretions, over which he has no control, profoundly influence his rôle in life.

Formerly the nervous system was believed to be the sole means of communication between the organs of the body; through the medium of the brain alone was co-ordinated and harmonic functioning thought possible. The discoveries relating to the ductless glands have proved the existence of another distinct means of inter-cellular communication. The thyroid, pituitary, pancreas, adrenals, ovaries, and testes elaborate substances which are absorbed directly into the blood stream. Hence they are called ductless glands in contra-distinction to those glands which pour their secretion by way of ducts into other organs or on surfaces. Their secretions are known as chemical messengers or hormones (excitants), and they form a chemical chain linking up groups of body cells. They are absolutely necessary for the continuation of life, and in this respect they are comparable to vitamins. The hormones of the thyroid and adrenal glands have been synthetised in the laboratory.

The ductless glands do not function as solitary organs; they are reciprocal, and in health maintain a balance peculiar to each individual—a glandular personal equation. Thus the thyroid and adrenals mutually excite to activity whereas the thyroid and pancreas are mutually inhibitory.

The exact contribution which each of these glands makes to the physical and mental make-up is at present uncertain, but the bodily configuration with regard to skeletal growth, texture of the skin, and distribution of hair, and the nature of the mind with regard to emotivity, sexual constitution (masculine or feminine predominance), energy display, moods and passions are basically determined in a general way by the interactions of the endocrine secretions.

THE THYROID GLAND

Much of the history of the endocrines is centred round the thyroid. Of all the glands it is the one most frequently diseased

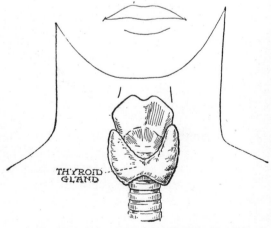

POSITION OF THE THYROID GLAND
The gland embracing the Adam's apple, whose secretion exercises so profound an influence upon all the body cells.

and the symptoms which result are most striking.

The thyroid consists of two lobes, on either side of the larynx, connected together by a bridge of tissue. It has a very rich blood supply. The gland produces the hormone thyroxin, a compound rich in iodine, which stimulates the activities of all the cells in the body and profoundly affects metabolism in general.

Absence or loss of function of the thyroid gland in infancy or from birth results in a species of idiocy known as "CRETINISM." In such a child, growth is arrested. The face looks prematurely aged. The eyelids are thick and baggy; the open mouth reveals a large protruding tongue and irregular decayed teeth. The skin, thick and coarse, with scanty hair, is usually cold and clammy. The abdomen is protuberant, and the development of the sexual organs is delayed. Mentally such children exhibit all degrees of deficiency; they are mostly stolid and apathetic.

Defective Secretion.

In adults the symptoms of thyroid deficiency reveal themselves gradually. Sufferers exhibit a bulky, ungainly appearance. The skin becomes dry, harsh, thick, and puffy; the hair is sparse, the reddish patches over the cheek bones give rise to a characteristic facies. There is marked mental deterioration; memory is very defective, and all intellectual processes are very slow.

This disease is called "MYXŒDEMA," and is twice as common in women as in men. Its onset usually coincides with the menopausal period and it may be associated with the failure of the sexual hormones. As with cretinism, all degrees of this affection occur.

Realisation that both cretinism and myxœdema were caused by a deficiency of the thyroid secretion led to an attempt to substitute extracts of the gland in order to alleviate the symptoms. Remarkable results were obtained; the obtuse stunted child became physically and mentally alert; the dull sluggish woman regained her normal vitality of mind and body. Thyroid admini-

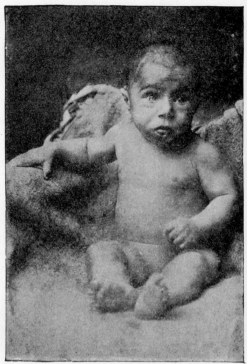

[*American Journal of Heredity*

EFFECTS OF THYROID DEFICIENCY (I)
A child showing the stunted growth and mental deficiency due to inactivity of the thyroid gland.

stration is one of the therapeutic marvels of modern medicine. The extract is prepared from the thyroid glands of sheep and is usually given in tablet form by the mouth. In order that the regained health may be maintained it is necessary that the extract be administered at regular intervals and for an indefinite period.

Excessive secretion of the thyroid results in the morbid state called EXOPHTHALMIC GOITRE. As might be expected, the symptoms are very much the reverse of those seen in cretinism and myxœdema. There is an acceleration of all the bodily processes. Enlargement of the thyroid and protrusion of the eyes are the prominent and constant signs of the disease. The patient has a frightened, startled expression; she is anxious, restless, tremulous, and hyper-excitable; in fact, she exhibits the facial and bodily characteristics of profound fear. There is marked rapidity of the heart action, anæmia and wasting, diarrhœa, and often profuse per-

Excessive Secretion.

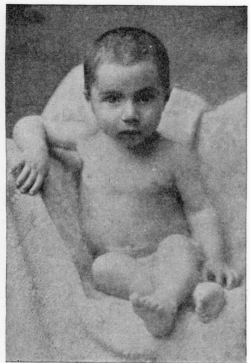

Photo., Courtesy]

EFFECTS OF THYROID DEFICIENCY (II)
The same child after several weeks' treatment with
thyroid extract from sheep.

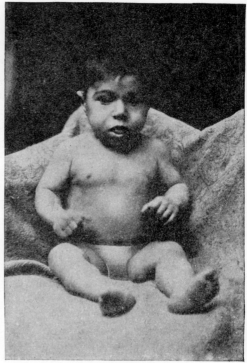

[*American Journal of Heredity*

EFFECTS OF THYROID DEFICIENCY (III)
A year later: the parents refused to continue the
treatment and the symptoms returned.

spiration. The disease is much more frequent in women than in men. Its causation is obscure. It may follow an emotional shock or prolonged mental stress. In essence the disease is an acceleration of all the functions of the body machine produced by a flooding of the circulating blood with the thyroid secretion. Consequently, rest of mind and body is the cardinal principle of treatment. At the same time the mental factor should not be overlooked.

In Simple Goitre there is a rounded swelling of varying size in the region of the throat due to enlargement of the thyroid gland. It is endemic, *i.e.* found locally, and is prevalent in parts of Derbyshire and in the Swiss valleys. As a rule it is not associated with abnormalities of the thyroid secretion and only produces symptoms from pressure on neighbouring organs. This affection appears to be due either to a deficiency of iodine in the food or an inability to utilise such iodine. Treatment of simple goitre with iodine rapidly

Simple Goitre.

relieves in most cases. Iodine is an essential element of our food, and is as vital to the healthy activity of the thyroid as iron is to the blood. The thyroid, as with all other organs of the body, may be a site of innocent or malignant tumours.

THE PARATHYROIDS

Attached to the thyroid are four small glands about the size of millet seed. Formerly they were regarded as part of the thyroid, but recent investigation has shown them to possess a separate function. Removal of the parathyroids (as sometimes happens in operation on the thyroid gland) produces " tetany," a condition where there is sudden, involuntary contractions of the muscles of the extremities. The hormone of the parathyroids is believed to play a part in metabolism by neutralising a nitrogenous poison (guanidine) and the symptoms after extirpation are thought to be due to the toxic effects of accumulation of this poison. The administration of calcium salts sometimes relieves tetany, and it is possible that the parathyroids are related to calcium metabolism.

THE PANCREAS

The pancreas is an example of a gland which has both an internal and external secretion. The external secretion is the pancreatic juice, a digestive agent, which passes via the pancreatic duct into the duodenum. The internal secretion is produced by certain isolated groups of cells, the " Islands of Langerhans," and it is a controlling factor of carbohydrate metabolism.

Disease of these special pancreatic cells is followed by the presence of sugar in the urine—in other words, the state of diabetes. The pancreatic hormone controls the utilisation of sugar by the body and its deficiency causes an increase of the blood sugar and consequently glycosuria. For many years attempts were made to substitute an extract of the pancreas in cases of diabetes after the manner of thyroid replacement in cretinism and myxœdema. Owing to inability to prevent the trypsin of the pancreatic juice destroying the hormone during its preparation, these attempts were unsuccessful. Recently a substance has been prepared by an elaborate process of extraction. It is called " insulin " and its injection into the blood stream of a diabetic tends to restore him rapidly to health.*

THE PITUITARY

The pituitary is a small pea-like body situated in a depression of the sphenoid bone at the base of the skull. It consists of an anterior and a posterior lobe, each with a separate function. The former is the growth promoting factor and influences sexual development ; the latter to some extent controls adiposity and the urinary secretion.

Over-secretion of the anterior lobe in early life produces giantism ; in later life it causes an overgrowth of the skeletal tissues —a disease known as acromegaly. Increased size of the features and of the hands and feet, necessitating larger hats, gloves, and

* See Diabetes Mellitus.

boots is the earliest sign of this disorder. The face is large and coarse : the hands are spade-like ; the skeleton may increase to huge proportions. Dimness of vision may result from pressure on the optic nerve and headache is usually a prominent symptom. The disease is very chronic ; operation may become necessary to relieve the intracranial pressure and to preserve vision. Under-secretion of the anterior pituitary lobe before puberty produces a species of infantilism.

Over-activity of the posterior lobe is not definitely recognised, but it is believed to cause certain forms of glycosuria. Diminished activity causes diabetes insipidus, a condition where the patient passes large quantities of urine. The loss of fluid causes thirst, constipation, and dry skin. As a rule there are no other symptoms. The disease is chronic and the polyuria may be temporarily diminished by injection of extract of the posterior lobe of the pituitary. This substance, known as pituitrin, when injected causes contraction of involuntary muscles (hence its use in obstetrics ; it promotes uterine contractions), raises blood pressure, and diminishes the urinary secretion.

It should be noted that when the pituitary is invaded by tumour growth, a mixture of symptoms referable to both lobes results.

The extreme importance of this tiny gland is revealed in its protean manifestations.

THE ADRENAL GLANDS

The adrenal or suprarenal bodies are two small cocked-hat-shaped glands which rest on the top of the kidneys. They consist of an outer cortex, firm and yellowish, and an inner medulla, soft and dark red. These parts are quite distinct in origin and in function. The medulla elaborates adrenalin, one of the most important and best known of all the hormones. Adrenalin has been prepared synthetically by the chemist and its effects on the body tissues are similar to those produced by the action of the sympathetic nervous system. It constricts the peripheral blood vessels, raises the blood pressure, quickens the heart, dilates the pupils, and increases the quantity of blood sugar. It is interesting to note that in emotional states of rage and fear there is a discharge of adrenalin into the blood. This is probably a protective response on the part of the body ; the extra adrenalin improves the efficiency of the heart and muscles, mobilises energy in the form of sugar, and thus defence and attack are rendered more effective.

Adrenalin has already taken its place as one of the most useful drugs in medical practice. Owing to its power of constricting the arteries it is an excellent styptic, *i.e.* it checks bleeding ; it is also used in conjunction with local anæsthetics to produce a relatively bloodless area and so give a clear field for operation. In shock and collapse it is invaluable ; in forms of asthma due to spasm of the bronchial muscle it rapidly gives relief.

Deficient secretion of the medulla of the adrenal glands produces an interesting disease characterised by profound weakness and a peculiar pigmentation of the skin and mucous membranes. It is known as Addison's disease, and in the majority of cases is caused by tubercular destruction of the adrenal glands. The onset is insidious, the initial symptoms being muscular and general weakness. Gastro-intestinal symptoms are nearly always present. Loss of appetite, nausea, vomiting, and diarrhœa make their appearance sooner or later. The pigmentation varies from a light brown to a dark bronzed colour. It is seen first in the parts normally pigmented. The mucous membranes are pigmented in a patchy manner. The cardiac weakness is very marked and death may result from heart failure or general tuberculosis. Unfortunately the substitution of the hormone adrenalin, as such, is of no value in this disease. Probably it is destroyed in the blood before its complete function can be performed. Grafting of the adrenal gland is still under trial.

With regard to the cortex of this gland, there is considerable doubt as to its function, but its hormone appears to be related to sexual development and activity. Tumours

Addison's Disease.

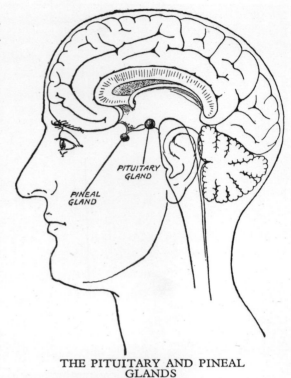

THE PITUITARY AND PINEAL GLANDS

The pituitary gland influences sexual development, adiposity, and the urinary secretion. The exact function of the pineal gland is not known.

of this portion of the gland produce a remarkable sexual precocity and their removal has resulted in a return to the normal. The specific hormone of the cortex has not been isolated, but it appears to be absolutely essential to life.

THE REPRODUCTIVE ORGANS
(OVARIES AND TESTES)

The ovaries and the testes, like the pancreas, produce an internal and an external secretion. The ova and spermatozoa are evidence of the external secretion ; they are responsible for the continuation of the species. The internal secretion moulds the sexual growth and development of the individual. The two secretions are produced by two different types of cells. The liberation of the internal secretion into the blood stream at puberty brings about the development of the secondary sex characters. In women the sex hormone or hormones are responsible for menstruation, lactation, implantation of the fœtus in the uterine wall,

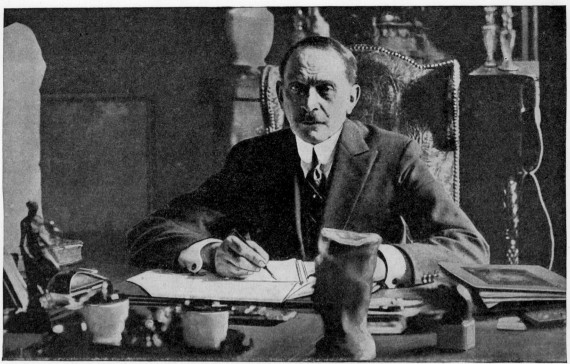

[Topical

A PIONEER OF GLAND-GRAFTING

Serge Voronoff, whose experiments in replacing senile sex-glands by young and active glands from other sources have revealed that a certain degree of rejuvenation is possible.

and many other phases of the reproductive process. In the menopause we see the hormone ceasing to function ; the bodily changes thereby induced are well known. So far the hormone of the sex gland (interstitial cells) has not been isolated, but its presence has been proved by the effects of the removal of the gland (by operation or disease) and subsequent grafting or replacement.

The removal of the sex glands, castration, inhibits the development of the secondary sex characteristics. This operation was extensively practised in antiquity to procure choir-boys and guardians of harems. Eunuchs are tall, flabby, beardless persons, with high-pitched childish voices. They are devoid of sexual desire, and possess none of the aggressiveness of the ordinary male. The excessive accumulation of fat is evidence of disturbed metabolism.

In old age the interstitial cells are diminished in size and number. This led to the belief that the physical and mental changes of advancing years were closely related to the waning in function of these cells. Consequently testicular extracts were injected in order to combat the senile processes— unfortunately with little success. Recently experiments have been tried with grafting or incorporating a young active sex gland, and accumulated evidence reveals that a certain degree of rejuvenation may be obtained. Another method is to tie the duct which leads from the testicle with the object of stimulating the interstitial gland at the expense of the generative function. This is a comparatively simple operation to perform and good results have been claimed for it. Senile subjects became virile; tremors disappeared ; memory and intellectual power returned and sexual potency was restored. If these experiments are confirmed it would appear that in the hormone of the sex glands, the elixir of life has at last been found. At the same time there would appear to be some danger in rejuvenating a person whose arteries are permanently hardened ;

THE HUMAN MACHINE

also it is questionable whether there are many who desire to live with all the vigour of youth beyond the allotted span. Probably the most useful application of this treatment would consist in arresting premature senility.

THE THYMUS

The thymus is a temporary structure which attains its maximum size about the second year of life, and then gradually disappears. The gland consists of two lobes situated in the lower part of neck and upper part of thorax. Occasionally the thymus does not undergo the normal atrophy, but persists into adult life. It is then associated with an overgrowth of the lymphatic tissue throughout the body and such a condition is important through being a cause of sudden death (Thymus Death). Subjects of this diathesis are pale and flabby and usually have enlargement of tonsils, adenoids, and spleen. They should be guarded against any sudden shocks or exertions.

There is considerable doubt as to the function of the thymus gland, but evidence is in favour of the belief that it is an internal secretory gland whose function is to check precocious development of the sexual organs.

THE PINEAL

The pineal is a small gland, about the size of a pea, situated at the base of the brain. It is usually regarded as a ductless gland, but there is considerable doubt as to its function. Tumours of the pineal gland produce signs of sexual precocity, hydrocephalus (water in the head), and paralysis of the eye muscles.

THE HYGIENE OF THE DUCTLESS GLANDS

In the present state of knowledge of endocrine physiology it is impossible to formulate precise rules for their maintenance in health. Nevertheless the damaging effects of over-stimulation of the ductless glands, notably the thyroid and adrenals, which follow severe emotional strains, can be avoided.

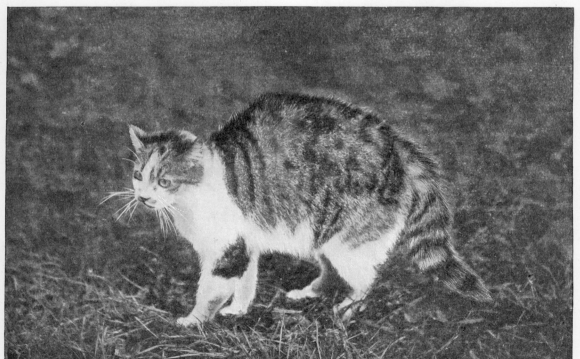

THE PHYSICAL EFFECT OF EMOTION [C. Reid

In a state of strong emotion, as rage or fear, the adrenal gland pours its secretion into the blood and brings about bodily changes (of which the hair-raising illustrated here is a familiar sign) which render defence or attack more effective.

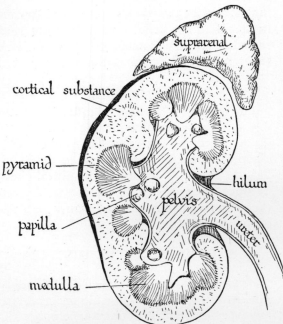

POSITION OF THE ADRENAL GLANDS
The adrenal or suprarenal glands rest on the top of the kidneys and are triangular in shape.

Anger, fear, prolonged anxiety and worry, grief and disappointment produce a temporary exhaustion of these glands which may become permanent. Nerve exhaustion or neurasthenia, with its morbid doubts and fears, is probably related in all cases to a disturbance of the endocrine function.

The toxic absorption from septic tonsils, teeth, appendix, or intestinal tract renders inadequate the thyroid secretion and generally upsets the endocrine balance. Radical cure can only be obtained by getting rid of the foci of infection. Diseased teeth or tonsils must be removed ; indigestion and constipation must be banished.

The climacteric in women is associated with a more or less sudden cessation in function on the part of the sex glands, and in many there is also a diminution of thyroid secretion. The endocrine balance is disturbed, and it is usually some years before a new adjustment is attained. Administration of small doses of thyroid and injection of raw ovarian extract may tide the woman over a difficult and trying phase. Similarly in men premature senile decay may be retarded by a rejuvenation operation.

To conclude, though the discoveries relating to the ductless glands mark one of the greatest medical triumphs, there is no method of treatment which has lent itself to greater commercial exploitation than endocrine therapy. Indiscriminate gland substitution is futile and nothing better than quackery : it only brings true scientific discoveries into disrepute.

PERSONALITY AND THE DUCTLESS GLANDS

By LEONARD WILLIAMS, M.D., Physician to the Legal and General Assurance Society ; formerly Physician to the Miller Hospital, Greenwich, and to the Metropolitan Hospital.

OF the glands endowed with a double function, internal and external, that which seemed to lend itself most readily to investigation was the male gonad or sex gland. Its anatomical position rendered it easy of access. The operation of castration, the oldest surgical procedure in the world, was known to present comparatively few dangers, and the results of this operation upon the general make-up of the individual had been observed and noted long before the question of internal secretion had ever been so much as suspected. The general consequences of a complete operation vary according to the age at which it is performed. When the organs are removed before the age of puberty, the results differ materially in degree from those which ensue when the operation is delayed until after the secondary sex characteristics have been developed. In the former case hair fails to grow, the larynx retains its puerile size and the voice consequently remains a soprano. The operation performed at this early age appears to influence the moral character. It weakens the intellectual faculties and renders the victim fainthearted, wanting in concentration, and incapable of sustained effort. When, however, the mutilation is delayed until after puberty, the results are much less striking. The secondary male characteristics, such as the beard and the bass voice, having already developed, in the majority of cases persist

Sex Glands.

unimpaired. Moreover, eunuchs of this adult type have often been very forceful in character. In Persia and under the later Roman emperors, such people were often promoted to high office and exercised considerable power. In eunuchs of both sorts the external conformation approximates to that of the female, and, like females, they seldom, or never, become bald.

That the female gonad, or ovary, is possessed of an internal secretion there is no manner of doubt ; but, inasmuch as the organ which secretes it is very inaccessible to experimentation, the hormone has not yet been isolated. It is nevertheless safe to speak of an interstitial gland in the ovary, whose secretion performs the same functions in the female as the corresponding glands have been shown to perform for the male. It is not necessary to refer to the effects of the removal of the female gonad. Physiological loss of this element occurs at the menopause with well-known results, and when a similar condition is prematurely imposed by surgical operation, the symptoms are the same in kind but more severe in degree. In both cases ultimate recovery is generally complete.

In elucidation of some points of considerable importance, it will

Sex Development. be necessary now briefly to consider the development of the interstitial glands in the two sexes. At the moment of conception two elements, a male and a female, combine to form an entity. Those elements are warring elements, each of them potentially charged with their characteristic interstitial glands, which develop very early in embryonic life. For several weeks this embryo is neuter, and we are to suppose that the male element and the female contained therein are striving for mastery, the one over the other. Then comes the time when one, say the male,

has definitely gained the victory. But the victory is never complete. The embryonic interstitial glands on both sides have been mobilised, the armies have been engaged, and albeit the one may win, the other though defeated, is by no means annihilated. Thus it comes about that in every child born there remain a certain number of these antagonistic interstitial gland cells which, entrenched opposite the victors, continue to glower at them, crouching for the next encounter. The two armies now cease firing and go into winter quarters.

Then, at the age of puberty, there ensues a second battle royal. The fact that the external evidences of maleness are firmly entrenched does not prevent the female interstitial cells from making one last desperate attempt to gain the mastery ; so that side by side with the secondary male characteristics there may appear some secondary female characteristics, such as a broad pelvis, high-pitched voice, together with female mentality and feminine tastes. There is no man but has some taint of the woman

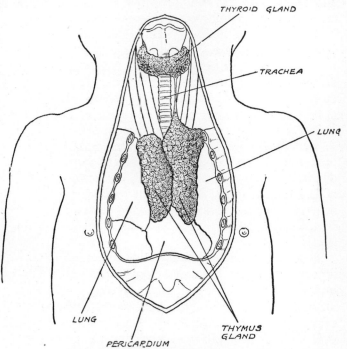

A TEMPORARY DUCTLESS GLAND

The thymus gland is present in a new-born child but normally begins to disappear about the second year of life. It is said to check the precocious development of the sexual organs.

623

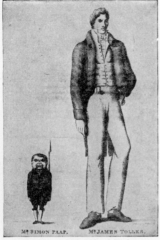

ABNORMALITY OF GROWTH

A well-known old print of Simon Paap and James Toller—a dwarf 2 ft. 4 in. high and a giant of 8 ft.

in him, and no woman without some taint of the male.

When the victory in favour of maleness is complete, the result is a cave-man, a Cæsar, a Napoleon, a Bismarck—active, resolute, ruthless. When less complete, there emerges the ordinary man ; respectable, hard-working, but with engaging weaknesses. With yet another dose of the female interstitial gland in his composition, you come upon the effeminate artistic male, who is usually homosexual at heart. Reverse the medal, and you are in the presence of such an eternal femininity as Josephine, or Mary Queen of Scots. With added male elements, in different degrees, you see Queen Elizabeth, Catherine of Russia, Madame de Stael, or the latter-day suffragette. It is more than probable that among the ranks of the last were a large proportion of women in whom the male and female elements were so nicely balanced as to render them frankly homosexual, and that their activities were directed, subconsciously, perhaps, to obtain, not so much a vote as the right to dispute on equal terms with their male adversaries in the gate of the forum and the market-place.

As the study of endocrine glands advanced it became evident that they determined other important factors besides sex. It was, for example, soon discovered that stature was dependent upon the pituitary ; in the sense that an excess of pituitary secretion in the growing period led to giantism in the adult and that insufficiency of the same secretion led to a particular type of dwarfism. A

study of the suprarenal showed that when this gland was active it produced a person of medium stature, inclined to be hairy, with a great deal of physical strength and force of character. The thyroid being very easy of observation, it was soon noticed that it was liable to become transitorily enlarged in certain physiological conditions, such as menstruation, sexual excitement, and the menopause. An increased activity of this gland produces restlessness, both physical and mental, a decreased activity gives rise to lethargy and hebetude. Now, although the general make-up of any individual is determined by the exact relative proportions in which his endocrine secretions are represented in his blood stream, in the present state of our knowledge it is not possible to do more than guess at the meaning of certain combinations. And inasmuch as these combinations are influenced by climate, by race and other factors of which we have as yet no certain knowledge, to attribute certain mental characteristics to the predominance of certain glands cannot yet be regarded as a scientific procedure.

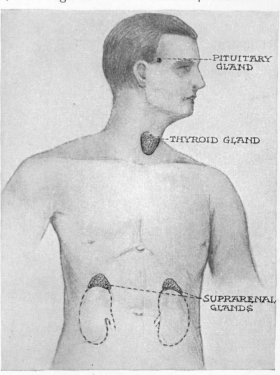

THE POSITION OF THE DUCTLESS GLANDS

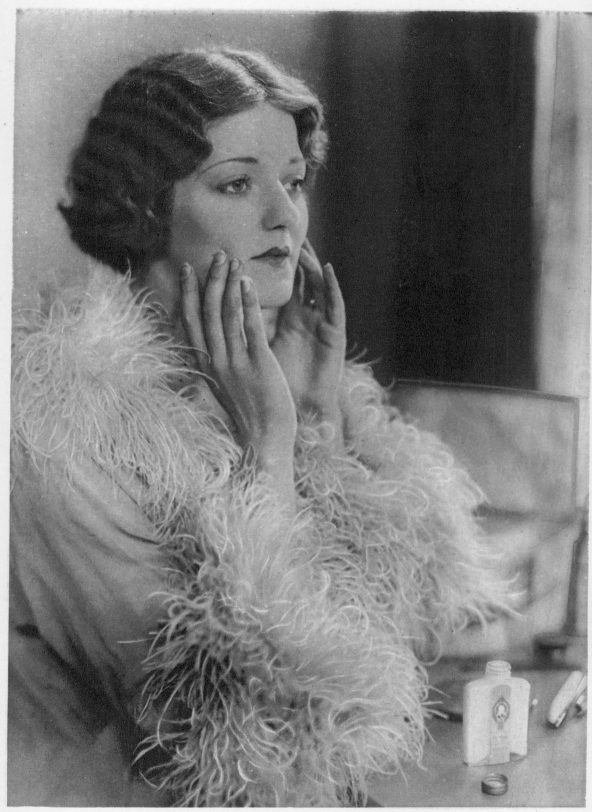

[Lenare

THE CARE OF THE SKIN

THE SKIN

By GEORGE SOMERVILLE, M.D., D.P.M., Deputy Medical Superintendent at the West Ham Mental Hospital.

THE skin is the external covering of the body. It consists of two main layers, namely, the epidermis or cuticle and the dermis or true skin.

The EPIDERMIS is the outer stratum, and is composed of several layers of cells. The surface cells are flat and scale-like and of a hard horny nature. They are especially abundant on the palms and the soles, which are the body areas subjected to most friction and pressure.

The cells of the deeper layers are round, soft, and highly vital. It is by their multiplication that the epidermis grows.

The epidermis is subjected to considerable wear and tear. Washing removes not only dirt but also the superficial cells. The " peeling " subsequent to infectious fevers like scarlatina and measles is simply an extensive shedding of the epidermis. A blister is a localised raising of the cuticle caused by an exudation of fluid from the dermis as a result of some form of irritation.

The DERMIS has a framework of fibrous tissue which becomes loose in structure in the deeper layers and imperceptibly merges into the fibrous supports of the fatty tissue under the skin.

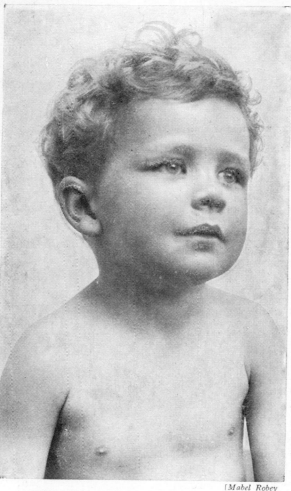

[Mabel Robey
THE HEALTHY SKIN OF BABYHOOD

The superficial layer is very vascular : it contains loops of blood capillaries which are arranged in finger-like projections called papillæ. Nerve fibrils and lymphatics ramify amongst the tiny blood vessels. Stimulation of the special endings of the nerves originates impulses which are interpreted in the brain as sensations on the skin.

The deeper layers are formed mainly by muscular, fibrous, and elastic tissue which permit the necessary movements of the skin. Situated in the true skin are the hair follicles, the sweat and sebaceous glands.

The HAIRS are epidermal growths which emerge from little pits called the " hair follicles." The part within the follicle is called the root. This is embraced by a network of capillaries which nourish the hair. Minute muscle fibres are attached to the hairs so that they are capable of movement. Hair " standing-on-end " is thus an anatomical possibility.

The SWEAT GLANDS consist of coiled tubes in the deep parts of the dermis. Their corkscrew-like ducts lead to cup-shaped depressions on the skin surface. The glands are most abundant on the palms and the soles.

The sweat glands are one of the main

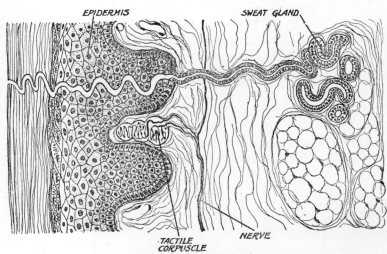

EPIDERMIS   SWEAT GLAND

TACTILE CORPUSCLE   NERVE

THE STRUCTURE OF THE SKIN

A section through the human skin, greatly magnified, showing the layers of cells composing the epidermis, the sweat glands deep in the dermis, and the network of nerves and blood vessels.

small quantities of a fatty secretion which softens the outer cuticle and prevents it from becoming harsh and dry. It is the natural lubricant of the hair and is responsible for its sheen and lustre.

The NAILS of the fingers and toes are modifications of the outer skin. They consist of hardened and horny epidermic cells.

The physiological functions of the skin may be summarised thus :—

(1) The skin is a protective organ. It affords a resistant and yet elastic covering for the softer structures below it.

(2) By virtue of the specialised nerve-endings it is an important sense organ. It renders us aware of pain, heat, cold and touch impressions. (Note that certain parts of the skin are more sensitive than others, *e.g.*, the finger-tips.)

The Skin's Functions.

(3) It helps to regulate body temperature. According to the state of dilatation or contraction of the superficial blood vessels, more or less blood is carried near the surface and consequently more or less heat is given off by radiation.

Body temperature is also related to the exudation and evaporation of the sweat. When the body becomes too hot, as in cases of fever, the superficial vessels dilate and the skin becomes flushed ; when it becomes heated through exertion, sweat is poured out, and as this evaporates the surface of the body is cooled. The average individual temperature is 98.4°F.

(4) The skin is an eliminating organ : its main excretory channels are the sweat glands, and to a lesser extent the sebaceous glands.

(5) The skin is an absorptive organ. Ointments are absorbed and general effects may be produced by local inunction, *e.g.*, mercury in syphilis.

excretory channels of the body. It is estimated that the average adult excretes one and a half pints of sweat in twenty-four hours. The greater part of the excretion passes off from the skin as invisible aqueous vapour. This is known as " insensible perspiration." When the glands act vigorously the sweat appears as drops upon the skin and this is known as " sensible perspiration."

The sweat contains organic matter, fatty acids, sulphur and a relatively large quantity of salts, notably sodium chloride and sodium phosphate. Small quantities of urea are commonly present.

When the kidneys are damaged, as in acute nephritis, the sweat glands can be made to take on their faulty functioning and relieve the body of the accumulating toxic products. This is obtained by stimulating the skin by hot-air baths and by certain drugs (pilocarpine). This transference of function allows the damaged organs to rest. This is the first principle in the treatment of any diseased organ.

The secretion of sweat is an integral part of the mechanism for maintaining a constant body temperature.

The SEBACEOUS GLANDS are small bag-like glands with ducts opening into the upper portion of the hair follicles. They produce

It is natural that the skin with its varied functions should be an important guide to

An Index to Health. the state of well-being of the body. Constitutional changes are quickly reflected in the appearance and functioning of the skin.

Pallor occurs in simple anæmic states and is of varying degree. In pernicious anæmia, however, the skin takes on a lemon-yellow tint. A yellow discoloration is also seen in jaundice, but it is accompanied by severe itching and the mucous membranes are similarly discoloured. Bronzing is seen in Addison's disease, a condition due to degeneration of the suprarenal glands and resulting in a gradually progressive physical deterioration. In grave wasting diseases, such as cancer or syphilis, an earthy hue is always present. A dusky, bluish colour is a common accompaniment of chronic heart disease and chronic bronchitis.

Most of the acute infectious fevers are associated with skin eruptions, known familiarly as rashes, and these, in their distribution and character, are significant of each special disease. The blotchy rash, first showing about the roots of the hair, is typical of measles. In typhoid fever successive crops of rose-pink spots make their appearance on the abdomen. Groups of papules and pustules are characteristic of chicken-pox. In such diseases the skin, acting as an eliminating organ, is endeavouring to rid the body of the poison.

The dryness or moisture and the quality of the skin are significant. In the diabetic, the skin is often dry and inelastic ; in the rachitic child, the perspiring brow is diagnostic. A thick, harsh skin with scanty, brittle hair, is related to deficiency of the thyroid secretion.

The shades of disease are reflected in the skin as surely as the bloom of health.

SKIN DISEASES

Skin diseases are important not only from the fact that they have a powerful influence on the general health but also because they are frequently the expression of constitutional morbidity.

Increased activity of the sweat glands is characteristically seen in the

Secretory Disorders. night sweats of phthisis and the profuse perspiration of rheumatic fever.

Excessive secretion of the sebaceous glands results in the depositing of greasy matter on the skin. Dirt and micro-organisms are entangled and eventually there is an accumulation of scales or crusts. This condition is known as SEBORRHŒA. It occurs commonly on the scalp where the nutrition of the hair is interfered with and baldness is the consequence. The thorough cleansing of the affected parts is the essence of prevention and of treatment. The crusts may be softened by olive oil or dissolved away by an ointment containing salicylic acid.

The blocking of the openings of the sebaceous ducts gives rise to BLACKHEADS or COMEDONES. These are commonly seen on the face, chest, and back of the adolescent. A careful skin toilette will prevent and cure. Blackheads may be removed by steaming the face and extracting the retained secretion by pressure.

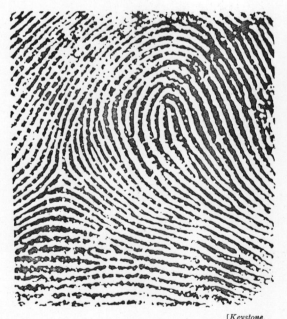

[*Keystone*

A TYPICAL " FINGER PRINT "
A print taken from the late President Harding's right middle finger. The arrangement of the ridges in the epidermis is unique for each individual.

Invasion of the blackheads by germs results in a papule or pimple. This may become pustular and cause inflammation of the surrounding skin. The hair follicles are also involved. This eruption is then known as ACNE. The main treatment is local. Individuals with greasy skins should wash thoroughly at least three times a day and dry with a rough towel to cause friction. Mor ing cold baths, with brisk rubbing afterwards, are excellent for those who react well to the cold. Any form of treatment must be regular and must be persevered in.

Untreated acne eventually leaves unpleasant pitting and scarring of the face.

Overgrowth of the cuticle, as a sequence to intermittent pressure, results in localised thickenings called CORNS. They generally occur on the toes—sometimes on the hands. The thickening is conical in shape, with the point pressing downwards on the true skin and so causing pain. Inflammation and suppuration may occur from misguided interference. Corns may be prevented by using sufficiently large and properly-shaped footwear. In their removal it is essential that the core should be extracted.*

Disorders of Growth.

Overgrowth of the papillary layer of the dermis produces the excrescences known as WARTS. Occasionally they disappear spontaneously, but more frequently require to be eradicated by some caustic. Exposure to X-rays is the simplest and most efficacious mode of treatment.

Loss of hair (BALDNESS —ALOPECIA) is a common senile change of almost universal prematurity. It depends upon atrophy of the hair follicles. When associated with definite scalp disease, as seborrhœa or ringworm, appropriate treatment may prevent further fallingaway of the hair. In the majority of cases the hygiene of the skin is the only palliative measure. The very multiplicity of the advertised cures is a certain sign of the incurability of this disease.

Persistent ulceration of the skin in the region

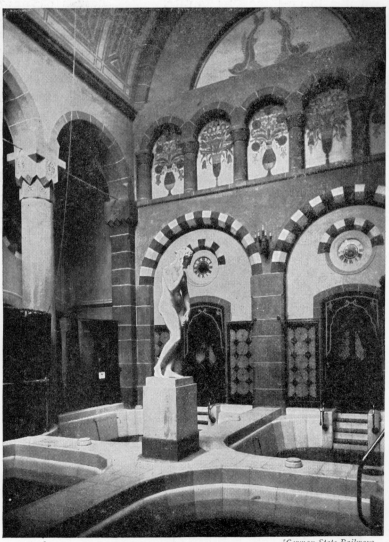

A BATH FOR SKIN DISEASES
A room in the bathing establishment at Wildbad, in the Black Forest, where many skin diseases are treated.

* See the section on The Feet.

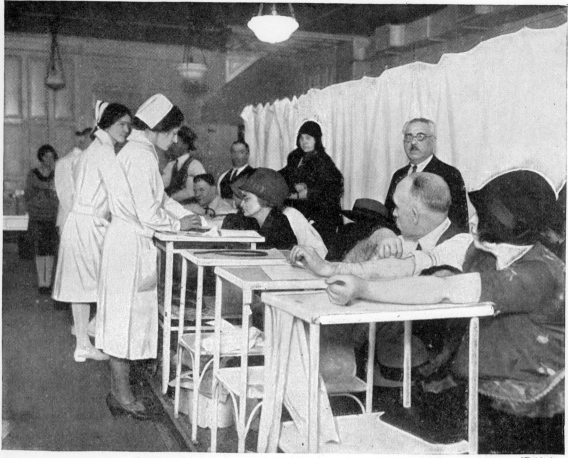

[Topical

A SKIN CLINIC IN NEW YORK
Nearly four hundred patients are often treated in one afternoon at this clinic—regarded as one of the busiest in America.

of the lips, nose, or eyes, which does not respond to simple treatment, is suggestive of malignant formations (Epithelioma : Rodent Ulcer). Treatment with antiseptics is dangerous. Excision or radium therapy are the sole curative methods. Medical advice should be sought immediately.

RODENT ULCER is a variety of cancer originating in the sweat glands or sebaceous follicles of the skin. Its seat of origin is remarkably constant, nearly always being located on the side aspect of the nose or in the neighbourhood of the lower eyelid.

Cancer of the Skin.

The disease commences as a small nodule in the skin which eventually ruptures through the epidermis and exposes a smooth raw ulcer with a well-defined " rolled " border.

The rodent cancer progresses very slowly—existing for many years—but tending to destroy every structure with which it comes in contact and producing unpleasant deformities.

In treatment, exposure to radium or X-rays results in cure in the majority of cases—with a minimum of disfigurement.

EPITHELIOMA is a variety of cancer originating from the flattened epithelium of the skin or mucous membranes. It reveals itself as a chronic indurated ulcer and frequently develops in relation to long-standing ulcers which have resulted from burns or lupus. The lymph glands are involved early in the disease and constitute a dangerous feature. Epitheliomas may arise in those who follow certain occupations, notably paraffin workers, chimney sweeps, and X-ray workers.

Epitheliomas vary in malignancy, but, as a rule, the outlook is unfavourable. Treatment is by excision, radium, or X-rays.

Diffuse inflammation of the skin is known as DERMATITIS. It is caused by various **Inflammatory Diseases.** agents—mechanical and chemical. Sunburn, heat, friction ; drugs such as belladonna, iodides and bromides are common causal factors.

Elevated dark-red spots or patches, appearing on the legs and backs of the arms, are often seen in relation to rheumatism.

ERYSIPELAS is a diffuse inflammation of the skin and subcutaneous tissue. It occurs commonly in alcoholics, diabetics, and sufferers from kidney disease. A virulent streptococcus is the causal germ.

The disease reveals itself as a spreading redness of the skin. There is considerable pain, heat and tingling in the affected part. The advancing edge is sharply marked and raised. The temperature varies with the severity of the inflammation. Erysipelas of the face is sometimes associated with delirium. Should the inflammation spread to the throat, suffocation may result from the swelling. The attack usually subsides in 7-10 days. Fatal forms occur.

A patient suffering from erysipelas requires careful nursing. It is regarded as an infectious disease and isolation is necessary. Antiseptic precautions must be employed. The strength must be maintained by a generous diet ; stimulants and tonics to be administered when occasion demands. Delirium, sleeplessness and high temperature require special treatment.

URTICARIA (NETTLE-RASH) is a diffuse redness of the skin accompanied by wheals, raised and pale in colour. It is set up by gastric disorder from the ingestion of peculiar articles of diet, e.g., shell-fish. It is attended with great irritation and itching.

The method of alleviation is to remove the cause by restricting the diet, and evacuating the bowels. Cooling lotions or dusting powder allay the skin irritation.

ECZEMA is a common skin disorder and consists of an inflammation of the true skin with the formation of papules, vesicles, or pustules. There may or may not be a watery discharge. Itching is always present. In essence the disease is the reaction of the skin to irritants, either from within or without. Intestinal intoxication is a common causal factor. Workers with irritant substances, flour, sugar, dyes, are often subject to this disease.*

This is a malady which tends to become chronic and which requires prolonged and patient treatment. The causal factor must be sought out and removed. Soothing ointments or lotions must be applied to allay the irritation. Constitutional remedies, iron or arsenic, are essential.

HERPES (SHINGLES) is an acute skin inflammation characterised by a rash of vesicles which makes its appearance over zones of the face or body. The eruption is usually preceded by stinging, neuralgic pains. At first the vesicles are full of clear fluid ; later they become turbid and in a few days they dry up and scale off. Inflammations of the respiratory organs are frequently accompanied by herpes of the lips.

When the vesicles have made their appearance, a soft sterilised dressing should be applied and the area kept dry by the use of dusting powder. The pain may be so severe as to necessitate the use of sedatives.

IMPETIGO is a skin inflammation of an infectious nature apt to occur in schools. It may assume epidemic proportions. Small pustules situated upon a reddened base appear over the face. They rapidly dry up and leave yellowish brown scabs which fall off and are a source of infection. No scarring is left subsequently. If untreated the eruption may last for months, but it rapidly disappears if treated with a dilute ammoniated mercury ointment. When nits are present in the hair treatment will be ineffective until these have been removed. The extreme contagiousness of this disorder renders it important.

BOILS (FARUNCLES) are localised inflammatory areas which commence in the hair

* See section on Occupational Diseases.

follicles. They are caused by a germ known as the staphylococcus. Aggregations of boils form an inflammatory mass called a CARBUNCLE.

Subjects exhausted by diabetes, chronic kidney disease, and chronic intestinal intoxication are very prone to this malady. The boil commences as a red pimple in connection with a hair. Eventually a vesicle forms which becomes pustular. This ruptures and discharges pus. A small slough separates and the boil heals. Owing to their infective nature and the tendency to self-inoculation, boils tend to occur in crops.

Treatment is directed to the reduction of the inflammation by the application of moist heat and of antiseptics. The pus should be evacuated by surgical means. Constitutional remedies are essential. When there is a tendency to recurrence vaccines may be employed.

Carbuncles are very exhausting and in old people may be fatal by originating a septic pneumonia.

PSORIASIS is an inflammatory involvement of the true skin attended by the formation of red patches which are covered by characteristic fine silvery scales. This is a family disease and is related to constitutional disorders. It makes its first appearance in youth and recurs throughout life. Psoriasis tends to appear at certain seasons of the year. It is not infectious. The eruption most frequently appears on the back of the elbows and the front of the knees.

The first essential of treatment is to attend to the general health. Gout or rheumatism must be appropriately remedied. Thyroid extract has been found valuable. Arsenic is given in chronic cases. Locally, tar and salicylic ointments are the chief applications. The tendency to recurrence of this disease renders it necessary to maintain therapeutic effort for considerable periods.

In relation to inflammatory diseases of the skin, it is well to remember that syphilis, tuberculosis and leprosy are productive of such lesions.

A chilblain is in some ways the opposite to a sunburn. The sun burns and browns the skin.

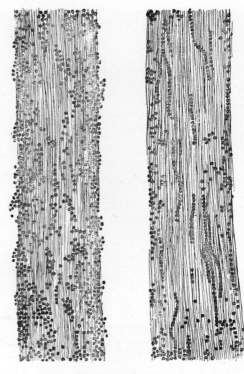

THE FUNGUS OF RINGWORM

Single hairs highly magnified to show the vegetable parasite which produces round bald patches, especially on children's scalps.

Cold first bleaches the skin and frequently reddens it subsequently by the chilblain which follows. A mild inflammation is set up in the true skin, and the well-known itching and pain attending the swelling are caused by the stretching of the nerve-ends in the swollen tissues. With chilblains the aphorism that " prevention is better than cure " holds doubly true, because prevention is as a rule not impossible. Tight gloves, tight shoes, tight stockings, all too thin for protection, should be discarded, their place being taken by articles fitted for comfort rather than appearance. Sedentary occupations should be exchanged for active ones. Warming of the chilled hands and feet at the fire is cultivating the trouble. Feeble circulation the result of heart or lung diseases, disordered digestions, certain nervous conditions, and general low vitality predispose to the development of chilblains. Excess of salt in the diet is to be avoided and also the use of alcohol. The numbers of

Chilblains.

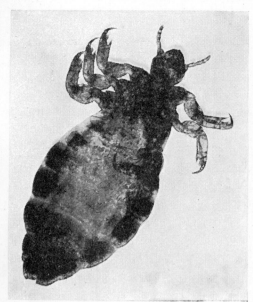

[*James's Press Agency*

THE BODY LOUSE
An enlarged view of the parasite which
thrives under dirty and insanitary conditions.

Tubercular disease of the skin, or Lupus Vulgaris, usually commences about the time of puberty. It most commonly affects the face, though the limbs and trunk may also be involved. It is about three times more frequent in females than males. The tubercle infection is probably conveyed through the mucous membranes, which may themselves be the site of disease, to the glands of the skin.

(Side note: Tuberculosis of the Skin.)

Lupus first shows itself as small nodules with a yellowish transparent appearance—described as " apple jelly nodules "—which aggregate and eventually form thickened infiltrated patches with an extending margin. As a rule there is no pain and little irritation. Destruction of the epidermis by the upward growth of the nodules is followed by ulceration. In the fully developed condition the area may be extensive : it shows an active edge with the typical nodules and the centre shows ulceration or scarring.

Lupus vulgaris runs a very chronic course ; at times stationary or even healing, at other times active and spreading. The disease may last a lifetime and much deformity may result due to the contraction of the scar tissue.

remedies suggested for the disease almost equal the numbers of the sufferers—a proof that no panacea exists. Painting the skin with collodion appears to lessen the irritation, and perhaps prevents the surface being scratched and ulceration occurring, thus converting the simple into the broken chilblain. The application of methylated spirit allays the itching for the moment but is not curative. The use of tincture of iodine is not desirable. Among the many remedies Paschki's Paint appears to deserve a place. It consists of tannic acid 30 grains, spirits of wine $1\frac{1}{2}$ drachms, collodion 6 drachms, tincture of benzoin 35 drops : to be applied twice daily with a brush. Where the yellow colour would be undesirable, as on the hands, an ointment may be used, such as chlorate of calcium 3 drachms, pure vaseline 3 ozs. This may be rubbed in frequently. Alternatively, Joseph and Veith's cold cream soap may be tried. This is put up in collapsible tubes and is rubbed into the skin until it disappears. The internal use of lactate of calcium in the form of an elixir taken two or three times a day in teaspoonful doses is said to be beneficial.

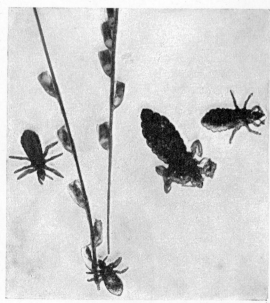

[*James's Press Agency*

HEAD LICE AND THEIR EGGS
The eggs or nits are laid on the hairs close to the
roots and, being small, are not easily detected.

In treatment attention to the general health is all-important. Ultra-violet rays, obtained through a Finsen lamp, in any of its modifications, or through a mercury vapour lamp, are extremely valuable as a means of local treatment, and produce excellent results.

LUPUS ERYTHEMATOSIS is a chronic, mildly inflammatory disease distinguished by the presence of pink patches covered with greyish-yellow scales and accompanied by fine scarring. In the face the condition assumes a characteristic butterfly or bat's wing distribution. Although microscopically no tubercle bacilli can be detected in the actual skin lesion it is the accepted opinion that the disease is associated with tuberculosis in the majority of patients.

The skin of the genitals is, in most cases, the primary site of the syphilitic infection. Syphilis of the Skin. The primary sore occurs from two to six weeks after infection, and shows itself as a small ulcer, relatively painless, and characterised by a peculiar " cartilaginous " hardness of the surrounding tissues. The neighbouring lymph glands become swollen and hard. The ulcer lasts for several weeks and then slowly heals.

In the secondary stage of syphilis, skin eruptions are prominent and constant symptoms. An evanescent measly rash widely diffused over the trunk usually appears within eight weeks of the infection and is followed by a scaly papular eruption similar to that seen in psoriasis. Later in the disease a pustular rash—acne-like—may appear, and superficial ulceration may result. The discharge tends to dry and form dark crusts resembling the shell of a limpet, and the term " rupia " is then applied. Disfiguring scars are left when the ulcers heal. Papules occurring on those parts of the body where the skin is habitually moist are called condylomata, and are characteristic of secondary syphilis. They are apt to ulcerate, and on healing leave fissure-like scars. The hair loses its gloss, becomes dry and brittle and readily falls out. The nail-folds occasionally reveal a pustular eruption and superficial ulceration.

In congenital syphilis all types of skin affection occur as in the acquired disease, but the most characteristic is the papular eruption which chiefly affects the buttocks, thighs, the genitals, and other parts which are constantly moist.

SCABIES (ITCH) is caused by a minute parasite—the acarus scabiei—which burrows Parasitic Skin Affections. into the skin between the fingers and on the wrists. Intense itching is caused, and the inevitable scratching leads to an eczematous condition. The arms, legs, and body may become secondarily infected.

Scabies is treated by the application of sulphur ointment or lotion after the skin has been softened and the burrows opened by hot baths. The clothes, bedding, and gloves must be disinfected (by heat), otherwise the mites left in them will renew the disease.

RINGWORM is caused by a vegetable parasite, a fungus, which especially attacks the scalp in children. Circular bald patches are produced. The skin becomes scaly, and the broken hairs are typical. The parasite may settle on the face and on the body. Scratching may lead to pustular inflammation and crusting. The disease is commonly spread by children using the caps, brushes, or combs of infected persons.

The disease stubbornly resists treatment. Exposure to X-rays is the most rapid and efficacious method of cure.

There are three species of ANIMAL PARASITE (PEDICULI—LICE) which vary in size and shape, and in the body area they infest. They are always associated with personal uncleanliness. The body louse really infests the under clothes, and lays its eggs there. Steam disinfection is the remedy. The head louse inhabits the scalp and lays its eggs (nits) on the hairs close to the roots. Enlargement of the glands of the neck is frequently associated. To remove the parasites the hair must be soaked with crude paraffin or oil of sassafras for three nights. The crab louse is found on the hairy parts of the body. It gives rise to great itching. It is got rid of by the application of antiseptic ointments or lotions.

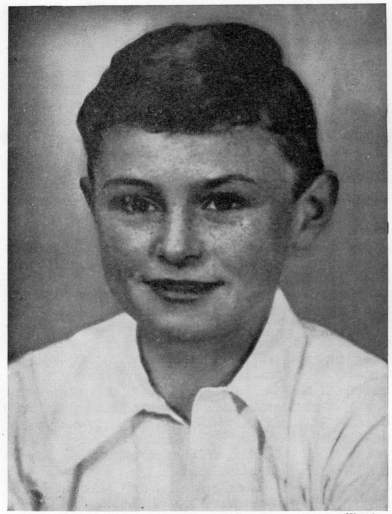

FRECKLES

[Hoppé

Showing the small brown spots, usually harmless, caused by exposure to the sun's rays.

COMMON FACIAL DISFIGUREMENTS

By W. H. HORNIBROOK, F.R.C.S., L.R.C.P., D.P.H. (Irel.), Late Medical Officer of Health to Mackenzie County, New Zealand.

FRECKLES are peculiar to the Northern white races, and are due to a localised deposition of the colouring matter in the superficial layers of the skin. This is caused by exposure to the sun's rays and is a hurried attempt by nature to provide a sunshade for the tissues underneath. They come with the summer and disappear when the leaves turn brown and fall. Occasionally they are permanent and they may by their size and colour cause real disfigurement, or blemish. Such extreme freckles are only to be dealt with by the dermatologist, any unskilled tampering with them being attended by considerable risk. The general bronzing which occurs in those who lead an open-air life is the more efficient means adopted by the body for its protection against the actinic rays of the sun, and is more marked in brunettes than in blondes. We see the greatest amount of freckles in young people of the auburn and rheumatic type, a type frequently presenting striking and attractive physical characteristics. The sudden occurrence of freckles in summer weather is often a cause of annoyance, their prevention a handicap on the freedom of the vain, who forego healthy pursuits in the attempt to evade the trifling penalty.

When freckles are numerous they are best left alone. The mere application of cosmetic washes and lotions can at best but mitigate the condition. Of all such applications perhaps Lergyel's Birch Balsam is one of the best :—

Carbonate of Potassium	-	30 grains.
Salicylate of Sodium	-	80 ,,
Pure Soap (Castile)	-	15 ,,
Mucilage of Gum Acacia	-	85 drops.
Glycerine	-	3 drachms.
Distilled Water	-	3½ ,,
Essence of Myrobalan	-	5 drops.
Oil of Neroli	-	2 ,,

This balsam is applied with a brush, or soft piece of rag, to the affected parts once daily.

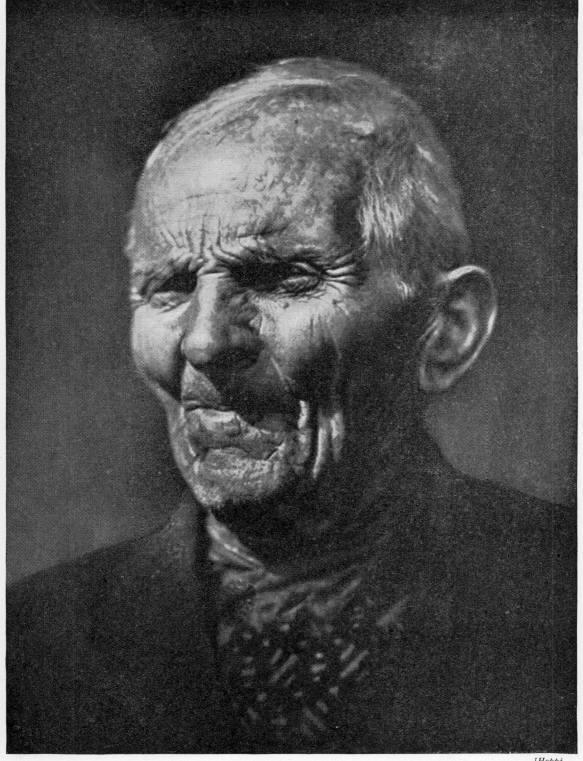

[Hoppé

THE WRINKLES OF AGE

It should be washed off in about half an hour with soft water and the skin carefully dried. Where the freckles call for removal the best means to attain that end is by cauterisation. Pure carbolic acid (the 90 per cent. carbolic acid of the chemist) is the caustic used, and is applied thus : Pare to a blunt point the end of a wooden match, dip it in the acid. Lightly touch a piece of clean blotting paper with the caustic-charged match to remove excess of the caustic. Then, exercising great care, press the blunted match point upon the freckle for a moment. It will immediately turn white, and after some time becomes reddened. This reddening is the evidence of inflammation which has been set up by the caustic, and without which removal of the living layer of skin cannot be effected. After a day or two the little patch turns yellowish brown and scaly, and then drops off, leaving a new and unstained skin in its place. Obviously such treatment is restricted in its application, and must be very carefully carried out. One point to remember particularly is that freckles on the eyelids must not be treated by this method unless by a skilled operator, because the skin of the eyelid is extremely thin, and also there is a risk of injury to the eye itself.

Cracks and slight abrasions of the lips are very common in winter, and are caused **Lip Cracks.** by the drying effect of cold easterly winds. Digestive disturbances are contributory factors, and at times the condition is the result of the unhealthiness of the mouth due to ill-kept and carious teeth. Common colds have as a usual accompaniment some soreness or stiffness of the lips, and the condition known as HERPES is almost an invariable part of a bad catarrhal cold. In this affection a sudden swelling and stiffness of part of the lip occurs which blisters, weeps and scabs, and is generally accompanied by some amount of pain. We see this lesion as part of some acute diseases such as pneumonia, typhoid, etc. Greasy applications protect the lips from weather effects to a certain extent, but most of the preparations sold by the chemist are highly coloured and perfumed. As neither the colouring matter nor the perfume contributes in any way to the virtue of the salve, their omission is desirable.

As one ages more rapidly than another, so one presents wrinkles from which the other **Wrinkles.** is free. Nothing known to science can finally arrest the processes of decay and age. Operations devised for the removal of wrinkles give but scars in place of lines. Materials pumped under the skin distend the spaces and fill the tissues with soft, shifting and unsightly tumours. Ill-temper, worry, malnutrition, the abuse of tea, coffee, alcohol and tobacco, constipation, late hours, bad general sanitation and lack of fresh air are contributing factors to early degenerative changes, which show themselves in the skin by flabbiness and wrinkling. The skin, covering that which is underneath it, participates in all the changes that take place there. Much quackery, humbug, and money have been interchanged in the vain pursuit by age of a youthful skin. Much credulity and delusion have attributed virtues to nostrums which in most cases are worse than useless. Any application that appears to lessen the depth or intensity of wrinkles depends upon its drying or astringent qualities. Paschki's Paste has earned for itself a place upon the prescription books of many, and is said to afford some measure of relief. It is made as follows :—

Sweet Almonds	-	-	-	-	1 ounce.
Bitter Almonds	-	-	-	-	110 grains.
Balsam of Peru	-	-	-	-	85 drops.
Honey	-	-	-	-	85 ,,

A piece of this about the size of a hazel-nut is rubbed up in about one quart of water. The face is then washed with the mixture.

Paschki also advises the use of a lotion :—

Salicylic Acid	-	-	-	-	45 grains.
Brandy	-	-	-	-	4 ounces.
Eau de Cologne	-	-	-	4	,,
Glycerine	-	-	-	-	1 ,,

In using this the face is first washed and the lotion then dabbed on with a soft rag. After a short interval the face is lightly dried and powdered. It must be emphasised that any measures recommended for the removal of wrinkles are at best merely palliative.

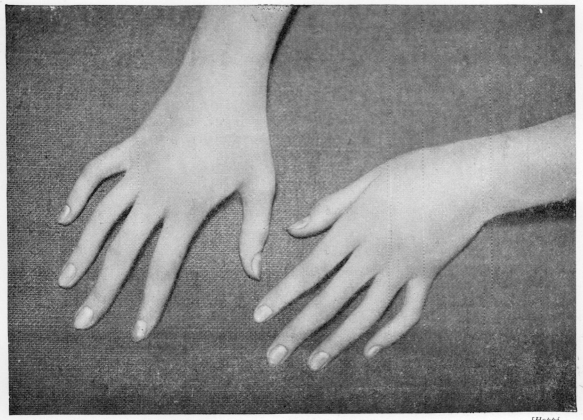

AN EXAMPLE OF MODERN MANICURING   [Hoppé

Over-manicuring is as bad for the nails as neglect. Nails should be rounded with a file and the cuticle should
not be separated from the base of the nail.

The blood vessels of the face at times become permanently enlarged causing a mottling, or reddish coloration, the depth of which depends upon age, complexion, and extent of the underlying trouble. In alcoholics of middle life this state of affairs is very marked. We are all familiar with the reddened and blotched face and the purplish and pimply nose betraying the intemperate habits of the individual. In much less degree dilatation of the facial blood vessels is seen in youthful subjects, especially females, and at times appears to have some sympathetic relationship with the menstrual function. A disfiguring disease characterised by enlarged blood vessels and occupying a definite area of both cheeks and the nose, the whole outline somewhat resembling a butterfly, is known as Lupus Erythematosis.

Mottled Complexions.

Chronic bronchitic cases frequently reveal facial congestion and in sufferers from chronic heart disease—especially the variety associated with defect of the mitral valve—mottling of the skin over the cheek-bones is characteristically present. The more frequently occurring groups of small vessels, seen especially on the cheek prominences and at the sides of the nose, are frequently the result of disordered digestion, especially constipation. The poisons developed in a loaded and sluggish bowel are absorbed into the circulation and by their continuous presence in the blood produce morbid changes, a faulty complexion being one of them. Sedentary habits, exposure to continual, strong electric light, and stooping postures are contributory causes. This latter group of cases will derive much benefit from attention to general hygienic conditions, namely, open air, exercise, attention to bowel action, avoidance of tea, coffee, alcohol, and

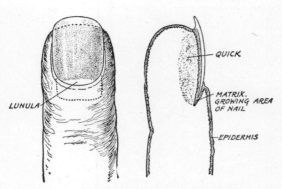

THE STRUCTURE OF THE NAIL
Showing how it springs from its bed under the folded skin at the base.

THE CARE OF THE NAILS

By W. H. HORNIBROOK, F.R.C.S., L.R.C.P., D.P.H. (Irel.), Late Medical Officer of Health to Mackenzie County, New Zealand.

THE nail springs from its bed under the folded skin at its base, and is a skin appendage in the same manner and analagous to a hair. In man it represents, in a changed and rudimentary form, the hoof of the quadruped. With many persons the care and cultivation of the nails occupy as much attention as that of the hair. Two errors prevail in connection with this. One, the over-frequent use of metallic instruments, cutters, scrapers, and polishers around the semi-lunar margin of the skin and the nail itself by the individual; the other, the too vigorous, usually quite uninstructed and far too dearly bought services of the so-called professional manicurist. The continual pressing back and paring of the skin cause minute cracks and bruising of its structure, and at the same time provide an entrance point for germs of infection; not infrequently we see whitlows as a result.

A well-trimmed and polished nail is an ornament. A somewhat casual inspection of the hands we see will convince us that the result sought is seldom attained. The shining, raised margin of skin surrounding the base of the nail and separated from it

tobacco, protection of the face from extreme climatic changes, and the adoption of a generous though simple dietary. Local measures are of secondary importance. The use of astringent washes will prove beneficial, various vinegars being both pleasant and efficacious. It is needless to state that these should be of the finest quality, and when combined with other substances their properties as cosmetic agents are enhanced. Of the following, the first may be taken as a good illustration of a suitable preparation for blonde subjects :—

(1) Camphor - - - - 180 grains.
Oil of Lavender - - - 2 drachms.
Oil of Cloves - - - 1 ,,
Oil of Rosemary - - - 1 ,,
Concentrated Acetic Acid - 8 ounces.

(2) Eau de Cologne - - - 8 ounces.
Concentrated Acetic Acid - 2 drachms.

while the second formula finds its sphere of usefulness among brunettes. Of either of these, two teaspoonfuls to two pints of pure water may be used for washing the face and hands. Water drawn from the tap frequently contains a certain amount of lime salts in solution. This lime has an antagonistic effect to the acetic acid, hence the necessity for pure water, and if the latter cannot be obtained the hard tap water should be boiled in order to precipitate the lime, subsequently decanted from its sediment and then used with the vinegar.

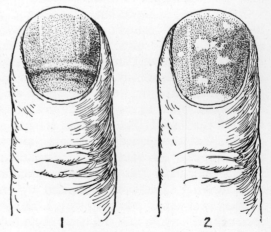

DEFECTS IN THE FINGER-NAIL
(1) Ridges across the finger-nail, caused by a severe illness. (2) White spots which are really air spaces between the cells composing the nail.

by a distinct groove presents evidence of the overdoing of the nail toilet. If a normal and unmanicured nail be examined, a thin margin of skin will be observed closely adherent to it around its base, no distinct gap was meant by nature to be maintained there. Fashion has decreed, however, that nature's pattern and design should be altered, and the result is frequently the unpleasing object that meets our view. The contour of the free end of the nail is best maintained by the judicious use of a file, and if the user will remember that the base of the nail presents a semilunar outline, and will content herself by copying nature's model, she will maintain an inverted semi-lunar outline at its free end. The pointed, claw-like weapon of offence is an eyesore.

White spots are frequently observed. These are the result of alterations in the arrangement of the cells which compose the nail, air spaces occurring between them, and so causing opacities. They appear frequently to be of familiar origin, and are possibly due to some faulty nutrition. It is not generally known that illnesses leave a record of their passing upon the nails. If the nails of a person who has suffered from a bad illness be examined within about a year from the date of its occurrence, a distinct ridge will be observable across them. We know that the hair falls off under such a condition; in a way we shed the nails also, but the process is more gradual.

The painful cracks that occur in the skin at the sides of the nails in winter-time are due to impaired blood supply consequent upon the effect of cold upon the blood vessels of the fingers. People of a rheumatic or gouty tendency are peculiarly liable to these. Avoidance of salt in the diet and the drinking of large quantities of pure water will help such people.

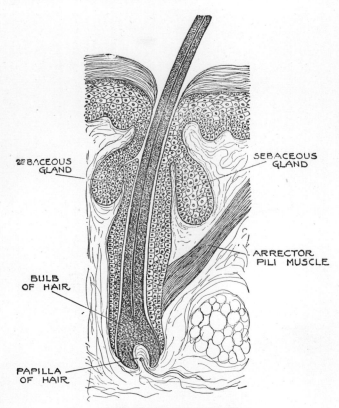

THE ROOT OF A HAIR

Hairs spring from little pits in the skin called hair follicles, and are nourished by the surrounding capillaries.

THE HAIR

By W. H. HORNIBROOK, F.R.C.S., L.R.C.P., D.P.H. (Irel.), Late Medical Officer of Health to Mackenzie County, New Zealand.

HUMAN hair is of three varieties, viz. : (1) long, as in the scalp, the beard, in the armpits and the pubes ; (2) short, as in the eyebrows, eyelashes, and limbs ; and (3) downy, or lanugo, which covers the whole body except the palms and soles.

If we examine a hair in its bed under the microscope we see that it begins as a bulb at the bottom of a little pit, called a follicle, formed by a prolongation inwards of the skin. Beyond the bulb it takes on its proper form, and terminates in a point. The bulbous end is hollow and fits closely over a little nipple of the skin which projects into the bottom of the follicle and is composed of skin cells, blood vessels and nerves. This little nipple is the true root of the hair. If

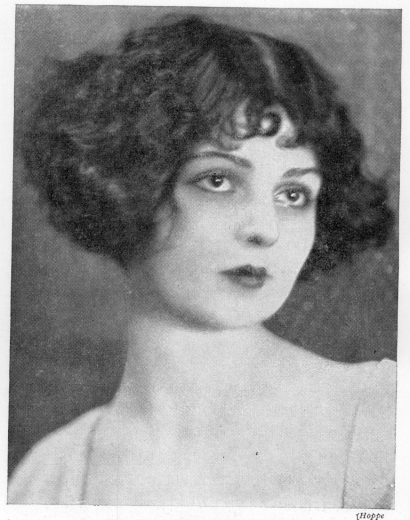

{Hoppe

THE BRUNETTE TYPE OF HAIR

Human hair varies considerably in shape and thickness. Straight hairs are round, while curly hairs are oval, and black hair is usually coarser than golden.

dition of this part depend the flexibility, elasticity, colour, and gloss of the hair. Running throughout the centre is a layer of soft cells known as the medulla ; but this is absent at times, and is never seen in downy hairs. Hairs are round, oval, and flattened on section, thus long straight hairs are round, the nigger's woolly hairs are flat, while curly hairs are oval.

Grease glands (sebaceous glands) open into the hair follicle and discharge their secretion (sebum) through that channel on to the surface of the skin. This discharge is facilitated by the compression caused by the contraction of little muscles attached to the outside of the follicle, the gland lying between the muscle and the follicle. The contraction of these muscles is strongly excited by cold or emotion. These effects are noticed in the "gooseskin" or "chicken-flesh" which results from exposure to chill, and in the "hair on end" which portrays fear and alarm.

a hair be pulled out, or is shed naturally, the bulb comes away from the nipple which in time produces a new hair. The part of the hair from the bulb to the skin surface is spoken of as the root, the remainder as the shaft.

A hair consists of cells, flat, smooth, and transparent on the outside, and overlapping in the same manner as the tiles on a roof, with their free edges upwards. These cells provide a transparent protection for the inner part, or cortex, where the cells are elongated and contain the colouring matter and oily substance. Upon the healthy con-

Hairs vary in thickness from the fine golden to coarse black and red. Of the former, 140,000 may find room on a scalp, while not more than 100,000 of the latter will be found on a similar area. The rate of growth of hair is not constant, it varies according to situation, health, climate, and individual peculiarity. The lifetime of hair is also variable, it may be a matter of months, or several years ; the long hair of women instances the latter, while the hair on the back of the hand is renewed frequently. An eyelash is said to live for about five months.

The hair has for long been an object of man's special attention. Its growth is said to be increased by cutting; this probably has some foundation in fact. The virtues attributed to pomades, washes, restorers, and lotions exist only in the advertisements of the vendors, and in the hopes of their dupes. When it is understood that hair is part of the skin, and derives its nutriment from the blood, blood that at one moment may be feeding the cells of a hair root and a few minutes afterwards is nourishing a brain cell, or absorbing food from the intestine, it will be evident that no application to the hair, or scalp, can have any renewing or strengthening action. It is well known that hair grows faster in the presence of heat, faster in summer than in winter; but it is almost equally not well known that heat in excess damages it. Sunlight is as beneficial to the hair as to the rest of the body, and on this is based the scientific use of artificial sunlight as a hair stimulant. Friction to the scalp by increasing the blood supply and loosening the underlying tissues improves the hair, and cleanliness is equally important.

The relation between the general health and Baldness. the hair is at once evident in the extreme cases where total shedding of it occurs, as in typhoid and scarlet fever, but since in lesser forms of illness this spectacular

effect is not produced the connection is not observed. Nevertheless the hair shares with the rest of the body all its departures from health, and we see in loss of lustre, thinning of the crop, and premature baldness the revolt of the hair against the poisons carried to it by the blood stream from the constipated bowel, the pus-infected tooth socket, the indolent and over-fed or the ill-nourished and overworked body, or perhaps from alcohol or chemical poisons introduced in certain trades. On the other hand, the blood may be healthy, but the quantity insufficient. The constant pressure of hard hats interferes with the nutrition of

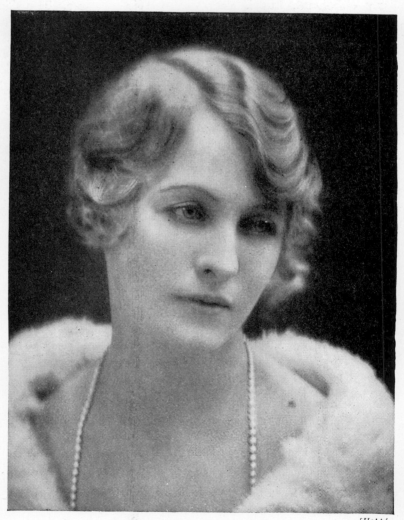

[Hoppé

THE BLONDE TYPE OF HAIR
A blonde head of hair may contain as many as 140,000 fine golden hairs —with the brunette this number would be reduced to 100,000.

the scalp, and the hair suffers. The loss of hair natural to old age has, as its forerunner, loss of colour with thinning of the individual hairs. Premature loss of hair is nearly always the result of a diseased condition of the scalp, seborrhœa. Dandruff and greasiness are the signals of its presence. In dry seborrhœa dandruff is excessive, while in the moist form of the disease greasy hat bands are the result of greasy hair.

The disease persists for years, is insidious in onset, and exceedingly difficult to cure. Generally much damage is done before it is noticed, and such baldness as has been caused is permanent. It is often seen in early childhood, but is very common in adults also. Caused by micro-organisms it is infectious, being conveyed by direct contact, by the use of infected brushes, combs, hats, towels, etc.

The treatment may be summarised in the words cleanliness and general bodily hygiene. Frequent washing of the scalp with bland, pure soap, the removal of all dead, scaly material, mild antiseptic and oily dressings, and massage. The use of the ultra-violet rays offers the best chance of cure. Attention to the general health is of the greatest importance.

A nervous type of baldness known as ALOPECIA AREATA in which sudden loss of hair in patches, or even all over the body, occurs is not uncommon. The loss may be permanent, but more frequently recovery takes place. Again baldness may be hereditary and is of course incurable.

RINGWORM of the scalp is a common infectious disease of childhood. It appears sometimes in epidemics in schools, is difficult to cure, and has a marked tendency to relapse. The X-ray is now the recognised treatment, and is very certain in its results. The bald patches caused by the disease become covered with hair on disappearance of the infection.

GREYNESS of the hair is due to absence of colouring matter and the presence of air in the cortex, the degree of greyness depending on the more or less total absence of the pigment. The condition is not curable, and may be the result of illness, worry, poisons, age, individual peculiarity, heredity and defective development (albinism). Dyeing the hair is to be deprecated ; it is dangerous, uncertain, and non-permanent.

In cases where hair growth is excessive or superfluous, the only method of permanent cure is by electrolysis. Every hair has to be treated separately. The process is tedious, painful, and apt to be followed by scarring.

THE HYGIENE OF THE BATH
By JOHN CAMPBELL, Ph.D.

THE bath and facial cleansing are most important factors in health and beauty culture. The skin is a subsidiary excretory organ and is constantly secreting perspiration even when there are no visible signs on the surface. Though mainly consisting of water, perspiration carries minute proportions of acid, salts, and other waste substances, which remain on the skin as an accumulating residue as the moisture evaporates. In addition, the outer skin is constantly shedding dead cells which are being gradually pushed up from the live lower multiplying layers.

There are also other glands which open into the hair sacs supplying an oily secretion serving as a natural dressing for the hair. These are most abundant in the scalp and under the arms, but are found generally over the whole dermic surface.

Part of this fatty secretion passes out on to the surface of the skin, mixing with the residue of sweat, the dead cells of the epidermis, air, and garment dust and particles, forming an accumulation on the cuticle, which if not periodically removed by bathing, clogs the pores, lessens the transparency of the outer integument, and may turn acid, producing considerable tenderness and irritation especially in the region of skin creases.

The equipment of the bathroom should include as essentials adequate means of ventilation without draught, a thermometer, and a cork mat. The last being a bad conductor of heat, prevents the feet from being chilled on leaving the bath.

Bathroom Equipment.

As the heat of the water cannot be properly gauged by the hands, a thermometer should be employed, the following table giving some useful data :—

Cold	-	-	-	-	33°— 65°F.
Cool	-	-	-	-	65°— 75°F.
Temperate	-	-	-	75°— 85°F.
Tepid	-	-	-	-	85°— 92°F.
Warm	-	-	-	-	92°— 98°F.
Hot	-	-	-	-	98°—112°F.

Should the heart be weak, a very hot bath is dangerous, a suitable maximum temperature being 95°F.

Should the district water be limey, the bath water should be softened by the addition of a little ammonia or bicarbonate of soda, or the use of good softening salts sold by most chemists. The latter are very refreshing, especially if they are of the variety that liberate oxygen in the water.

The kind of soap used is also of great moment. A good toilet soap is neutral in reaction, though

Soap. it probably liberates minute quantities of alkali on lathering, which help to dissolve the fatty matrix holding the accretion on the skin. But an inferior soap has usually more or less free alkali already present, which leaves the skin harsh and tender. Choose an uncoloured super-fatted soap, which while cleansing has a soothing and emollient action, leaving the skin smooth and soft.

A good transparent soap is also excellent for bathing purposes, representing a further refining process on ordinary soap, and in the case of very tender skins a glycerinated brand is to be recommended. Of late years the soaps made from vegetable oi are deservedly growing in popularity. They lather very freely, and for the most part are neutral in reaction.

Where the skin is very sensitive, the lathering process should be very short. After the cleansing action,

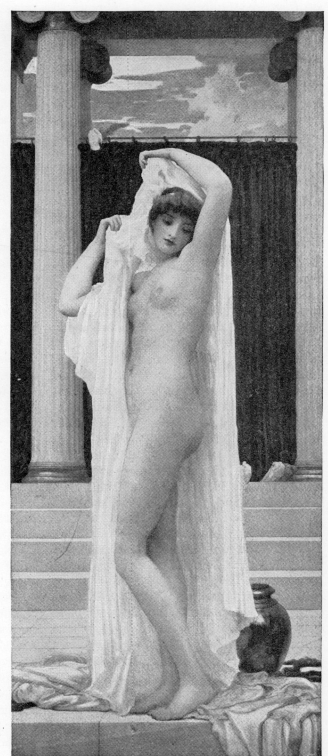

THE BATH OF PSYCHE
Lord Leighton's famous picture in the Tate Gallery.

well lave the body in order to remove all traces of lather from the skin, and gradually cool the water down to the tepid stage. This will lessen the risk of chill.

If a tepid shower bath is available that is the ideal method of finishing off a bath. Dry thoroughly but gently with a soft towel. Brisk friction after a hot bath is not necessary or desirable.

When the bath is taken merely for a restorative effect after a strenuous time, or a long journey, use only a fragrant oxygenating bath salt.

The cool, plain water bath, either ordinary or shower, is not cleansing but is very refreshing as a bracing tonic in hot weather to the skin and system to those who are vigorous enough to stand it. The sudden shock of the cold water tones up the nerves and by constricting the blood vessels stimulates the heart to more powerful action. It should be short and in this case calls for brisk rubbing and friction during drying.

After a cold bath the body should glow with a circulatory reaction. If this is not evident the cold bath has failed in its most important function. As a rule, the cold bath is perhaps best left to the young and robust and those who possess vigorous circulation.

Facial ablution calls for more care and discretion than the body bath, as it is complicated by the universal use of face creams and powders, and the effect on the skin and complexion may be disastrous if carelessly carried out with inferior or unsuitable cleansing materials.

Care of the Face.

In the first place soft water should invariably be used, and nothing is better than strained rain water if available.

Failing that, always use a softening agent as previously indicated as limey water is ruinous to the complexion.

The most important ablution is the nightly one before retiring. It is absolutely necessary, if the natural complexion is to be preserved and the formation of enlarged pores and blackheads prevented, to leave the facial and neck skin soft and free from all accretions, and in a favourable condition to perform its natural functions during the hours of sleep.

A famous French beauty specialist gives the following formula :—

First treat the face and neck with a good soft fatty cream or lanolin, using the fingers very gently for the application. Let the cream remain for a few minutes and then gently smooth off with a soft fabric. Next lave the face in warm softened water and use a superfatted or transparent soap with a soft face cloth, forming the lightest of lathers. Wash off the lather by laving with soft clean warm water and gently dry by dabbing with a soft towel. Finally apply rosewater to which a few drops of simple tincture of Benzoin has been added.

In special cases where there is a decided tendency to dryness and perhaps desquamation of the surface cells, the merest trace of a good night cream may be used after the rosewater.

This formula leaves the skin soft and in a natural condition, and cleans off the day's accumulation of waste matter, powder, and facial cream. It helps to keep the outer skin transparent, and thus allows the delicate pink tinge of the dermic blood to manifest itself, giving that radiant effect which every woman seeks.

Should facial massage be practised for any special purpose, the correct time is after the last laving with clean water, the skin and muscles being then in the best condition to benefit by the action. The next best time is in the morning as soon as is practicable after rising.

Except in special cases the use of a night cream is not only unnecessary but undesirable, for the facial skin requires this period for action and recovery, free from the clogging effect of surface artificial coverings.

In special cases where soap is found to be unsuitable, fine oatmeal may be used as a substitute in the form of a paste, or added to the washing water. In the latter case, place a tablespoonful of the oatmeal in a small muslin bag, and move to and fro in the basin, using the fingers to work the

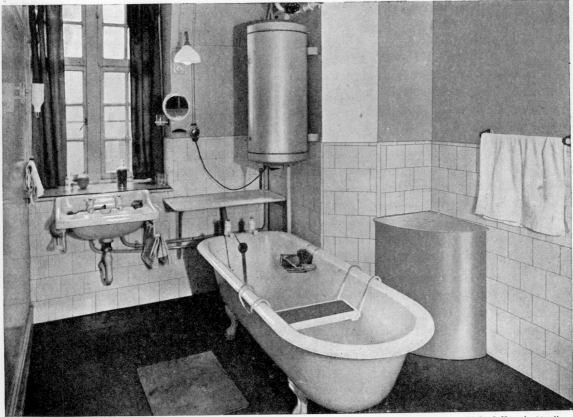

A MODERN BATHROOM

soluble contents into the water. When the latter becomes cloudy the water is ready for use.

After the use of oatmeal it may perhaps be best to finish up with a very slight application of a night cream, especially if the skin is inclined to be dry. It is not necessary to use soap more than once a day for the face, and so the morning ablution may be carried out with soft warm water only, followed by the customary toilet operations.

TOILET SOAPS FOR HEALTH AND BEAUTY

By JOHN CAMPBELL, Ph.D.

THE skin is not only a protective organ guarding the body against external infection, but is to some extent a channel for excretion of waste material. It performs also a vital function in regulating the loss of heat from the body through the secretion and subsequent evaporation of sweat from its surface.

It is thus of the utmost importance that it should be kept in such a condition that its work may be carried out freely and efficiently. When the skin is not functioning properly, health is adversely affected and the radiant glow of the facial skin which is the foundation of an attractive complexion is absent.

The main excretion of the skin is sweat, in the form of water, containing small proportions of acid and other waste material which remains in the skin in the form of a deposit as the moisture evaporates. Some of these excretory substances are volatilised by the heat of the body, giving rise to a faint characteristic odour.

Skin Excretions.

The perspiration is secreted by myriads of tiny glands which open on the surface of the skin by minute pores, and any condition which clogs these seriously interferes with the normal function.

In addition small quantities of oil from special glands which open out into the hair follicles accumulate on the skin, giving the skin surface deposit a greasy character.

The outer integument is also constantly shedding its surface coat in the form of squamous dead cells which still further increase the accretion.

Minute particles of aerial dust and dirt from contact with external substances and articles, cotton and wool fibres from the clothing, also rest on the skin surface. The tendency of these accretions is to clog the pores and to thicken the outer dermis, producing a dull lifeless tone by masking the natural tint of the skin which is partly due to the glow of the blood in the lower layer. The keynote to skin health is cleanliness without irritation. The clogging accretions must be regularly removed, without hardening the cuticle, leaving the pores open and free to act.

As the binding medium of the deposit is partly fat, water alone will not effect its thorough removal. It is necessary to have a water soluble medium which in its turn dissolves the fatty basis of the dirt, and soap fulfils this function.

Toilet soaps are known as " soda " soaps, and are very soluble in water. In a good soap, the soda or alkali is exactly neutralised by the fatty acids. This is a most important point. Uncombined soda is injurious and irritating to the skin, and the aim of the manufacturers is to produce soaps without free alkali.

Varieties of Soap.

This result can only be achieved by using the finest and best ingredients and by a strict scientific supervision and control over every stage of the process. It is false economy to buy cheap unbranded soaps. They usually contain excess of water and are more or less alkaline in character, and much harm may be done to the complexion and skin by their use. Such soaps are irritating and leave the skin dry and harsh. For toilet purposes the guaranteed branded soaps of reputable makers are best and safest.

Inferior soaps are usually unbranded and are often highly coloured and crudely scented to mask the low quality, and should never be used for toilet purposes. The best toilet soaps are " superfatted," that is to say, they contain in addition to the actual soap basis a percentage of pure neutral fat, and are delicately scented, pleasing the æsthetic sense and leaving the skin faintly fragrant. Concurrently with the cleansing process, which even in neutral soaps is accompanied with a slight dissociation of soda, the neutral fat soothes the skin and counteracts the tendency to dryness.

The transparent soaps are prepared from ordinary neutral soap by a further refining process and are most emollient and soothing even to the most sensitive skins.

Recently the vegetable fat soaps have had a great vogue. They are manufactured from palm olive oil, and dissolve into a very soft and bland lather, particularly soothing in its effect.

Glycerine soaps are most valuable for harsh and dry skins, and where there is much exposure to the air. The glycerine prevents minute cracking of the external layers and thus tones down the tendency to roughness and uneven colour.

Medicated soaps have their place in ablutions, the most common being the antiseptic brands. There are also special varieties intended for abnormal conditions of the skin. Generally they are not needed, and should only be used under medical advice. The carbolic and allied brands have, however, a certain value in counteracting surface infection and may be occasionally used as conditions arise which indicate the possibility of tactile contamination.

The choice of a shaving soap is of great importance to the mere man. The habitual use of an unsuitable kind roughens the skin and leaves it tender and sensitive. Most of the well-known shaving creams and sticks are superfatted and soft to use, but the writer has found that an ordinary cake of a high-class toilet soap is excellent for shaving purposes and minimises in a marked degree the usual unpleasant after effects of shaving.

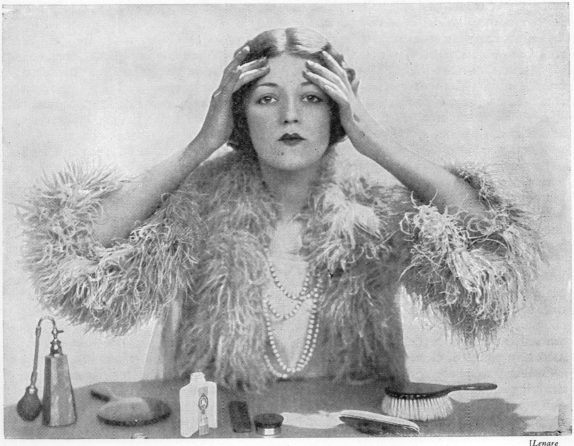

[Lenare

THE DAILY SKIN TREATMENT
Applying the day cream after carefully washing and massaging the face. For normal skins a night cream is not necessary.

Soap lathers best in soft water, and filtered rain water is excellent for the ablutions. In hard water, part of the soda soap is used to neutralise the lime which is in solution, forming an insoluble lime soap which remains suspended in the water as a fine curd. Until all the lime is so neutralised lathering is impossible. The lime curd is irritating and nullifies in some degree the cleansing and emollient action.

Soft Water Best.

This undesirable effect may be entirely obviated by softening the water in the basin before washing by the use of a little ammonia or a small teaspoonful of one of the softening powders usually sold by the chemists of the district.

Hard water can easily be distinguished by the fact that after washing there remains at the bottom and side of the basin a soapy deposit.

Facial washing requires just a little care and attention to detail. As a preliminary to the morning ablution gently lave the face in the plain softened warm water, using a very soft and fine texture cloth, sponge, or cotton wool. Next form a lather on the face sponge or cloth and gently massage the face and neck surface with circular movements. When finished lave the lather off with the basin water and finally with clean soft water.

How to Wash.

Thoroughly dry with a very soft towel, avoiding hard rubbing. The skin is now ready for the usual application of the day cream. It is most important that the face should be thoroughly cleansed at night from the stale day cream and powder, and the same procedure may be followed as outlined for the morning wash. It must be a matter for individual preference and needs whether a night cream is used. For normal skins a night cream is not necessary, indeed it may be even harmful. The writer believes that it is beneficial to the complexion and the facial skin to allow them to rest and function naturally during the night free from surface applications of any kind.

The same care should be exercised in the choice of a bath soap. It should be of the best quality and superfatted, but may be used with advantage in conjunction with one of the many excellent bath salts that are available for bathing purposes.

Where the skin is super-sensitive and ultra thin, the morning ablution with soap may be dispensed with, and the face cleansed with a gentle laving with warm soft water, followed by the use of a cleansing cream, the soiled application being removed with successive pieces of clean cotton wool.

Ordinary soaps are not well suited for the cleansing of the scalp and hair. It is best to use one of the reputable shampoo powders, carefully following the directions given in the sachet.

ACTINOTHERAPY AND SKIN DISEASE

By PERCY HALL, M.R.C.S., L.R.C.P., Honorary Actino-Therapeutist to the Mount Vernon Hospital.

ULTRA-VIOLET Radiation, or Actinotherapy, is a comparatively recent addition to the practice of dermatology, but one which has abundantly proved its value in a wide range of skin diseases. Many physiotherapeutic methods are now employed by dermatologists, including X-rays, luminous and heat rays, the gamma rays of radium, ionisation, and many forms of electro-therapy, but it may be stated that of all the available methods ultra-violet radiation is the most universally useful form, and applicable to the greatest number of different skin affections.

The technique of administration, and the particular ultra-violet wave-lengths employed, must necessarily vary according to the particular disease to be treated. Skin diseases fall roughly into groups, some being of parasitic origin, others due to infective organisms, others again being the outward manifestation of some internal constitutional disorders, and finally, some being due to disturbances of the nervous system.

The wave-lengths of ultra-violet available for therapeutic purposes vary from the long and more penetrating radiations to short rays which exert a powerful local action on the superficial layers of the skin, but have practically no penetrative power. It is essential therefore that the physics and physiological effects of the various rays to be employed be fully understood by those essaying to treat disease by this means. Several different sources of ultra-violet light are now available, each giving off ultra-violet rays, heat rays, and luminous rays in different amounts and relative proportions. They are each valuable in certain cases, according to the result desired.

Ultra-violet radiation applied to any part of the body exerts its effects initially through its action on the skin. The radiations are absorbed to a varying extent into certain layers of the skin, the depth of penetration varying in direct proportion to the length of the waves of light employed, and set up chemical effects in the tissues. The products of this chemical process are absorbed into the numerous blood vessels in the skin, carried into the general circulation of the blood, and hence throughout the body as a whole. They therefore produce effects at a considerable distance from the site of irradiation, or exposure to the ultra-violet rays. When the wave-lengths employed are of the longer and more penetrating variety, greater constitutional and slighter local effects are obtained than in the case of the short, less penetrating rays, which, on the other hand, exert profound local changes on the superficial layers of the skin, but are not absorbed to the same extent into the blood stream. The innumerable tiny nerve-endings in the skin

Effects of Radiation.

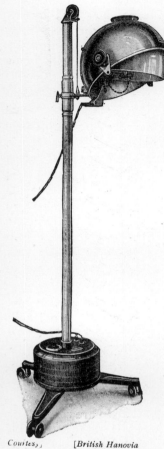

Courtesy] [British Hanovia
Quartz Lamp Co.

**A MERCURY QUARTZ
LAMP**
Designed for general irradiation as well as for the special irradiation of small areas.

are stimulated by the action of the light falling upon them, and set up nervous impulses which are transmitted through the brain and central nervous system to every organ and part of the body.

Alterations in the composition of the blood are produced by irradiation. The red corpuscles are increased in number, these being diminished in various states of ill-health, such as anæmia. Iodine, phosphorus, calcium and iron are all present in normal blood, but are diminished in amount in debilitated conditions. These essential organic salts are all increased in amount after suitable exposure to ultra-violet rays. The red colouring matter of the blood is increased in amount also. The power of the blood for dealing with infective organisms is increased after irradiation, thus enabling the body to deal more effectively with infective diseases either of the skin or elsewhere.

The internal secretory glands of the body are all stimulated by ultra-violet radiation, and these glands exert an influence upon the condition of the skin.

From the above brief description of certain of the effects of actinotherapy, it will be seen that when a local stimulation of tissue is aimed at, exposures to short, non-penetrating wave-lengths are required, a small area of skin at a time being treated. On no

account should large areas of skin be given *severe* doses simultaneously, as the products of destruction of the tissues are absorbed into the blood, and exert harmful effects upon the general health ; also the excessive stimulation of the local nerve-endings is not beneficial. In cases of extensive burns or scalds similar harmful effects may often be noted, shock, collapse, and even death possibly resulting in severe cases, or in weakly individuals. When the skin condition being treated is chiefly due to some constitutional defect or disorder, then longer wave-lengths, smaller doses over large areas of skin, are indicated. The tonic effects of the radiations will often suffice to clear up the condition, without requiring much local treatment.

Apparatus for the generation of ultra-violet rays is of three main types, viz.: carbon arc lamps, tungsten arc, and mercury vapour quartz lamps. All of these find a use in certain skin disorders, but, on the whole, the various types of quartz mercury vapour lamps are most generally employed in dermatology. These lamps give off a large proportion of the short rays, which stimulate the skin, and exert profound local effects upon it. The erythema or reddening of the skin which follows exposure to an adequate dose of ultra-violet light is most readily produced by this type of lamp.

X-rays have been used for many years in the treatment of skin disorders, and are still employed to-day. The combined effects of

Varieties of Lamps.

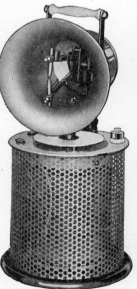

Courtesy] [*Ajax, Ltd.*

**A CARBON ARC
LAMP**
A portable lamp providing ultra-violet light for home use.

X-rays and ultra-violet will sometimes produce results which cannot be gained from either source alone. On the other hand, the dangers of X-rays are much greater than those of actinic rays, and these latter have therefore superseded them in the treatment of some obstinate and recurrent skin conditions, where the prolonged use of X-rays might be injurious.

For years the author has requested manufacturers to provide him with a modified form of Coolidge (X-ray) tube, made of quartz instead of glass, to be activated by a current so that the emission would be in the neighbourhood of one Ångström unit, the point where X-rays begin and ultra-violet rays end. It was thought that this type of radiation would be likely to be particularly beneficial in many skin disorders. Such manufacturers always stated their inability to produce this. However, such a tube has now been manufactured, and is, I believe, available from German sources. So far, its use has met with quite wonderful success.

The first disease of any kind to be treated with actinotherapy was a skin disease, Lupus. The pioneer of the science of actinotherapy was the late Niels Finsen of Copenhagen, who, after finding that lupus could be benefited and often cured by exposure to natural sunlight, devised the first lamp for the artificial production of the most beneficial solar rays. This lamp, the "Finsen Lamp," was installed in the London Hospital nearly thirty years ago, and is still used in the local treatment of lupus. It has, however, been superseded for many reasons, as the scientific basis of actinotherapy has been investigated since. Finsen believed that the good results obtained were due to local destruction of organisms at the site of irradiation, and his lamp is designed merely to treat about one inch of skin at a time, giving powerful doses which result in local destruction and death of the superficial layers of the skin. This method is slow and painful, and is now shown to be unnecessary. Indeed, with modern methods of treating the body as a whole, and relying upon the effects upon the

blood stream, lupus may be cured by exposing the rest of the body to the ultra-violet radiations, and actually covering up the diseased area! By combined local and general treatment with actinic rays, nearly all cases of lupus can be cured, even when extensive, and when other methods of treatment, including X-rays and radium, have failed.

Lupus Erythematosis, a disease of different and obscure origin, can also be successfully treated by this method.

In a very great number of skin affections some constitutional factor is at fault, and general tonic treatment in addition to local exposures is required to effect a cure. This corresponds to some extent to the older dermatological methods, when ointments were the principal method of treatment. In addition, various drugs were given for internal administration, to overcome the underlying fault. Actinotherapy is, as a rule, more successful both in its local and general effects, and has not the disadvantages of sticky greasy ointments.

Skin affections of the scalp are remarkably benefited by ultra-violet irradiation. Seborrhœa, whether localised to the scalp, or extending to the body, can be cleared up most successfully. Alopecia responds extremely well in a very large proportion of cases. When the bald areas have resisted all other methods of treatment for years, it is often possible to get an extensive growth of hair in a short space of time. When the baldness is local only, local irradiation alone is required, but when aggravated by poor general health, additional tonic body doses may require to be given. It may be stated with confidence that of all methods of treating baldness, ultra-violet radiation is the best.

Psoriasis is a troublesome condition, very apt to recur after apparent cure. The older method of X-radiation was fraught with dangers for this reason, as X-rays do not manifest any harmful results immediately, but after prolonged and repeated doses injurious effects may result years later. Ultra-violet radiation may be repeated without fear of ill results at a later date. The effects are good in a large majority of cases, either permanent benefit resulting, or at the worst, longer intervals and less extensive eruptions occurring.

URTICARIA (NETTLE RASH) can be successfully dealt with in most cases by treating the body as a whole, a constitutional defect being present. This also applies to Chilblains (Erythema Pernio), where the calcium content of the blood is deficient, and the body cannot absorb it in sufficient amounts from the blood. The ultra-violet radiation, as has been already stated, enables the body to absorb and retain additional calcium from the blood. Very rapid and lasting improvement is obtained in such cases. ACNE, IMPETIGO, and FURUNCULOSIS (BOILS) respond excellently to this treatment. A local infective eruption is present, with an underlying cause which usually requires investigation and treatment in acne and boil formation especially.

Various curious conditions of the skin where pigment is laid down irregularly and in excessive amounts can be modified and often cured by actinic rays, viz. : LEUKODERMA. This condition, although not harmful, is distressing, and the pigmented areas may often be removed or altered in character to resemble the normal surrounding skin.

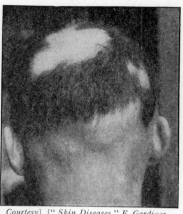

Courtesy] [" *Skin Diseases,*" *F. Gardiner*
(*E. & S. Livingstone*)

A CASE OF PATCHY BALDNESS

Alopecia, a scalp disease which benefits under treatment with ultra-violet rays.

ECZEMA of most types responds well to this treatment, and in a relatively short space of time. PRURITIS can, as a rule, be relieved, the duration of treatment varying according to the cause of the condition. It is important in all cases of skin disorders to eliminate grave inherent disease before commencing local treatment alone, otherwise failure will result. HERPES ZOSTER (SHINGLES) is a most painful condition in which the posterior nerve-roots of the spinal cord are involved. The older methods of treatment were ineffective, and chiefly directed to the symptomatic relief of pain. Ultra-violet radiations clear up this condition speedily, with disappearance of both local lesions and pain in a short space of time.

There are but few skin affections in which actinotherapy fails to give helpful results, and speaking generally, it is an inestimable boon to the dermatologists and their patients. In the treatment of X-ray burns, strikingly successful results have been obtained. These burns were till recently incurable, and progressive lesions and destruction of affected parts occurred. Suitably applied, however, is is now

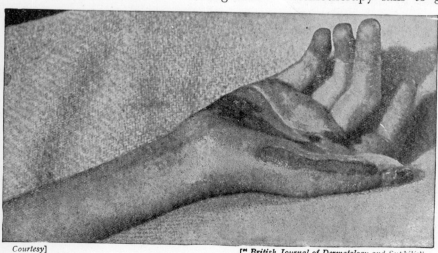

Courtesy] [" *British Journal of Dermatology and Syphilis*"

BURNT BY X-RAYS

A case of radio-dermatitis—severe burning produced by injudicious exposure to X-rays—a condition formerly considered incurable but now successfully treated with ultra-violet rays.

possible not only to arrest the progress of this condition, but actually to restore the parts to normal, by ultra-violet therapy. Keloids, excessive scar formation, and similar resistant conditions, also respond favourably.

As our knowledge of the subject increases and our technique and apparatus improve, it will no doubt be possible to achieve even more striking results in the future, but enough has been said to show that at the present time, actinotherapy holds an eminent position in the field of dermatology.

THE REPRODUCTIVE SYSTEM

THE MEANING OF SEX

By MARY G. ADAMS, M.Sc. (Cantab.), Tutor in Biology to Cambridge University Board of Extra Mural Studies.

THE nature of the sexual organs and the general organisation of the reproductive process are factors of supreme importance in evolution. For an effective method of reproduction is one of the guarantees of survival, and on the whole the high animals have specialised in efficient, economical methods. Few well-tended offspring, nourished and protected before birth, fed and taught after birth, become one of the essential conditions of life on the high levels of evolution. Man, as a mammal, is viviparous, suckles his young, and is highly sexually differentiated. Naturally attention is directed to the last of these characteristics, for the distinguishing marks of men and women have been emphasised by all the arts of civilisation.

From the crown of her head to the sole of her foot woman's body differs from man's; she buttons her dress differently, she walks, speaks, and breathes differently. The differences may be thought of as additional devices of nature for making each sex easily recognised by and more attractive to the opposite sex. Over bodily characters there can be little difference of opinion, for such differences as exist are relatively unmodified by the environment. About mental and emotional differences, however, there is no such agreement. Nevertheless, it seems fair to infer that even these more changeful and impressionable characteristics are not exempt from the general specialisation. In a general way it is true that healthy conditions of living are the same for both sexes, but it must not be forgotten that male and female will react differently to these conditions on account of their bodily differences. The optima are not the same for both sexes.

Although the sex of the young child is probably determined at conception by the

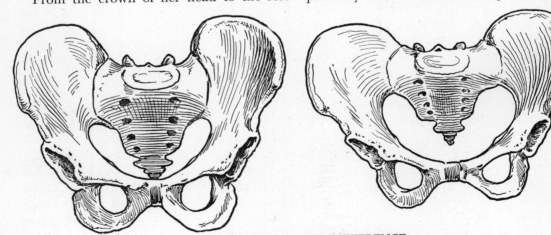

AN IMPORTANT SEX DIFFERENCE
The male pelvis (*left*) is stronger, deeper, and narrower than the female (*right*). The latter has the wider opening necessary for child-birth.

presence or absence of a chromosome, it is not possible to distinguish the sex of the embryo until practically the end of the second month of development. Before this time the basal parts of *both* sexes are present : two reproductive glands are connected with four parallel tubes passing to a common opening, the cloaca. After the sixth week the glands become either male (testicles) or female (ovaries), and throw into the blood stream appropriate hormones, which cause certain parts to grow and certain parts to atrophy. In the female the two inner ducts become the oviducts, fusing in their lower parts to form the uterus, while only vestiges of the two outer ducts remain. In the male the two outer ducts develop, the inner being reduced to vestiges. This same principle can be observed in the presence at birth of rudiments of breasts in both sexes. At a much later period female hormones seem to cause the development of breasts in the female, while male hormones appear to inhibit their growth in the male.

Differences not directly affecting the organs of reproduction themselves are known
Sex Differences.
—as secondary sexual characteristics —differences in breasts, massing of hair, and voice which frequently become manifest at puberty. There are many less obvious differences, however, which to greater or less degree distinguish male and female from birth, or even before birth. A brief survey will indicate their range and importance. Differences in the pelvis are, perhaps, fundamental. The pelvis of man is stronger, deeper, narrower in proportion to the thorax than in woman. The birth of the child clearly is conditioned by the width of the pelvic opening in woman. The shape of the pelvis gives to woman broad hips (*i.e.*, compared with man), and thigh bones set farther apart. The thigh bones are also "set" in the pelvis at a slightly wider angle than in man, and

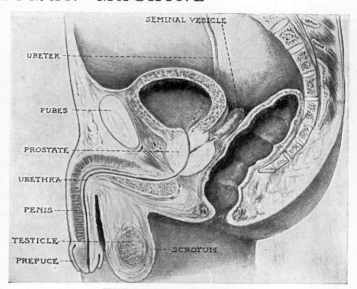

THE MALE SEX ORGANS
A diagram of the male pelvic region showing the different organs in section.

woman consequently tends to be slightly knock-kneed by nature. She also runs less able for the same reason. As well as average differences in height and weight, bodily proportions differ in the two sexes. Compared with men, women have larger, rounder heads, shorter necks, longer trunks and shorter limbs. These are child-like proportions. The rate of growth is different ; girls grow faster and mature earlier, although puberty also depends to some extent on stature and climate ; short persons mature earlier, a hot climate causes precocious puberty. Metabolism varies, men run to muscles, women to fat ; woman's blood is less dense, on account of fewer red blood corpuscles ; her pulse beats more rapidly ; she breathes more quietly, is less susceptible to some poisons (*e.g.*, carbon dioxide), and is more susceptible to others (*e.g.*, lead).

One of the most striking differences is in the thyroid gland, which is not only relatively, but absolutely greater in women. If it is the " gland of emotion," then here may be a partial explanation of woman's greater emotionalism. She is certainly more liable to other nervous manifestations—hysteria, flushing, crying, etc. It is almost impossible to estimate the nature of the mental differences between the sexes. Woman's brain is,

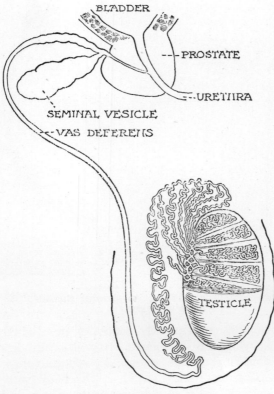

THE MALE SEX GLAND

Showing the long gland tubes, coiled up inside the testis, in which the male element of reproduction is formed.

compared with her body weight, not less than man's ; there seems to be no reason for supposing that her *innate* mental capacity is less than man's, but she has a capacity which manifests itself in different ways, and civilisation has not, on the whole, allowed for her development and self-expression. "There are no women of genius : women of genius are all men " is clearly a man-made epigram. Nevertheless, certain details stand out. Women are quicker in thought and speech, attentive to detail, perceptual rather than conceptual, deductive rather than inductive. They may resort to subterfuge to gain their ends ; hunters always complain that female animals are more cunning and difficult to trap than the male. In an uncertain realm it seems true to say that women tend to " play for safety " much more than man ; experiments, either physical, mental, or sociological, are too dangerous for the mother and nurse of the race ;

women are natural conservatives except where the interest of the race is at stake.

All these secondary and " tertiary " sexual characters are caused by the presence of the primary sexual characteristics—the sex organs and their accessories—their development is brought about by the secretion of the sex hormones produced by special tissue in ovaries and testes. This can be clearly demonstrated by removing the sex organs completely. If this operation is done before puberty none of the normal " signs " of sex develop ; if after puberty they may be altered in such a way that a " neuter " sex having some of the characteristics of male and female is produced. Moreover, if in guinea-pigs, for instance, ovaries are removed and testes successfully implanted— not only male physical characteristics but male behaviour as well are developed.

THE REPRODUCTIVE ORGANS
By W. H. HORNIBROOK, F.R.C.S., L.R.C.P., D.P.H. (Irel.), Formerly Medical Officer of Health to Mackenzie County, New Zealand.

THE male reproductive or genital organs consist of the penis, testes, seminal vesicles,
Male Sex Organs.
ejaculatory ducts, the prostate, and Cowper's glands.

The penis is composed of erectile tissue arranged in three parallel columns, two on the back whose spaces communicate with each other towards the front end, and one below which contains the urethra, and ends in an enlargement, the glans penis, which fits over the extremities of all three like a cap. This erectile tissue is made up of a fibrous network into which the arteries open, and wherein the veins have their beginnings. Two muscles attached to the back part of the penis and to the ischial bones control the return flow of the blood through the veins. When the muscles contract they compress the veins, the blood continues to be poured into the spaces through the arteries and the organ becomes erect. The skin of the penis is very thin, loose and without fat. It folds back upon itself at the end of the organ to be attached closely behind the glans. It thus forms the foreskin or prepuce. This doubled back hood, or cover, is the part removed in the rite of circumcision, a measure probably originating as a sanitary rather than a distinctive mutilation.

A certain degree of contraction, at times amounting to a slight malformation, is very common (phimosis); the prepuce in these cases is apt to become irritated owing to accumulation of its gland secretion. This is especially the case if the foreskin becomes adherent to the surface of the glans. Epileptic attacks may possibly be caused by this as well as minor disturbances of health. Circumcision can never do harm if properly performed and in after life it saves trouble. The presence of an irritating foreskin frequently sets up the evil practice of self-abuse. The penis may become affected with cancer, necessitating amputation of the organ, and it is the common site of the primary sores of venereal disease.

Testes. The testes secrete the semen which is conveyed to the seminal vesicles for storage until discharge. They also secrete a hormone which, absorbed into the blood, determines the sex characteristics, modifies the physical development and shapes the mind of the individual. The testis is from one and a half to two inches in length, an inch in breadth and rather more than an inch in thickness. It is oval in shape, and hangs freely in the scrotum (where it is separated from its fellow by a median partition) by the epididymis which is attached to its upper and back part. The surface of the testis is covered with a serous coat which also lines the scrotum. A small quantity of fluid in the cavity acts like the fluid in a joint and enables the testes to move about with great freedom. Under its serous coat the testis has a strong fibrous shell which sends parti-

tions throughout the organ, dividing it into lobules.

The gland tubes of the testis are coiled up in these places. These little tubes are of great length, and within them are formed the male element of reproduction. The gland tubes become collected into from ten to twenty ducts which pass out of the upper end of the testis and enter the epididymis where they open into a common tube. This coiled up tube forms the epididymis which, when opened out, is over twenty feet in length. At its lower extremity begins the ductus deferens which conveys the semen to the seminal vesicles situated below the prostate and under the trigone of the bladder. The semen reaches the urethra through two minute orifices in its prostatic part. The seminal vesicles are two tubular reservoirs for semen placed under the bladder and behind the prostate gland. This gland, which is about the size of a chestnut, surrounds the outlet of the bladder, the urethra passing through it. It is composed of muscle and gland tissue, and has, together with Cowper's glands which lie near it, some accessory sexual function.

Descent of Testes. Before birth the testes lie in the abdominal cavity, from whence they pass into the scrotum through clefts in the abdominal wall just above the groins. These passages are called inguinal canals. Under normal conditions the canal closes after the testis passes out of it on its way down to the scrotum, except

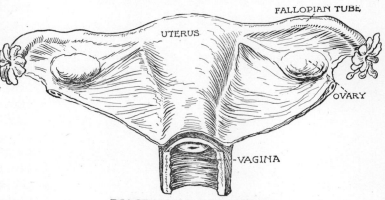

DIAGRAM OF THE WOMB

Showing the uterus or womb in relation to its connected organs.

for a small channel occupied by the spermatic cord which is made up of the duct of the testes, blood vessels, nerves, and lymphatics. It sometimes happens that one or both testes remain in the abdomen, or the organ may stick somewhere during its descent, or it may miss the scrotum and get lodged somewhere else. When both testes remain in the abdomen the individual, known as an anorchid, is sterile, though perhaps not impotent. When one organ only descends (monorchid) the person is not sterile. If a testis remain in the canal the canal cannot close behind it, and a hernia develops on top of the undescended testis. Weakness of this canal, or imperfect closure of it, is a necessary condition for the occurrence of inguinal hernia. By hernia is meant the escape of an organ, or part of an organ, from its natural cavity. Owing to the special anatomical conditions, hernia in the inguinal regions is of great frequency. A hernia extending into the scrotum is usually of sufficient size to attract attention. Occasionally when very small the person may be unaware of its existence until

strangulation or some other accident attracts attention to the part. On the other hand, persons suffering from hernia often complain of a sense of weakness and disability ; occasionally pain is present. The condition may exist from birth, or may occur at any subsequent period in life. It frequently follows upon strains, equestrians being particularly prone to it.

The external reproductive or genital organs of the female are the mons veneris, the labia majora, the labia minora, **Female Sex Organs.** and certain accessory structures.

The mons veneris is the eminence over the pubic bone which becomes covered with hair at puberty, and is composed of fatty tissue. It extends backwards on each side of the pudental cleft, or rima, as the labia majora. The outer surfaces of the labia are pigmented and covered with hair : the inner smooth and studded with grease glands. The labia minora are two folds of the skin within the labia majora which lie outside the vaginal orifice. In front they embrace the clitoris, forming a prepuce for it. The clitoris is a small erectile structure analogous to the penis. The space behind the clitoris and between the labia minora is called the vestibule, and contains the orifices of the urethra in front and the ducts of Bartholin's glands farther back. The vaginal orifice is a slit, partially closed by a membrane—the hymen—in virgins. This membrane may be of various shapes, *i.e.,* crescentic, ringlike, fringed, or even imperforate. Presence of the hymen is no proof of virginity, nor its absence the negation of it. In the rare cases where it is imperforate, the menses cannot escape, and a tumour develops which requires surgical treatment. Bartholin's glands are situated one on each side of the vaginal orifice. Occasionally their ducts become blocked, producing a small tumour, or

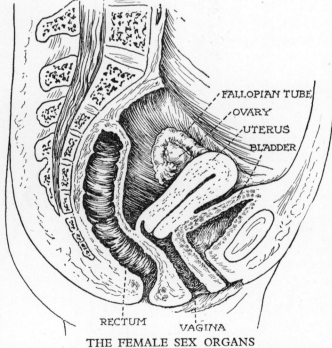

FALLOPIAN TUBE
OVARY
UTERUS
BLADDER

RECTUM   VAGINA

THE FEMALE SEX ORGANS
A diagram of the female pelvic region showing the different organs in section.

cyst, or become inflamed and produce an abscess.

The internal genital organs are within the pelvis, and consist of the vagina, the uterus, Fallopian tubes, and ovaries.

The presence of the vaginal and rectal openings in the floor of the pelvis would constitute a danger of prolapse (falling down) of the whole of the abdominal contents, were it not for the strong muscular sling stretched across the space from one point to another. This muscular floor is so arranged that the openings in it are slit-like and are maintained in a condition of closure, except when functioning, by the constant tone of the muscles. Anything which tends to weaken or lessen this support produces corresponding symptoms. General want of muscle tone, the result of ill health or sedentary habits, also causes weakness of the pelvic floor. Lacerations of the perineum at childbirth, which have not been properly repaired, weaken the floor by removing some of its support.

The vagina extends from the vestibule to the womb, to the lower end of which it is attached in such a manner that the womb appears to project into the vagina for a short distance. In front it is in close contact with the bladder and urethra, and here measures from two and a half to three inches in length. Behind it is three and a half inches long, and has intestines resting on it above, whilst below it is in contact with the rectum. It consists of a muscular and a mucous coat with a vascular layer between. The mucous coat is corrugated transversely and is provided with numerous mucous crypts.

The uterus (womb), which is freely movable in the pelvis, lies between the bladder and rectum. It is pear-

The Womb. shaped, and measures three and a half inches long, two inches wide by one inch thick ; the narrow end or neck projects into the vagina, while its upper end, or fundus, has the Fallopian tubes springing from its sides. They pass outwards to be attached loosely to the ovaries. They convey the ova from the ovaries to the womb. In close association with the tubes are two muscular cords, the round ligaments, which extend upwards to the brim of the pelvis, and pass out through the inguinal canals to the labia majora, where they end. The uterus has six other supporting ligaments composed of folds of the peritoneum. Inside, the uterus presents a flattened triangular cavity, into which the Fallopian tubes open above, and which becomes prolonged below into the cavity of the neck under the name of the cervical canal. This opens into the vagina, the opening being called the external os, to distinguish it from the constricted part (internal os), where the cervical canal joins the cavity of the body.

The womb consists of an outer, or serous coat, a middle, or muscular coat, which forms its chief bulk, and an inner, or mucous coat. The mucous coat is rich in glands and of peculiar structure. During the child-bearing period of life it undergoes certain changes which culminate in destructive hæmorrhages at the menstrual periods. On the occurrence of pregnancy it alters its character completely, and after the birth of the child, when restored to its normal condition, it usually remains quiescent until lactation has ceased. During pregnancy the womb increases in size to accommodate itself to its contents, but returns to its normal dimensions about a month after the pregnancy terminates. Owing to its movability the womb is constantly being elbowed about by its neighbours, especially by the bladder, the varying size of which necessitates an accommodating movement of the womb.

The ovaries are two glandular organs analagous to the testes. They lie close up against the bony wall of the pelvis, and are attached to the womb and the Fallopian tubes by the layer of peritoneum which covers all three. Each ovary is an inch and a half long, three-quarters of an inch wide, and three-eighths of an inch thick. Their function is to produce the ova, the cells which, when fertilised by the male cells (spermatozoa), develop into the fœtus. They also supply a hormone to the blood which has similar developmental and regulating qualities to that produced in the testis.

The mammæ or breasts are accessory glands of the reproductive system whose **The Mammary Gland.** function is to provide food for the infant. The mammary gland is present in both sexes, but is rudimentary in males. The glands increase in size at the onset of puberty and wither in age. The right mamma is usually a little smaller than the left. The gland consists of bundles of lobules embedded in fat and fibrous tissue. The ducts unite to form fifteen to twenty main ducts, which open on to the nipple. This is situated in the centre of an area called the areola. In virgins it is pink, but begins to darken and enlarge in the second month of pregnancy. In brunettes it is darker than in blondes, and during pregnancy it may become almost black, but reverts to a paler hue after lactation ceases.*

* For Diseases of the Female Reproductive Organs, see " Woman and Her Health."

DISEASES OF THE REPRODUCTIVE SYSTEM

By GEORGE SOMERVILLE, M.D., D.P.M., Deputy Medical Superintendent at the West Ham Mental Hospital.

THE VENEREAL DISEASES

IN the category of the Venereal Diseases are included syphilis, gonorrhœa and the soft sore or chancroid. They are so called because for the most part they are acquired during the congress of the sexes.

Syphilis is a specific constitutional infectious disease caused by an organism, the **Syphilis.** treponema pallidum or the spirochæta pallida. Strictly speaking, it is not a disease of the reproductive organs *per se*, but as its presence and spread are chiefly related to the sexual function it is conveniently dealt with in this section.

It is generally believed that syphilis was unknown in the Old World before the year 1493, when it was introduced into Spain by Columbus's crew, who had been infected in Haiti. To-day syphilis is widespread throughout the whole world—particularly the civilised portions—and its ravages account for a tremendous amount of human sickness and suffering. Its prevention is one of the most pressing of all social problems.

When syphilis is communicated from one person to another by direct contact, it is spoken of as " acquired syphilis." Those who have thus acquired the disease may then transmit it to their children, who are described as suffering from " congenital syphilis." Acquired syphilis may originate venereally, *i.e.* during sexual intercourse when easily abraded surfaces are brought into contact, or it may arise accidentally in those who are in close contact with syphilitics, viz., doctors, nurses, or members of the family. A diseased wet nurse may infect a healthy child, and vice versa a diseased child may infect a healthy wet nurse. The infection may be conveyed indirectly through the medium of articles contaminated by a syphilitic, such, for example, as smoking pipes, wind musical instruments, table utensils, towels or clothing. These extra-genital sources of infection must never be lost sight of, for there is a danger of a failure to recognise the initial sore of syphilis should it appear in such unusual situations as the finger, lip, or nipple.

The interval between the infection and the appearance of the primary sore or chancre, *i.e.*, the incubation period, varies between two to six weeks—the average being twenty-one to twenty-eight days.

The course of the disease is conveniently divided into three stages.

The primary stage is characterised by the appearance, at the site of inoculation, of the **Primary Syphilis.** primary sore or hard chancre. It commences as a painless, small red papule; enlarges to the size of a pea, and then ulcerates. The ulcer has sharply cut edges with a hard base and on palpation feels like a nodule of cartilage. It exudes a scanty discharge. As a rule there is little pain or discomfort, and the

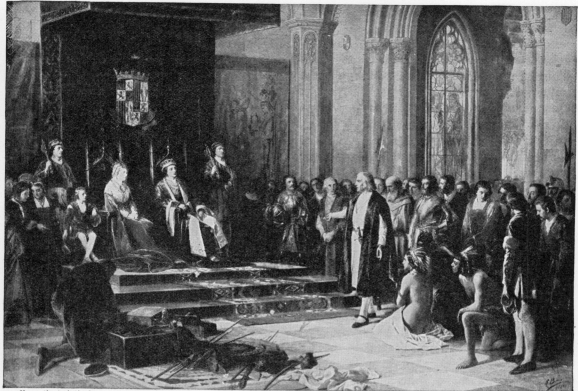

From the painting]
[By R. Balaca

THE TRIUMPH OF CHRISTOPHER COLUMBUS

" It is generally believed that syphilis was unknown in the Old World before the year 1493, when it was introduced into Spain by Columbus's crew, who had been infected in Haiti."

sufferer may be unaware of its presence. The commonest sites of the lesion in the male are the inner aspect of the foreskin, and the glans, while in the female the labia are the chief sites. About the same time as the appearance of the sore, the lymph glands in the groin become enlarged and " shotty." If there is superadded septic infection they may suppurate and discharge through the broken skin. Should the sore be situated within the sac of a prepuce which cannot be retracted, it is described as a " concealed chancre," and, as it is impossible for the infected person to keep the parts clean, septic inflammation arises and there is a copious discharge of pus.

With the onset of constitutional symptoms, six to twelve weeks after infection, syphilis enters its secondary stage. The
Secondary Syphilis. manifestations are a sequel to the entrance of the syphilitic poison into the general circulation. As a rule the general health is disturbed. The patient becomes feverish, anæmic, and complains of lassitude and headache. Skin affections are a constant feature of this stage. The rash of syphilis is very mixed—consisting of rose-coloured spots, papules and pustules : it is roughly symmetrically disposed over the body : it does not itch, and as it fades it tends to leave behind brownish stains. Where the skin is moist, raised thickened patches appear which have a highly infective discharge and are called " condylomata." The hair loses its natural gloss ; becomes dry and brittle and readily falls out. The nails also tend to become brittle—and often show ulceration at the nail fold. Changes occur in the mucous membranes, particularly of the throat : the tonsils and soft palate show mucous patches and there may be a number of small, superficial " snail track " ulcers. Wandering pains in the bones—worst at night—are sometimes complained of, and these originate from an evanescent perio-stitis. Iritis may occur in one or both eyes,

in which case the sufferer complains of impairment of sight, frontal pain, undue sensitiveness of the eyes to light, and discoloration of the iris. In such cases immediate treatment is imperative or permanent impairment or loss of sight will result. Occasionally a painless synovitis may arise in the knee joints ; more rarely, an acute inflammation of the spinal cord —myelitis—may lead to a sudden muscular paralysis.

The diagnosis of secondary syphilis can nowadays be established with certainty by means of the " Wassermann Reaction." A positive reaction is usually obtained between the fifteenth and thirtieth day after the appearance of the primary chancre, and during the secondary stage the reaction is always positive—as is the case in the tertiary stage unless the course of the disease is modified by treatment. In the post-syphilitic affections—general paralysis and locomotor ataxy—the reaction is positive in nearly every case, and in inherited syphilis a " positive Wassermann " is always to be obtained. A positive reaction indicates spirochætal activity and repeated testing gives a valuable means of estimating the efficacy of treatment—the object of which is

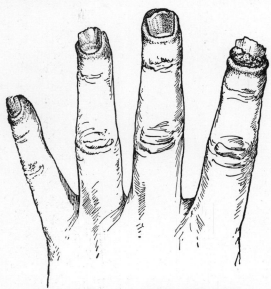

HOW SYPHILIS AFFECTS THE NAILS
Brittle finger-nails with ulcers around their base are common symptoms of syphilis in its secondary stage.

to alter a persistently positive reaction to a permanently negative one.

The secondary symptoms persist for varying periods, depending largely upon treatment, and may be followed in certain cases by the tertiary manifestations. The onset of tertiary symptoms is usually within two to ten years after infection, but they may appear within six months, and there is no absolute upper limit. They are particularly liable to arise in those who have had their powers of resistance lowered by privation, alcoholic excesses, or tropical disease.

Tertiary Syphilis.

The general nature of tertiary syphilis is a chronic inflammation which affects cellular tissue, bones, muscles, or organs. Granulation tissue arises and forms a tumour-like mass which, from its peculiar elastic consistence, is known as a " gumma." In the early stages, the gumma is a firm greyish-red localised mass of tissue, but later it becomes yellow and with a tendency to soften and liquefy. If treatment is instituted before destructive changes arise, gummata are remarkably quickly dispersed.

No tissue or organ is immune to gummatous disease, but the skin, mucous membranes, muscles, and bones are peculiarly susceptible. A firm, painless swelling develops rapidly, softens, ruptures, discharges its contents, and an ulcer results. Tertiary ulcers—often multiple—are most frequently met with in the leg, especially in the region of the knee : their edges have a punched-out appearance and their bases are occupied with granulation tissue which discharges thick purulent matter. When the ulcers heal, they leave behind a round oval depressed scar which is often pigmented. Gummata or gummatous infiltrations occurring in the tongue, nose, and larynx are very apt to lead to the formation of ulcers which are highly destructive and which, in such situations as the larynx, may prove dangerous to life. The tertiary manifestations of syphilis occurring in the bones, joints, muscles, and the various internal organs have been described under the diseases of the appropriate systems as also the part played by syphilis in the production of cardio-vascular and nervous disease.

Inherited Syphilis. Congenital syphilis is likely to arise in children according to the recency of the parental disease: thus in secondary syphilis the infection is transmitted with almost absolute certainty. The mode of transmission is not definitely known, but in the case of the syphilitic mother, infection is probably transmitted through the placental circulation, while in the case of the syphilitic father, the infection is thought to be conveyed in the seminal fluid to the ovum at the time of conception.

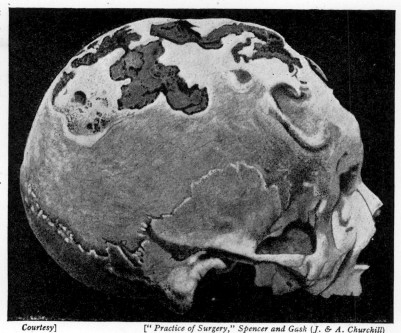

Courtesy]   [" *Practice of Surgery," Spencer and Gask (J. & A. Churchill)*

SYPHILITIC DISEASE OF THE SKULL
Syphilitic necrosis of the skull, in which the bone is eaten away in patches by the disease.

In congenital syphilis, the disease is generalised from the beginning. Spirochætes are found in enormous numbers in practically all the internal organs. In many cases the developing child dies within the womb so that miscarriage results. As the virus tends to become attenuated, should further pregnancies ensue, the date of miscarriage becomes later, until eventually a full-time but still-born child arrives, or it may be born alive and exhibit syphilitic manifestations.

Where the symptoms are obvious at birth, the child is emaciated and feeble; shows bulbous skin eruptions and has an enlarged liver and spleen. Death occurs in a few days. On the other hand, the child may appear healthy at birth, but in a few weeks manifests characteristic symptoms. The child ceases to thrive, becomes emaciated and sallow, and suffers from eruptions on the skin and mucous membranes. "Snuffles" —a syphilitic rhinitis—makes its appearance, giving rise to a contagious discharge. Destruction of the nasal bones results and later leads to the characteristic "saddle-nose"

deformity. Enlargement of the liver may be associated with jaundice. Inflammation of the growing ends of the long bones— syphilitic epiphysitis—may arise and be confused with rickets. Joint swellings are common. The bones of the skull may become thin and soft—" craniotabes "—or there may be " bossing "—a heaping up of new spongy bone beneath the pericranium.

Should the child survive, symptoms show up later during the second dentition or at puberty. Affections of the eyes—interstitial keratitis, iritis and choroiditis*—are frequently observed. Permanent. bilateral deafness of labyrinthine origin sets in in a limited number of cases. Changes occur in the permanent teeth: the upper central incisors become peg-shaped and present a deep semi-lunar notch at their cutting margin (Hutchinson's Teeth). Gummata, though not common, may occur as in acquired syphilis. Juvenile general paralysis may arise about the age of sixteen years, but this condition is fortunately rare.

* See section on The Human Eye.

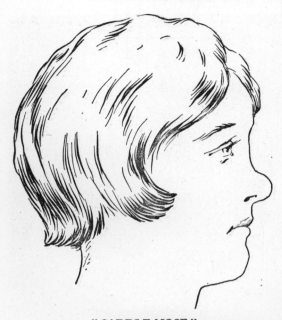

"SADDLE-NOSE"

A deformity showing an extreme snub-nose, which is due to inherited syphilis.

The treatment of syphilis must be commenced immediately, but not before the diagnosis has been established by the demonstration of the spirochæte or by a positive Wassermann reaction. The object of treatment is to maintain the general health at a very high level and to introduce into the circulation agents which will destroy the invading parasite. The latter is accomplished by injections into the blood stream of certain arsenobenzol preparations (originally elaborated by Ehrlich) such as salvarsan or "606," neo salvarsan or "914," kharsivan, or novarsenobillon.

Treatment of Syphilis.

Mercury, the drug originally used in the treatment of syphilis, is used to supplement the arsenical injections, but its administration requires to be carefully controlled according to the idiosyncrasies of the patient. Arsenical injections cause the outward manifestations of the disease to disappear with remarkable rapidity—within weeks—with the unfortunate result that frequently the sufferer imagines he is cured and neglects to continue treatment. Here lies a great danger, for the spirochætes have not been completely eradicated : they are merely quiescent and sooner or later the disease will renew its activity and make rapid progress. It cannot be too strongly emphasised that treatment of syphilis must be maintained *under expert guidance for at least two years* : even then the word "cure" can only be pronounced by the expert after the performance of certain clinical and laboratory tests.

If syphilis is radically treated, tertiary symptoms should never arise. Their frequency to-day, however, is evidence that complete cure is not attained in many cases.

Only the general scheme of treatment has been described here : all details have been avoided. We strongly insist that the person infected or who suspects infection should *immediately* seek expert advice and guidance.

The soft sore, soft chancre, or chancroid, is a common form of venereal disease which is caused by a virulent pus-forming organism called Ducrey's bacillus. Soft sores are contracted by direct contact. The incubation period varies from two to five days. The sores originate as pustules which soon develop into painful ulcers with sharply cut margins, bleeding readily and causing a copious yellow purulent discharge. Infection of the glands of the groin (bubo formation) follows in most cases and suppuration may result. The soft sore yields rapidly to antiseptic treatment. Eusol is particularly useful in such cases. If the sore is concealed under a tight prepuce incision becomes necessary in order to gain access. Painful glands in the groin may be alleviated by ichthyol and glycerine fomentations.

The Soft Sore.

Although, by itself, the soft sore is a comparatively minor ailment, the possibility that it may be combined with and mask syphilitic infection renders it important from a diagnostic point of view.

Gonorrhœa is an acute infection caused by a micro-organism—the gonococcus—and it is practically always contracted during sexual intercourse. Occasionally, however, it may result—especially in women and children—from contact with linen, towels, sponges, etc., which have been

Gonorrhœa.

contaminated with gonorrhœal pus. After an incubation period varying from three to five days, a feeling of heat and itching is experienced about the opening of the urethra : there is smarting on passing urine and a discharge—at first mucous but later purulent—appears. As the inflammation extends up the urethra, the discharge becomes abundant and consists of thick, greenish pus : there is severe pain on passing water and painful erections disturb the sleep. The acute phase of the disease lasts about ten days and then it gradually abates : the discharge from the urethra persists for about five to eight weeks after infection, but towards the end of this time it becomes thin, watery, and intermittent. Finally it ceases entirely, or it may remain indefinitely as a mucoid discharge known as "gleet." The diagnosis of gonorrhœa is rendered definite by the microscopic demonstration of gonococci in pus from the urethral discharge.

The treatment of gonorrhœa requires expert direction. Gonorrhœa is not a trivial disease and self treatment is highly dangerous. Also it should be remembered that the discharge is *highly infective* and there is danger of conveying the infection to the eye where it may set up a dangerous inflammation. Therefore great care should be taken in carrying out antiseptic precautions, and all contaminated dressings should be burned at once.

The principle of local treatment is to wash out the urethra with antiseptic solutions, *i.e.*, permanganate of potash, or silver salts, by means of an irrigating apparatus or a large glass syringe. In general treatment, the patient should be confined to bed for the first ten days. Large quantities of diluent fluid should be taken and the diet should consist of milk and light foods. The bowels should be kept well open by means of saline laxatives.

Gonorrhœal affections of the seminal vesicles, prostate, epididymis, bladder and inguinal glands may arise at any time during the course of the disease but are most liable to complicate the acute phase.* Acute blood-

Complications.

* See Diseases of Individual Organs.

poisoning, or septicæmia associated with endocarditis is an occasional complication. Gonorrhœal rheumatism and involvement of the joints and tendons are of fairly common occurrence and are difficult to eradicate.*
GLEET is a sequel rather than a complication of gonorrhœa. The discharge is scanty and is chiefly observed in the morning. It tends to occur mostly in neurotic individuals and it may be associated with various neurasthenic symptoms. Its treatment is difficult : the general health should be improved and, as some prostatic catarrh is frequently present, massage of the prostate is of some value.

STRICTURE of the urethra is one of the commonest and most important complications. It is due to contraction of the scar tissue which may follow a severe and persistent urethritis, along with superadded congestion and spasm. The stricture is generally situated at that portion of the urethra called the " bulb." Gradual difficulty is experienced in passing urine : the stream is found to be smaller in size and less forcible and straining is found to be necessary. Exposure to cold or indulgence in alcohol aggravates these symptoms owing to the induction of congestion and spasm, and may lead to retention of urine—a serious

* See Diseases of the Locomotory System.

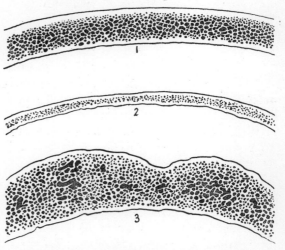

DEGENERATION OF THE SKULL BONE
(1) A normal skull bone in section ; (2) the bone in a case of craniotabes ; and (3) with " bossing " —two degenerative changes due to syphilis.

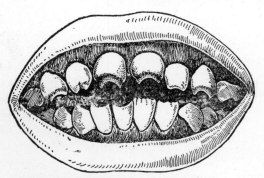

" HUTCHINSON'S TEETH "
A result of inherited syphilis—some of the permanent teeth become notched and peg-shaped.

condition which requires immediate attention : a hot bath may relieve but catheterisation or bladder puncture is often necessary. Other complications which may arise in connection with stricture are peri-urethral cellulitis and abscesses, extravasation of urine and urethral fistulæ : all these conditions call for immediate surgical treatment. In uncomplicated cases strictures are treated by the method of intermittent dilatation, which consists in the passage of bougies into the urethra at intervals of two or three days. Even when the urethra is fully dilated it is necessary for this operation to be performed at intervals which, however, can be gradually lengthened until once a year may suffice. The sufferer should carefully avoid exposure to cold : alcohol should be abstained from, but Vichy or Contrexéville waters should be freely taken.*

Venereal diseases take a foremost place in the category of preventable diseases. They are an almost inevitable concomitant of sexual promiscuity unless means of self-disinfection are adopted whenever the risk of infection is taken.

Prevention.

Within the first few hours after exposure to gonococcal infection the organisms can be exterminated and the disease prevented by washing the glans penis with spirit, irrigating the urethra with a 1 in 3000 solution of potassium permanganate and instilling a 2 per cent. solution of argyrol which should be retained for twenty minutes. Thorough inunction of the penis and urethral orifice

* For Gonorrhœa in Women, see " Woman and Her Health."

with calomel cream or ointment is a preventive measure against syphilis. Should these methods be unemployable, then ordinary cleanliness, with the plentiful use of soap and water *may* prevent infection. Finally, on the first suspicion of disease, expert advice should be sought immediately. In no other disease are such beneficial results of early treatment observable as in the case of venereal disease.

DISEASES OF THE SCROTUM AND TESTES

The scrotum is liable to become the seat of acute inflammation (cellulitis) as a result of extravasation or escape of urine following stricture or rupture of the urethra. The inflammation may spread to the penis and the abdomen. Sloughing is apt to ensue and lead to involvement of the testes. In treatment, the pelvis should be raised and ichthyol fomentations applied. If improvement does not rapidly follow, incision becomes necessary. In patients who suffer from incontinence of urine, an eczema may be induced by the dribbling urine, and in chimney-sweepers and paraffin workers a chronic eczema is fairly common. This latter condition is important, for it may be the starting point of a cancer or epithelioma. The disease commences as a scaly patch or wart on the skin and progresses slowly over a number of years until it ulcerates. Attention to personal cleanliness prevents this affection ; when fully developed, treatment is by excision.

The testes are subject to abnormalities in their development—especially in their transit from the abdomen to the scrotum.* Any portion of the spermatic tract—testes, epididymis, ductus deferens, or seminal vesicles—may become involved by the inflammatory process which, when acute, most commonly arises from gonococcal infection and, when chronic, from tubercular or syphilitic infections.

Acute Epididymitis is most frequently met with during the second or third week of gonorrhœal infection. It is caused by a

* See section on Congenital Deformities.

direct spread of the gonococci from the urethra by way of the ductus deferens. The attack commences with swelling and tenderness of the spermatic cord ; the scrotum becomes red and œdematous, and involvement of the epididym is revealed by the presence of a C-shaped swelling behind the body of the testis. There is fever and malaise : the pain is severe and constant. The inflammation reaches its highest in from four to six days and then gradually subsides. As a rule there are no serious after effects, but, should the ductus deferens become occluded, sterility results.

Acute Epididymitis.

In treatment, the patient should be confined to bed with the scrotum supported by a pillow. Fomentations of ichthyol should be frequently applied. A purge of calomel followed by a saline is advisable. During the acute stage all local treatment of the gonorrhœa should be suspended. When the acute inflammation has subsided, oleate of mercury ointment should be well rubbed into the affected part in order to disperse any induration.

Orchitis, or inflammation of the testis, is liable to complicate the course of certain infectious fevers—notably mumps, scarlet fever, and enteric. It may also arise during the course of gout and chronic rheumatism. Most characteristic is orchitis complicating mumps. It is met with chiefly in young men and shows itself towards the end of the first week of the parotitis. The testicle—usually only one side is affected—becomes suddenly swollen, firm, tense, painful and exceedingly tender. The condition may be associated with a slight muco-purulent discharge from the urethra. The inflammation remains for about four or five days and then gradually abates. Atrophy of the testis may follow, and should both organs be involved, then sterility results. The orchitis which occurs during the course of the other infectious diseases is similar but as a rule is not so severe and may be overlooked. In gouty subjects an inflammation of the testes often manifests itself just before the onset of one

Acute Orchitis.

of the regular attacks. Treatment is the same as that indicated for acute epididymitis.

Tuberculosis of the testis may be a first manifestation of the disease, but, in the majority of cases, it follows pulmonary phthisis or other tubercular affections. The disease usually commences in the epididymis of one testis : small tubercular nodules develop, increase in size and run together until the whole epididymis is involved. Subsequently the disease spreads to the body of the testis, and, unless the active process is arrested, ultimately destroys the organ. Other parts of the genito-urinary system may be invaded, or generalised tuberculosis may ensue.

Tuberculosis.

The onset of the condition is usually between the ages of 20 and 30. As a rule there are no marked constitutional symptoms. Should the prostate be involved, there is pain with micturition of increased frequency.

In the very early stages the disease may be successfully arrested by the usual methods adopted to combat tuberculosis. If the condition is advanced, the question of adopting operative measures arises. Abscesses may require to be evacuated or it may be deemed advisable to remove the whole organ. Modern practice, however, tends towards conservative methods as opposed to extirpation.

Syphilitic disease of the testis may occur during the tertiary stage—as a rule some years after the primary infection. There may be a diffuse involvement of the body of the organ, or the disease may be localised in small nodules or gummata. The body of the testis slowly and painlessly becomes enlarged until it may reach twice its natural size. On palpating the organ, it feels hard and has a characteristically " wooden " consistence. There is no tenderness. In the later stages the syphilitic tissue may break down, invading the skin and causing ulceration with discharge.

Syphilis.

Anti-syphilitic treatment will rapidly alleviate the condition and the testis regains its function. If ulceration has resulted, then mercurial lotions should be applied.

It is to be noted that the testis may be a site of disease in the inherited form of syphilis.

Tumours of the testis are important because almost without exception they are **Tumours.** of a malignant type and also they may arise at any age—even in children. Embryonic tumours, cancers and sarcomata are the most common varieties of new-growth found in the testis. Swelling of the organ is the first sign, and it is usually accompanied by a dragging sensation. The testis slowly enlarges—frequently to three or four times its natural size—and in the later stages becomes irregular in shape and varying in consistence. The skin of the scrotum, at first free, is eventually invaded by the growth, and a fungating ulcer arises. Lymph gland involvement takes place early —and rapid dissemination leads to secondary growths in the lungs, skin, and other organs. The outlook is thus grave owing to the rapidity with which the disease becomes generalised. Treatment is by radical surgical excision.

Neuralgia of the testis is a condition occurring in adolescents—usually of neurotic **Neuralgia.** disposition, in which recurrent attacks of paroxysmal pain are experienced in the region of the testis. It is often associated with local trouble such as inflammation of the testis or ductus deferens, irritation of the prostatic urethra or neck of the bladder, kidney stone, anal fissure, or persistent constipation; frequently, however, the origin is quite obscure. In treatment it is essential that the possible cause should be sought out and remedied. Every effort should be made to improve the general health. Warm fomentations are helpful during the actual attacks, and in the intervals a suspensory bandage should be worn.

Hydrocele is the term applied to describe a collection of fluid within the serous sac which envelops the testis (tunica **Hydrocele.** vaginalis). In inflammatory affections of the testis or epididymis, some exudation of fluid is usual—the so-called "acute hydrocele," but the commonest variety is that known as the "chronic hydrocele." In this condition the cause is obscure, although occasionally it is related to some injury, and, in the majority of cases, the testis remains healthy.

The affection comes on insidiously in middle-aged men and shows itself as a smooth, uniform, and pear-shaped swelling —tense and elastic in consistence. No pain is felt, but the weight of the fluid causes a dragging sensation. Most often only one side is involved, but sometimes it is bilateral.

It is an unsightly and inconvenient condition and calls for surgical treatment. This consists of the simple operation of "tapping"; a fine trocar and cannula are introduced and the fluid withdrawn; a pad of wool is applied over the scrotum and pressure kept up by means of a bandage. This operation is seldom curative and requires continued repetition.

A congenital form of hydrocele is met with in children and is often associated with the presence of a hernia or rupture. It presents similar features to the adult condition except that the fluid can be slowly pressed back into the peritoneal cavity when the patient is recumbent. The treatment is surgical— the same operation as for congenital hernia being performed.

Varicocele is the term applied to a varicose condition of the veins of the spermatic cord. **Varicocele.** It results from factors which are operative in producing this condition in other parts of the body. Deficiency of the valves and weakness of the walls of the veins are probably the fundamental causes, but habitual constipation, liver trouble and malignant disease of the kidney are believed sometimes to act as contributory causes. As a result the veins become dilated, elongated, twisted and thickened.

Varicocele is a disease of adolescence : it tends to disappear with manhood. Frequently it remains undetected until some medical examination for insurance or entry into the services reveals its presence. Examination shows the scrotum to be lax and pendulous and on palpation a soft mass of distended veins is found to occupy the scrotum. The dark blue vessels are usually rendered visible when the skin is stretched, but on lying down the veins slowly empty and the swelling practically disappears. The health of the testis is not impaired to any obvious degree and the affection seldom gives rise to any trouble apart from a slight dragging feeling on prolonged walking or standing. Neuralgic pains may complicate certain cases and occasionally a sexual hypochondriasis, with fears of impotence and sterility, arises.

It must be emphasised that varicocele is a comparatively unimportant ailment and is not liable to lead to any undesirable disability. In treatment, it is necessary to maintain the general health at a high level, to correct constipation and to apply a cold spray to the affected part in order to brace up the skin and muscle. Discomfort may be relieved by wearing a suspensory bandage.

DISEASES OF THE PENIS

Phimosis is a common malformation of the penis in which the foreskin (prepuce),

Phimosis. owing to the small size of its aperture, cannot be retracted over the glans, with resulting interference with micturition. Phimosis may be inherited or acquired. In the inherited form occurring in children the interference with passing urine may lead to dilatation of the urethra and bladder. It is also believed to be a cause of micturition during sleep, and, if the prepuce is adherent to the glans, it may lead to balanitis or inflammation of the skin lining the glans. The constant straining during the act of passing urine is thought to be a factor in producing hernias and in causing prolapse of the anus. In later life, phimosis renders the individual more liable to acquire venereal disease owing to the pouch forming a suitable site for the lodging and growth of the infecting organisms ; also, as the discharges are likely to be retained within the prepuce, the severity of the disease is apt to be aggravated. Acquired phimosis is found in adults and results from the congestion arising from gonorrhœa, syphilis, or eczema.

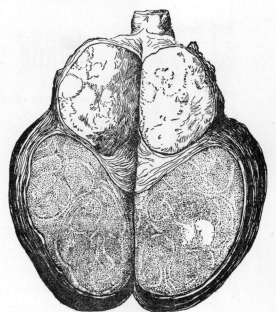

TUBERCULOSIS OF THE TESTICLE
The organ dissected to show an advanced stage of the disease which, if not arrested in time, ultimately destroys it.

If there is any suspicion that the phimosis is interfering with micturition in children, the operation of circumcision should be performed. The slighter degrees of phimosis tend to disappear spontaneously.

Paraphimosis is the term applied to the condition which arises when the glans penis

Para-phimosis. is constricted by a narrow foreskin which has been drawn back and which cannot be pulled forward again. The foreskin is thus turned inside out and consequently it becomes congested and swollen. Later, if the condition is not rectified, the glans also becomes swollen, and ulceration may arise at the constricting ring. Paraphimosis is attended with considerable pain. In adults it frequently accompanies venereal infection.

To remedy the defect the application of firm and persistent pressure to the parts is necessary. If this fails, after the application of a cocaine solution, the glans is well vaselined and the penis is grasped between the index and middle fingers of both hands and steady pressure is made on the glans with both thumbs. In severe cases it may be necessary to divide the constricting band by means of incision.

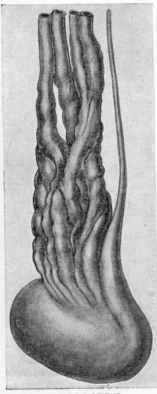

VARICOCELE
A disease in which the veins of the spermatic cord become dilated and varicose.

Balanitis. Balanitis is the term used to describe an inflammation of the skin which lines the prepuce and covers the glans. It is most frequently associated with phimosis. It may also occur in gouty and diabetic subjects owing to decomposition of the urine. The most grave form is that which arises in cases of concealed chancre.

The affection is revealed by an itching, burning sensation which is most marked during micturition. The prepuce becomes red and swollen and there is an offensive discharge. It is always advisable in all cases of balanitis to exclude the possibility of venereal infection.

In treatment it is necessary to cleanse the parts thoroughly with an antiseptic such as hydrogen peroxide. If phimosis is marked, circumcision is indicated.

Herpes. Herpetic eruptions are often found on the foreskin and glans. They commence as small vesicles containing clear fluid : they aggregate and recur in crops. Herpetic eruptions are liable to be mistaken for venereal sores, but bacteriological examination will decide the diagnosis. Cleanliness and the application of mild antiseptics will remedy the affection.

Tumours. Innocent tumours—papillomas or warts—are sometimes found in the glans penis as a result of venereal infection. They take the form of red, cauliflower-like masses, and give off a foul discharge. Cancer of the penis—rarely found in the circumcised—commences as a wart or fissure and finally develops into an ulcer with a hard base. The tumour bleeds easily and there is usually an offensive discharge. Neighbouring lymph glands are invaded and the cancer implicates adjacent organs. Free removal by operation is the only method of treatment.

DISEASES OF THE PROSTATE AND SEMINAL VESICLES

Acute Prostatitis. Acute prostatitis is usually of gonorrhoeal origin and occurs towards the end of the third week of the disease. Alcoholic indulgence or exposure to cold may be the exciting factors. The condition is shown by a feeling of weight and discomfort in the perineal region associated with pain on micturition and defecation. If suppuration ensues, the pain becomes throbbing in character and the sufferer becomes feverish and obviously ill. Blood may be passed in the urine or there may be retention. As a rule the abscess finally ruptures into the urethra and the symptoms rapidly abate.

In treatment it is necessary to confine the patient to bed, the foot of which should be elevated. The bowels should be kept freely open and a fluid diet is best. To relieve the pain, hot fomentations should be applied to the perineum or the patient should make use of a sitz bath. Should abscess formation take place, incision becomes necessary.

Chronic Prostatitis. Catarrh of the gland follicles—most frequently a sequel to gonorrhoea—is found in young adults and is manifested by the escape of milky, viscid discharge from the penis—usually observed in the morning. Examination of the gland through the rectum reveals it to be irregularly enlarged, being nodulated like a bramble.

A feeling of weight and fullness is experienced in the perineum and thighs, and there may be some irregularity of micturition, but —apart from these—there are no other symptoms, except that many sufferers are apt to become troubled in mind over the affection—believing it to be a serious drain on their health.

A regular, quiet, open-air life, with a non-stimulating diet and avoidance of all forms of excitement are the main indications for treatment. Massage of the gland from the rectum is very helpful, and favours a return to the normal. This, of course, must be performed by a physician.

Tuberculosis of the prostate seldom occurs alone : it is usually an accompaniment of tuberculosis of the testicle or **Tuberculosis.** seminal vesicles. The condition is revealed by pain and frequency of micturition, and the last drops of urine are often stained with blood. Examination shows the presence of a number of nodules, or, if abscess formation has taken place, a boggy fluctuating swelling can be recognised. In treatment, the application of the usual general measures is indicated : surgical removal of any disease of the testis or epididymis frequently leads to an arrest of the prostatic condition.

Enlargement of the prostate is a condition occurring in men after middle-life—the **Enlargement of Prostate.** distinguishing feature being an irritability of the bladder and a progressive incapacity to empty it. The middle lobe of the gland is especially involved, and the enlargement leads to an alteration in length, direction, and calibre of the urethra, with the result that there is obstruction to the out-flow of urine, and, owing to urine accumulating behind the enlarged middle lobe, the bladder cannot be completely emptied. Dilatation and hypertrophy of the bladder are liable to follow from the increased difficulty in voiding urine, and, owing to decomposition of the retained urine along with superadded pyogenic infection, cystitis or bladder inflammation arises as a common complication. The kidneys are apt to exhibit chronic degenerative changes.

Although an enlarged prostate is compatible with good health and an absence of symptoms for some time, ultimately the disability shows itself by the sufferer requiring to rise at night to pass urine, and it is noticed that the flow is slow and less forcible than previously. He may require to strain, and this straining is liable to induce piles or prolapse of the anus. As time goes on, the frequency of micturition increases until the patient is passing water every half-hour, and this condition may merge into actual incontinence owing to the bladder being filled to its utmost. At this stage the general health suffers, and symptoms of chronic urinary poisoning arise. Bleeding may occur at any stage, but this is helpful rather than otherwise, for it relieves the condition temporarily. Cystitis and stone are important complications which influence the outlook considerably.

The treatment of enlarged prostate consists either in removal by operation (which is to be preferred unless there are valid contra-indications) or in palliative measures for the relief of the symptoms and complications.

The latter alternative means a " catheter life " : in other words, the patient himself must learn to pass a catheter regularly in order to draw off the residual urine. He should possess at least two soft rubber catheters (No. 7 or No. 8 English), and should thoroughly boil them before use in order to render them aseptic. Before introducing the catheter, it should be dipped into an antiseptic lubricant. It may be

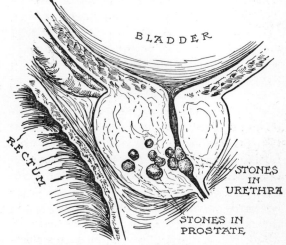

OBSTRUCTION OF THE URETHRA
Stones in the prostatic urethra can always be detected by means of X-rays.

necessary to catheterise up to three or four times daily. Urinary antiseptics should be administered by the mouth regularly. The occurrence of severe cystitis or stone usually necessitates surgical intervention.

Cancer of the prostate occurs in men between the ages of fifty to seventy. The symptoms are similar to those observed in ordinary enlargement of the organ, but they progress more rapidly. Pain is a marked symptom, and there is often an escape of blood and mucus from the urethra apart from micturition. Rectal examination reveals a stony, hard, irregular swelling. Radium is of particular value in cancer of the prostate. It is applied by means of special instruments by the urethra and rectum, and encouraging results have been obtained.

Cancer of Prostate.

Stones may form in the prostatic urethra from the deposition of phosphates, or they may be arrested there in their transit from the kidney and bladder. The presence of stone is revealed by a constant aching pain with purulent and hæmorrhagic discharge from the urethra, and pain is experienced during and after micturition which is referred to the point of the penis. By means of X-rays the diagnosis can be rendered certain. Treatment is by means of operation.

Stone.

Acute Vesiculitis, or inflammation of the seminal vesicles, usually results from an extension of gonococcal infection. The condition is revealed by pain and tenderness in the groin with frequent and painful micturition. Sleep is disturbed by painful erections. Considerable fever is present. With the escape of pus into the urethra the condition abates, but abscess formation may take place or (rarely) infection may spread to the peritoneum, setting up local peritonitis. To treat the affection the patient should be confined to bed, and the pain may be relieved by hot-water enemata or the application of poultices to the perineum.

Vesiculitis.

Chronic Vesiculitis may follow the acute type, or it may develop independently. The symptoms are similar to those of the acute form—only less severe. There is often a discharge of clear fluid from the urethra, and this symptom is apt unduly to worry the sufferer, who becomes apprehensive of his sexual functions. The seminal vesicles may be a seat of tuberculous disease in connection with tubercle in the prostate and testis.

FUNCTIONAL DISTURBANCES OF THE MALE SEX ORGANS

Priapism is the term applied to persistent and painful erection of the penis, unaccompanied by sexual desire. It is a symptom which frequently accompanies bladder or urethral stone, stricture or cystitis, and is sometimes present in gonorrhœa, when the penis becomes curved downwards (known as chordee). If the exciting cause is removed this troublesome symptom soon disappears. " Essential priapism " is the expression employed when the erection cannot be accounted for by any of the causes named above. It occurs in young, virile men—often after a drunken sexual debauch. The penis assumes a wooden hardness and is exquisitely sensitive. The affection may last for days or weeks, and there is usually difficulty in passing urine. Sedative drugs—morphia, bromides, chloral—are given to alleviate priapism, but are often ineffective.

Priapism.

Impotence signifies inability to perform the sexual act : sterility is the inability to procreate or beget children. Impotence may result from deformity of the sexual organs, but the most frequent cause is psychological in origin. It may be met with in young men on the eve of marriage who fear inability to perform the sexual act. In other cases it may arise from exhaustion due to sexual excesses : in certain diseases of the nervous system (e.g., locomotor ataxy) and after the excessive use of drugs such as opium, cocaine, or alcohol, the power of erection may be lost.

Impotence and Sterility.

Sterility is caused either by absence of spermatozoa from the seminal fluid or absence of the fluid itself. Absence of spermatozoa may result from atrophy or disease of the testes. This condition may also arise

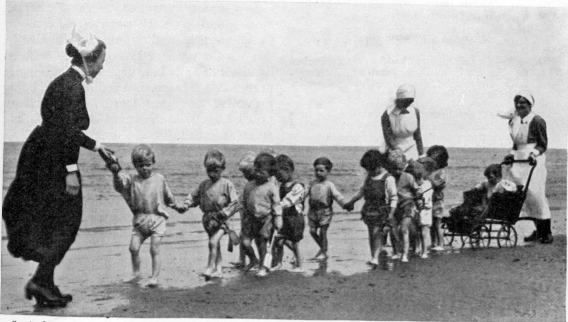

Courtesy]   *[National Institute for the Blind*

BLIND CHILDREN AT THE SEASIDE

A large proportion of the blindness in the world, and especially that existing from early childhood, is due to inherited syphilis.

subsequent to prolonged exposure to X-rays, and if the testes remain undescended spermatozoa are frequently absent from the semen. When no fluid is ejaculated, although the sexual act is performed, the condition is usually due to some obstruction of the seminal tract from gonorrhœal inflammation or the presence of stone.

The treatment and outlook in these cases naturally vary with the cause. If they are a result of anatomical defect or of disease of the nervous system, they are for the most part incurable : if psychical in origin, attention to the general health along with persuasion and suggestion will remedy the affection in most cases.

THE SOCIAL PROBLEM OF VENEREAL DISEASE

By Mrs. ETTIE A. HORNIBROOK, Author of " Exercises for Women," " Practical Birth Control," etc.

SYPHILIS is the most horrible of all poisons. It is not a dead poison, *e.g.*, like cocaine, but a living poison—a poison which creeps insidiously from husband to wife, from mother to child, from brothers and sisters to each other, from one friend to another. Much we hear about preventing the sale of cocaine ; but syphilis is bought and sold and given away with the utmost freedom —inside marriage and outside marriage. On the sale of the venereal poisons there is practically no restriction : it is only on the sale of the antidotes to these poisons that we place our ban. In England those who sell venereal disease preventatives as such are liable to the penalty of seven years' imprisonment.

" Syphilis of the Innocent " may sound a contradiction in terms to the uninformed. To those who know the facts, it is the worst of all our social tragedies. From a book thus entitled, published by the United States Inter-departmental Social Hygiene Board, Washington, I take the following typical cases :—

CASE 27.—Jennie's mother had syphilis. Both Jennie and the other daughter had juvenile paresis, with paralysis and dementia, and were certain to eventuate in early death.

CASE 34.—Bertram infected his wife with syphilis. The first child was a blind syphilitic who died of marasmus at the age of five months. The second child was a living syphilitic.

CASE 38.—Francis (age 15) had been in an institution for the blind since about 7 years of age. This boy was blind as a result of congenital syphilis.

CASE 40.—Albert became blind at the age of 5 years. He was placed in a school for the blind but was incapable of making progress, and it was found that in addition to his blindness he was feeble-minded. The blindness was definitely caused by congenital syphilis, as was probably the feeble-mindedness.

CASE 41.—Lucia was brought to the hospital by her teacher because of headaches, pains in her back, and defective vision. Examination showed that she was a congenital syphilitic. Her visual difficulty was due to syphilitic choroiditis.

CASE 72.—Patrick's son was syphilitic. His mother has had to take him to hospital for treatment over a period of sixteen years.

CASE 129.—Philip undoubtedly infected his brother by sleeping in the same bed with him when he was in a contagious stage of syphilis.

CASE 130.—Frances N. had a lip chancre as a result of kissing her fiancé.

CASE 131.—Jack, a three-months' baby, had a chancre on the eyebrow—it was thought the child was infected by a syphilitic relative kissing it. The father and mother were perfectly healthy.

And so one might go on quoting case after case of innocent infection—genital infection in marriage ; extra-genital infection ; congenital or heriditary infection. Altogether it is calculated that about 80 per cent. of the women who attend the venereal clinics are married women, and nearly all of these are innocent infections. Naturally all the children are innocent victims.

The ravages of gonorrhœa are no less serious to the nation and the individual—above all to women and children. Over half the women who go on the operating table for abdominal section are put there by gonorrhœa. For every one brought to operation there are many chronic invalids, made such from the same disease, spending painful, weary lives wondering why they have been so afflicted ; and many a barren and childless woman owes her loss to gonorrhœa acquired in marriage.

And apart from the floods of mental, moral, and physical anguish suffered by men, women, and children individually, there is the needless loss of money suffered by the nation. The venereal diseases are preventible diseases, and yet instead of being prevented they are treated at enormous public expense in numerous hospital clinics ; and from half to three-fourths of these clinic patients disappear before being cured—the majority of them probably dropping back into the community in an infective condition.

Those of us who have studied the venereal problem most carefully are convinced that no headway can be made in preventing disease till the medical and moral issues are completely separated, and that, generally speaking, the world will be neither better nor worse morally by the elimination of venereal disease.

Those who pretend to believe the " punishment for sin " theory should consider this picture :—

A tiny baby sitting all day in its chair before the window, waving its little hands to and fro—to and fro—to and fro—between the light of heaven and what should have been its own bright eyes. Just a blur was all the babe could see. Blind from birth. Its father—syphilitic !

It cannot be too often repeated that the venereal diseases are dirt-diseases—due to lack of cleanliness rather than to lack of morality. They will indeed continue to afflict the nation till we realise that morality is based on the promotion of virtue and not on the maintenance of disease and the ruin of women and children ; and so long as the venereal diseases do continue to poison the national blood stream, so long will there be physical disablement, mental anguish, moral torture, and the vast, perhaps ultimately overwhelming, tide of national deterioration and degeneration expressed statistically in the rising percentage of lunacy and feeble-mindedness. On the other hand, once we realise that the way to prevent venereal disease is to stop it before it begins, we shall have taken the first step towards national regeneration and the restoration of social and family health and happiness.